Dermatopathology

Editor

STEVEN D. BILLINGS

CLINICS IN LABORATORY MEDICINE

www.labmed.theclinics.com

September 2017 • Volume 37 • Number 3

ELSEVIER

1600 John F. Kennedy Boulevard • Suite 1800 • Philadelphia, Pennsylvania, 19103-2899

http://www.theclinics.com

CLINICS IN LABORATORY MEDICINE Volume 37, Number 3
September 2017 ISSN 0272-2712, ISBN-13: 978-0-323-39569-4

Editor: Stacy Eastman
Developmental Editor: Colleen Dietzler

Reprints. For copies of 100 or more, of articles in this publication, please contact the Commercial Reprints Department, Elsevier Inc., 360 Park Avenue South, New York, New York 10010-1710. Tel. 212-633-3874, Fax: 212-633-3820, E-mail: reprints@elsevier.com.

Clinics in Laboratory Medicine (ISSN 0272-2712) is published quarterly by Elsevier Inc., 360 Park Avenue South, New York, NY 10010-1710. Months of issue are March, June, September, and December. Business and Editorial offices: 1600 John F. Kennedy Blvd., Suite 1800, Philadelphia, PA 19103-2899. Periodicals postage paid at New York, NY and additional mailing offices. Subscription prices are $258.00 per year (US individuals), $488.00 per year (US institutions), $100.00 per year (US students), $314.00 per year (Canadian individuals), $593.00 per year (Canadian institutions), $185.00 per year (Canadian students), $402.00 per year (international individuals), $593.00 per year (international institutions), $185.00 (international students). Foreign air speed delivery is included in all Clinics subscription prices. All prices are subject to change without notice. POSTMASTER: Send address changes to *Clinics in Laboratory Medicine*, Elsevier Health Sciences Division, Subscription Customer Service, 3251 Riverport Lane, Maryland Heights, MO 63043. **Customer Service: 1-800-654-2452 (US). From outside of the US and Canada, call 1-314-447-8871. Fax: 1-314-447-8029. E-mail: journalscustomerservice-usa@elsevier.com (for print support) or journalsonlinesupport-usa@elsevier.com (for online support).**

Clinics in Laboratory Medicine is covered in *EMBASE/Exerpta Medica, MEDLINE/PubMed (Index Medicus), Cinahl, Current Contents/Clinical Medicine, BIOSIS* and *ISI/BIOMED.*

Contributors

EDITOR

STEVEN D. BILLINGS, MD
Professor, Department of Pathology, Cleveland Clinic Lerner College of Medicine, Cleveland Clinic, Cleveland, Ohio, USA

AUTHORS

STEVEN D. BILLINGS, MD
Professor, Department of Pathology, Cleveland Clinic Lerner College of Medicine, Cleveland Clinic, Cleveland, Ohio, USA

THOMAS BRENN, MD, PhD, FRCPath
Department of Pathology, Western General Hospital, The University of Edinburgh, Edinburgh, United Kingdom

DARYA BUEHLER, MD
Assistant Professor, Department of Pathology and Laboratory Medicine, University of Wisconsin-Madison School of Medicine and Public Health, Madison, Wisconsin, USA

MAY P. CHAN, MD
Departments of Pathology and Dermatology, University of Michigan, Ann Arbor, Michigan, USA

JONATHAN L. CURRY, MD
Associate Professor, Section of Dermatopathology, Departments of Pathology and Dermatology, The University of Texas MD Anderson Cancer Center, Houston, Texas, USA

KATHARINA FLUX, MD
Labor für Dermatohistologie und Oralpathologie, Munich, Germany; Department of Dermatology, University of Heidelberg, Heidelberg, Germany

KAREN J. FRITCHIE, MD
Consultant, Division of Anatomic Pathology, Assistant Professor, Department of Laboratory Medicine and Pathology, Mayo Clinic College of Medicine, Mayo Clinic, Rochester, Minnesota, USA

PAUL W. HARMS, MD, PhD
Assistant Professor, Departments of Pathology and Dermatology, University of Michigan, Ann Arbor, Michigan, USA

CHARITY B. HOPE, MD
Fellow in Dermatopathology, UCSF Dermatopathology Section, University of California San Francisco, San Francisco, California, USA

JENNIFER S. KO, MD, PhD
Department of Anatomic Pathology, Cleveland Clinic, Cleveland, Ohio, USA

URSULA E. LANG, MD, PhD
Departments of Pathology and Dermatology, University of California San Francisco, San Francisco, California, USA

TIMOTHY H. McCALMONT, MD
Departments of Pathology and Dermatology, University of California San Francisco, San Francisco, California, USA

VISHWAS PAREKH, MD
Department of Pathology, City of Hope Comprehensive Cancer Center, Duarte, California, USA

LAURA B. PINCUS, MD
Associate Professor, Departments of Dermatology and Pathology, UCSF Dermatopathology Section, University of California San Francisco, San Francisco, California, USA

VICTOR G. PRIETO, MD, PhD
Professor and Chair, Section of Dermatopathology, Department of Pathology, Professor, Department of Dermatology, The University of Texas MD Anderson Cancer Center, Houston, Texas, USA

MELISSA PULITZER, MD
Associate Attending Pathologist, Department of Pathology, Memorial Sloan Kettering Cancer Center, Assistant Professor, Department of Pathology and Laboratory Medicine, Weill Cornel Medical College, Cornell University, New York, New York, USA

ALEXANDRE REUBEN, PhD
Post Doctoral Fellow, Department of Surgical Oncology, The University of Texas MD Anderson Cancer Center, Houston, Texas, USA

RYAN C. ROMANO, DO
Dermatopathology Fellow, Department of Dermatology, Mayo Clinic, Rochester, Minnesota, USA

JOHN T. SEYKORA, MD, PhD
Department of Dermatology, Perelman School of Medicine, University of Pennsylvania, Philadelphia, Pennsylvania, USA

WONWOO SHON, DO
Associate Pathologist, Department of Pathology and Laboratory Medicine, Cedars-Sinai Medical Center, Los Angeles, California, USA

EMILY H. SMITH, MD
Departments of Pathology and Dermatology, University of Michigan, Ann Arbor, Michigan, USA

ANTONIO SUBTIL, MD, MBA
Associate Professor, Departments of Dermatology and Pathology, Yale Dermatopathology Laboratory, New Haven, Connecticut, USA

MICHAEL T. TETZLAFF, MD, PhD
Associate Professor, Section of Dermatopathology, Departments of Pathology and Translational and Molecular Pathology, The University of Texas MD Anderson Cancer Center, Houston, Texas, USA

PAUL WEISMAN, MD
Assistant Professor, Department of Pathology and Laboratory Medicine, University of Wisconsin-Madison School of Medicine and Public Health, Madison, Wisconsin, USA

IWEI YEH, MD, PhD
Departments of Pathology and Dermatology, University of California San Francisco, San Francisco, California, USA

ARTUR ZEMBOWICZ, MD, PhD
Professor, Department of Clinical and Anatomic Pathology, Tufts Medical School of Medicine, Boston, Massachusetts, USA; Senior Staff, Lahey Clinic Foundation, Inc, Burlington, Massachusetts, USA; Medical Director, www.DermatopathologyConsultations.com; Founder, www.Dermpedia.org

Contents

Cutaneous T-cell lymphomas comprise a heterogeneous group of diseases characterized by monoclonal proliferations of T lymphocytes primarily involving skin, modified skin appendages, and some mucosal sites. This article addresses the basic clinical, histologic, and immunohistochemical characteristics of this group of diseases, with additional attention to evolving literature on dermoscopy, reflectance confocal microscopy, flow cytometry, and molecular data that may increasingly be applied to diagnostic and therapeutic algorithms in these diseases. Select unusual phenotypes or diagnostic examples of classic phenotypes are demonstrated, and flags for consideration while making a pathologic diagnosis of cutaneous T-cell lymphoma are suggested.

B-cell lymphomas represent approximately 20% to 25% of primary cutaneous lymphomas. Within this group, most cases (>99%) are encompassed by 3 diagnostic entities: primary cutaneous marginal zone lymphoma, primary cutaneous follicle center lymphoma, and primary cutaneous diffuse large B-cell lymphoma, leg type. In this article, the authors present clinical, histopathologic, immunophenotypic, and molecular features of each of these entities and briefly discuss the rarer intravascular large B-cell lymphoma.

The classification of myeloid neoplasms has undergone major changes and currently relies heavily on genetic abnormalities. Cutaneous manifestations of myeloid neoplasms may be the presenting sign of underlying bone marrow disease. Dermal infiltration by neoplastic cells may occur in otherwise normal skin or in sites of cutaneous inflammation. Leukemia cutis occasionally precedes evidence of blood and/or bone marrow involvement (aleukemic leukemia cutis).

This article focuses on primary cutaneous sweat gland carcinomas with basaloid differentiation, including cribriform apocrine carcinoma, endocrine mucin-producing sweat gland carcinoma, mucinous carcinoma, adenoid cystic carcinoma, spiradenocarcinoma, and digital papillary adenocarcinoma. These tumors are rare and pose a significant diagnostic challenge. Their clinical presentation is nonspecific and there is significant overlap of their histologic features. Confident diagnosis is necessary because their clinical behavior ranges from indolent, nonrecurring, nonmetastasizing tumors to those with potential for disseminated disease and mortality. They should be separated from cutaneous metastases of primary visceral

CLINICS IN LABORATORY MEDICINE

FORTHCOMING ISSUES

December 2017
Flow Cytometry
David M. Dorfman, *Editor*

March 2018
Global Health and Pathology
Dan Milner, *Editor*

RECENT ISSUES

June 2017
Emerging Pathogens
Nahed Ismail, James W. Snyder,
and A. William Pasculle, *Editors*

March 2017
**Risk, Error and Uncertainty: Laboratory
Quality Management in the Age of
Metrology**
James O. Westgard, David Armbruster,
and Sten A. Westgard, *Editors*

RELATED INTEREST

Surgical Pathology Clinics, June 2017 (Vol. 10, Issue 2)
Dermatopathology
Thomas Brenn, *Editor*
http://www.surgpath.theclinics.com

THE CLINICS ARE NOW AVAILABLE ONLINE!
Access your subscription at:
www.theclinics.com

Preface

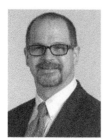

Steven D. Billings, MD
Editor

Dermatopathology remains one of the most difficult areas in anatomic pathology given the broad scope and diversity of disease processes that present in the skin. In this issue, leaders in the field of dermatopathology have written excellent reviews that span the spectrum of critical issues in dermatopathology for the general surgical pathologist and dermatopathologist. Not only does it provide practical information for approaching individual entities, it provides an update on new developments in dermatopathology. Difficult melanocytic lesions are covered with an emphasis on histologic features as well as relevant molecular and immunologic aspects of Spitz tumors and melanoma. In addition to melanocytic tumors, there are updates on cutaneous adnexal tumors, squamous cell carcinoma, Merkel cell carcinoma, cutaneous T-cell and B-cell lymphoproliferative diseases, myeloid diseases, soft tissue tumors, and finally, an overview of common and critically important inflammatory lesions of the skin. I truly believe that this issue should find a place on the bookshelf of any pathologist who deals with dermatopathology.

Steven D. Billings, MD
Cleveland Clinic Lerner College of Medicine
Department of Pathology
Cleveland Clinic
9500 Euclid Avenue, L25
Cleveland, OH 44195, USA

E-mail address:
billins@ccf.org

Clin Lab Med 37 (2017) xiii
http://dx.doi.org/10.1016/j.cll.2017.06.007
0272-2712/17/© 2017 Published by Elsevier Inc.

labmed.theclinics.com

Blue Nevi and Related Tumors

Artur Zembowicz, MD, PhD[a,b,*]

KEYWORDS

- Blue nevus • Cellular blue nevus • Atypical blue nevus • Malignant blue nevus

KEY POINTS

- The family of blue nevi and related dermal dendritic melanocytic proliferations includes common blue nevus, cellular blue nevus, atypical blue nevus, and malignant blue nevus.
- Genetically, as uveal and leptomeningeal melanoma, blue nevi harbor mutations in G-protein–coupled receptors subunits GNAQ and GNA11.
- Malignant blue nevi acquire additional mutations including in BAP1 on chromosome 3 and multiple losses or gains of chromosomal material involving multiple chromosomes.
- Molecular techniques, such as mutational analysis, fluorescence in situ hybridization, and array-based comparative genomic hybridization, are emerging diagnostic adjuncts.
- BAP1 mutations and loss of BAP1 locus are associated with more aggressive behavior of malignant blue nevus.

OVERVIEW

Blue nevi (BN) and related dermal dendritic melanocytic neoplasms are considered together as a group because of common clinical and histologic features. They present as pigmented papules, plaques, or nodules with dark-bluish or blue-black coloration. Under the microscope, they contain pigmented dendritic dermal melanocytes combined with other types of melanocytic cells. BN are derived from neural crest cells migrating ventrally along the developing nerves during embryogenesis, which also give rise to glial and Schwann cells.[1] The bluish color of BNs is caused by preferential scatter of the short wavelength component of visible light by melanin

This is an update of the originally published article that appeared in *Clinics in Laboratory Medicine*, Volume 31, Issue 2, June 2011.

The author has no relationship with a commercial company that has a direct financial interest in subject matter or materials discussed in article or with a company making a competing product.

[a] Lahey Clinic, 41 Mall Road, Burlington, MA 018056, USA; [b] www.DermatopathologyConsultations.com, C/O Harvard Vanguard Medical Associates Laboratories, 152 2nd Avenue, Needham, MA 02494, USA

* c/o Harvard Vanguard Medical Associates Laboratories, 152 2nd Avenue, Needham, MA 02494.

E-mail address: dr.z@DermatopathologyConsultations.com

particles, so-called Tyndall effect. Diagnostic entities in the BN family include the following:

- Common BN
- Cellular blue nevus (CBN)
- Malignant blue nevus (MBN)

The term atypical BN is applied to cellular BN, which show some but not all features associated with MBN. BN are also related to developmental hamartomas/dermal melanocytoses such as Mongolian spot, nevus of Ota, and nevus of Ito. These entities are congenital macular deep dermal proliferations of dendritic melanocytes confined to areas supplied by different cutaneous nerves. Common and cellular BN are benign. MBN is a variant of malignant melanoma. Atypical BN is a borderline diagnostic category including lesions of uncertain biological potential.

Common Blue Nevus (Jadasson-Tieche-Type)

BN was described by Jadasson-Tieche in 1906.[2] It is most common in children and young adults, especially girls, but can occur at any age or as a congenital lesion.[3,4] The most typical sites are the dorsal aspects of extremities, scalp, and buttocks.[5–7] BNs have been also reported in the oral and nasal mucosa, female genital tract, prostate, and lymph nodes.[8–12]

BN presents as a small (<5 mm) dark blue or blue-black macule or papule. Most BN can be diagnosed easily by clinical observation or with help of dermoscopy.[13] Clinical variants of BN include the following:

- Eruptive[14–16]
- Plaquelike[17–19]
- Agminate[20,21]
- Linear[22]
- Satellite[23]
- Disseminated[14,24]
- Familial[25]
- Targetoid[26]

Microscopically, BN are usually symmetric mid and/or upper dermal proliferations of pigmented dermal melanocytes with an inverted wedge-shaped configuration. The base of the lesion is parallel to the surface of the epidermis, and the apex points to deep reticular dermis or subcutaneous tissue (**Fig. 1A**). BN can extend deep into reticular dermis along adnexal structures and/or neurovascular bundles. In most cases, tumor-associated stroma is dense and fibrotic. BN are dermal tumors and lack junctional component. BN contain dendritic spindle-shaped pigmented dendritic cells with slender branching network of dendritic processes (see **Fig. 1B**). Their nuclei are small, elongated, and hyperchromatic. A variable number of spindle or epithelioid melanocytes, some resembling type A and B cells of common nevi, are also present in many BN (see **Fig. 1C**). Nuclear pleomorphism and mitotic activity are exceptionally rare. Rarely, pigmented BN may include melanophages. Immunohistochemically, dendritic melanocytes of BN stain positively with S100, Sox10, HMB-45, and MART-1.[27,28] BN can be a component of a combined nevus.[29,30]

Cellular Blue Nevus

Cellular blue nevus (CBN) was established as a distinct entity by Allen and Spitz,[31,32] who realized that CBN is a benign neoplasm related to BN. CBN can present at all ages, although adults less than the age of 40 are the most commonly affected. The

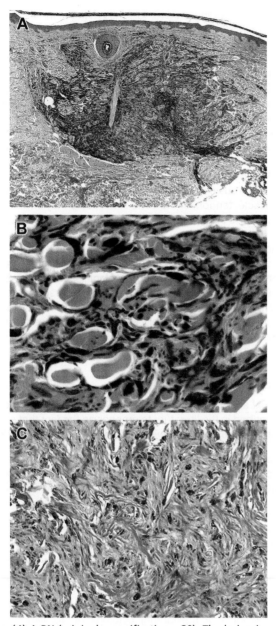

Fig. 1. Blue nevus. (*A*) A BN (original magnification ×20). The lesion is wedge shaped and associated with stromal fibrosis. (*B*) BN dendritic cells from lesion (original magnification ×600) illustrated in (*A*). (*C*) shows BN with epithelioid cells (original magnification ×400; epithelioid and fusiform cell BN).

most common sites of occurrence are the buttocks and the sacrococcygeal region, followed by the scalp, face, and extremities. Other locations include male and female genital tract, breast, subungual mucosa, orbit, and conjunctiva.[6,7,33] Clinically, CBN is a firm bluish-black to bluish-gray dome-shaped nodule. Although most lesions are small

(1–2 cm), large tumors, including giant tumors measuring more than 10 cm, were documented. Large long-standing lesions can degenerate, ulcerate, and become painful.

Histologically, CBN is a biphasic pigmented dermal tumor with a component of a classic BN and distinct cellular areas composed of spindled to oval melanocytes with clear or finely pigmented cytoplasm. Rarely, precursor common BN cannot be identified. Most CBN are well circumscribed, and the cellular is component sharply demarcated from the common BN forming nests, cohesive sheets, or nodules (**Fig. 2A, B**). In many cases, the cellular areas emerge from the deep portion of BN and extend vertically into deep reticular dermis and subcutaneous tissue following adnexal structures or neurovascular bundles, sometimes forming a dumb-bell–shaped outline. In some lesions, the cellular areas are entirely surrounded by the BN component. Multiple nests can form an alveolar pattern and be surrounded by collagen and dense fibrous septae. Involvement of the subcutaneous and soft tissue such as skeletal muscle, tendon, or the bone of the scalp may occur.[34] Myxoid degeneration, hemorrhage, and stromal hyalinization can occur in larger tumors. These features have to be distinguished from tumor necrosis typical for MBN.[35,36] The cells forming cellular nodules of CBN are oval to spindle (see **Fig. 2B**). They have moderate amounts of clear or lightly pigmented cytoplasm. Their nuclei are usually vesicular with finely stippled chromatin and inconspicuous nucleoli (see **Fig. 2C**). Sometimes multinucleated wreathlike giant cells may be seen. In most cases, only minimal nuclear pleomorphism or hyperchromasia is observed. Although mitotic activity in cellular nodules can usually be found, it is typically low and rarely exceeds 1 to 2/mm^2. Immunohistochemically, the cells stain positively for S100, Sox10, MART-1, and HMB-45. CD34 expression was reported in a subset of CBN.[37]

Histologic Variants of Blue Nevi

Benign BN and CBN are usually easy to diagnose. Several rare histologic variants of BN have been described in the literature to emphasize the fact that some BN have unusual features and may be confused with other benign or malignant entities.

Sclerosing (desmoplastic) blue nevus

Sclerosing/desmoplastic BN is a histologic variant of BN with prominent dermal fibrosis. Clinically, sclerosing BN is usually a firm solitary variably pigmented papule or nodule. Dendritic melanocytes may be rare but are usually more abundant at the periphery. In many cases, diagnosis may be aided by architectural features typical of BN, such as inverted wedge-shaped configuration of the lesion, extension into deep dermis along adnexal structures, and neurovascular bundles and lack of epidermal hyperplasia. Rare cases will require immunohistochemistry to confirm the diagnosis. Desmoplastic BN must be distinguished from desmoplastic melanoma. Both lesions share the presence of spindled melanocytes and desmoplastic stroma. In contrast to desmoplastic malignant melanoma, BN lacks atypical junctional proliferation (observed in 50% of cases of desmoplastic melanoma), cytologic atypia, lymphoid infiltrate at the periphery of the lesion, or mitotic activity.[38] S100 and Sox10 are typically the only immunohistochemical stains expressed by desmoplastic melanoma, while expression of HMB-45 is exceptionally rare.[39,40] In contrast, strong expression of HMB-45 is an expected feature in all BN.[41–43] Desmoplastic BN may also be confused with dermatofibroma, other desmoplastic spindle cell soft tissue tumors, and scars.

Hypomelanotic/amelanotic blue nevus and cellular blue nevus

Rare BN and CBN produce little melanin. Such amelanotic lesions are not suspected clinically.[44,45] Histologically, it is difficult to appreciate dendritic processes of BN in

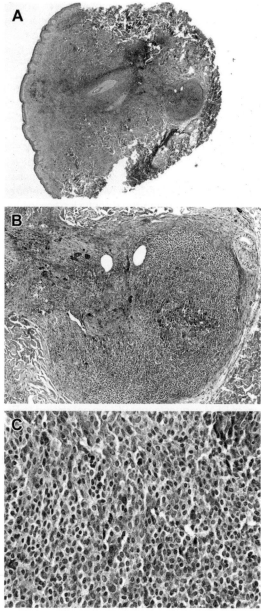

Fig. 2. Cellular blue nevus. (*A*) A low magnification view of an CBN (original magnification ×20). Cellular area extends deep into subcutaneous tissue. (*B*) Cellular nodule (original magnification ×100). (*C*) Cytologic features of from cellular nodule (original magnification ×400).

amelanotic lesions without immunohistochemical stains, such as HMB-45 (always positive) and S100, Sox10, and MART-1 (expressed in most but not all cases).[44,45] The diagnosis often has to rely on architectural features, such as inverted-wedge shape and extension into deep reticular dermis along adnexal structures or biphasic appearance (in the case of amelanotic CBN). An example of amelanotic CBN is illustrated in **Fig. 3**. Entities to be considered in histologic differential diagnosis of hypomelanotic/amelanotic BN/CBN are scar, neurofibroma, perineurioma, and desmoplastic melanoma. Amelanotic CBN has to be distinguished from clear cell sarcoma.

Epithelioid blue nevus

The term "epithelioid blue nevus" was first used in the literature for distinctive pigmented melanocytic lesions occurring in patients with Carney complex.[46] Histologically, indistinguishable lesions occurring in patients without Carney complex were described under the rubric of pigmented epithelioid melanocytoma (PEM).[47] Thus, PEM is a melanocytic proliferation occurring in a sporadic and familial cancer syndrome setting. The term "epithelioid blue nevus" is also frequently used descriptively for common BN containing increased number of epithelioid cells, but not necessarily fulfilling strict criteria for PEM. In the literature, such lesions were recently referred to as epithelioid and fusiform BN (see **Fig. 1**C).[48] In order to avoid confusion associated with different applications of the term epithelioid BN, it seems most logical to apply the term PEM also to Carney complex–associated epithelioid BN. Importantly, PEM may not be even related to BN despite casual microscopic resemblance. Unlike BN, PEM often has a junctional component. The key diagnostic feature of PEM is the presence of distinctive large epithelioid cells with vesicular nuclei and prominent nucleoli resembling Reed-Sternberg cells. Such cells are not found in BN. Dendritic cells of PEM contain slender vesicular epithelioid nuclei with nucleoli rather than small and hyperchromatic nuclei of dendritic cells of BN. Genetic studies did not show GNAQ and GNA typical mutations typical for BN in PEM. In contrast, many PEMs show mutations and loss of expression of Carney complex–associated gene protein kinase regulatory subunit R1 alfa.[49] Recently, a fusion of an adjacent gene located on chromosome 17, protein kinase C alfa, was identified in PEMs.[49] Finally, unlike BN, PEM frequently metastasizes to local lymph nodes but rarely spreads beyond lymph nodes. This unique clinical, histologic, and molecular feature of PEM suggests that PEM is not related to BN family of lesions.

Malignant Blue Nevus

MBN is defined as a melanoma arising within a preexisting BN or CBN or as a melanoma histologically reminiscent of BN.[50–54] MBN typically presents as a large darkly pigmented ulcerated plaque or nodule on the scalp or, less often, on extremities. Men and boys are affected more often than girls and women. MBN is a locally aggressive tumor and frequently metastasizes.[54,55] Earlier studies suggested that MBN may be more aggressive than conventional melanoma.[51,52] However, this may not be true and may simply reflect the fact that most MBN are deeply invasive tumors. A recent study reported 23 patients with MBN and found no difference in clinical outcome in comparison to conventional melanoma when the patients were matched for Breslow thickness, Clark level, and ulceration.[56] Histologic diagnosis of MBN is best established relying on standard cytologic criteria of malignancy,[51] such as:

- Large epithelioid or spindled cells
- Nuclear pleomorphism
- Large eosinophilic nucleoli
- Destructive sheetlike growth pattern
- Tumor necrosis
- Brisk mitotic activity, including atypical forms

An example of amelanotic CBN is illustrated in **Fig. 4**. MBN may lose HMB45 staining and have high Ki67 proliferation index.[57]

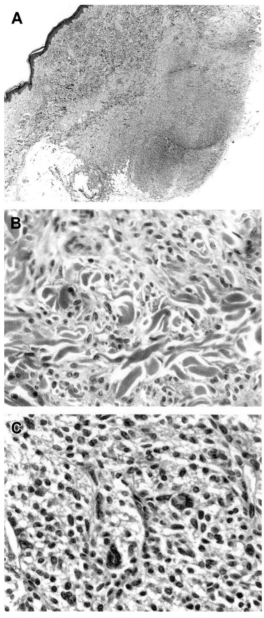

Fig. 3. Amelanotic cellular blue nevus. (*A*) A low magnification view of an amelanotic CBN with biphasic alveolar growth pattern (original magnification ×20). There is a sharp demarcation between the common BN area in the superficial dermis and cellular nodules in the deeper dermis. (*B*) Cytologic detail of subepidermal area (original magnification ×600). It is impossible to appreciate dendritic nature of spindle BN cells in the absence of melanin. (*C*) Cellular area of CBN (original magnification ×600). Of note are uniform oval nuclei with small nucleoli and occasional wreathlike multinucleated giant cells.

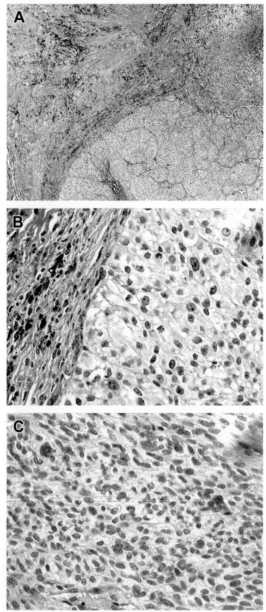

Fig. 4. Malignant blue nevus. (*A*) MBN arising in BN (original magnification ×20). (*B*) Malignant component characterized by severely atypical epithelioid cells with nuclear pleomorphism, eosinophilic macronucleoli, and atypical mitotic activity (original magnification ×400). The same lesion also had area of CBN visualized in (*C*) (original magnification ×40).

Atypical Cellular Blue Nevus

Rare CBN showing histologic features intermediate between CBN and MBN are usually reported as atypical cellular BN.[7,58–62] There are no consensus criteria regarding this diagnostic category, and concordance among melanoma experts in assigning lesions to this category is low.[63] However, this term is useful to convey uncertainty about the biological potential of CBN with insufficient cytologic atypia to warrant outright diagnosis of MBN but concerning features, such as:

- Large size (>5–10 cm)
- Ulceration
- Areas of nuclear pleomorphism
- Increased mitotic activity (up to 3–4/mm^2)
- Infiltrating margins

Early clinicopathologic studies emphasized that atypical mitoses and tumor necrosis are the most specific features favoring MBN.[59] Nevertheless, these features are not always present in MBN, and when present, they have to be interpreted in the context of other features. Misinterpretation of degenerative changes and hemorrhage in large atypical CBN as tumor necrosis is a potential diagnostic pitfall to avoid. Five-year follow-up in atypical CBN is favorable,[58,59,62] even in cases with sentinel lymph node metastases.[62,64–66]

Key histologic features helpful in differentiating between BN, CBN, atypical CBN, and MBN are summarized in **Table 1**.

Genetic Basis of Blue Nevi and Related Tumors

Genetically, BN and other dermal dendritic melanocytic proliferations are more related to uveal and leptomeningeal melanoma than common acquired melanocytic nevus.

Table 1 Key histologic features	
Common BN	• Mid and upper dermal melanocytic proliferations • Symmetric, wedge-shaped • Variably fibrotic stroma • Composed of dendritic melanocytes with elongated cytoplasmic processes and darkly staining hyperchromatic nuclei • Frequently admixed with type B melanocytes
CBN	• Biphasic, usually with a component of common BN • Extension along adnexal structures and neurovascular bundles into the subcutaneous tissue • Cellular areas forming distinct nests, sheets of alveoli composed of uniform nest pale-staining oval, spindled, or epithelioid melanocytes. • Wreathlike multinucleate giant cells • Infrequent mitoses can be found in cellular areas
Atypical CBN	• Features of CBN, but: • Large size (up to 10 cm) • Increased mitotic activity (<3–5 per mm^2) • No abnormal mitoses • Increased pleomorphism • Hemorrhage and degenerative changes (but not frank tumor necrosis) • Severe cytologic atypia
MBN	• Preexisting common or CBN • Severe cytologic atypia • Tumor necrosis • Atypical mitoses • High mitotic activity • Large expansile nodules • Diffuse infiltration of subcutis

Mutations in BRAF and NRAS, MAPK signaling pathway genes found in most acquired nevi[67–69] are present only in 5% to 15% of BN or cellular BN.[70,71]

Defining feature of BN family of lesions is the presence of activating mutations in the G protein a-subunits, GNAQ and GNA11, which can be identified in up to 90% of BN and CBN.[69,71–73] GNAQ or GNA11 mutations are also found in unusual variants of BN and dermal melanocytoses[69,71,72,74] and 50% to 90% of malignant BN.[69,73]

These somatic mutations occur in exon 5 (Q 209) or less frequently exon 4 (R 183). They result in loss of GTPase activity and subsequent activation of MAPK pathway signaling. The net result is similar to that caused by mutated BRAF and NRAS in acquired nevi. As melanocytes with BRAF and NRAS mutations, GNAQ-mutated melanocytes are not able to form malignant tumors in in vivo models.[69] These findings are consistent with the benign nature of BN.

Progression of a BN to MBN requires additional genetic events,[73,75–79] which are similar to those occurring in uveal melanoma.[80] The key molecular events are loss of chromosome 3p21 locus associated with BAP1 gene, BAP1 mutations, and gains in chromosomes 6p and 8p. Other frequent abnormalities found in MBN include loses on chromosomes 1p, 4q, 6q, 8p, 16q, and 17q and gains of chromosomes and 11q, 21q.[74,75,77,79,81] Unusual concomitant gains/losses involving the same chromosome (1p–/1q+ and 4p+/4q–) were reported in aggressive MBN.[77] Sixty-five percent of MBN show loss of BAP1 expression on immunohistochemical studies. As in uveal melanoma, loss of BAP1 expression correlates with more aggressive behavior of MBN.[73] Loss of whole or part of chromosome 3 was the only aberration shared by 3 metastatic MBN in another study.[77] It was recently suggested that, as in uveal melanoma, presence or absence of BAP1 expression may separate MBN into class 1 and class 2 tumors associated with more or less favorable prognosis, respectively. As in uveal melanoma, MBN with GNAQ and BAP1 mutations have a predilection to liver metastases.[82] In addition to chromosomal instability, MBN may contain mutations in genes involved in progression of melanoma, such as PT53.

Molecular features may be helpful in differentiating MBN from atypical CBN. In contrast to MBN, CBN does not show loss of BAP1 expression. Cytogenetic techniques such as array CGH typically show normal chromosomal pattern or loss of only isolated chromosomal segments or whole chromosomes in atypical CBN.[73,77] In contrast, most MBN show many (often 4 and more) different chromosomal aberrations involving multiple chromosomes.[77] Thus, array CGH may be helpful adjunct in differential diagnoses between atypical CBN and MBN.

Melanoma fluorescence in situ hybridization (FISH) using RREB1 (6p25), MYB (6q23), MYC (8q24), and CCND1 (11q13) is also an excellent tool to differentiate between CBN and MBN.[83] However, judging from the prevalence of chromosomal aberrations targeted by this assay in MBN, one may expect that this FISH assay may miss some MBN.[77]

Key genetic features helpful in differentiating between BN, CBN, atypical CBN, and MBN are summarized in **Table 2**.

Prognosis and Management

BN and CBN are benign lesions, and local excision is curative. BN is a very common lesion, and most cases are diagnosed clinically and not biopsied. Even though MBN can rarely supervene in a benign BN, preventive removal of BN is not recommended. CBN should be excised with clear margins to assure evaluation of the entire lesion and to prevent recurrence, which can sometimes mimic locally aggressive disease.[84,85] MBN typically supervenes in a long-standing BN or CBN. Therefore, any sudden changes in size or color in a previously stable BN should prompt biopsy. The

Table 2
Key molecular and genetic diagnostic adjuncts

Common BN	• Immunohistochemistry: HMB45[+], BAP1[+] • Normal melanoma FISH and cytogenetics
CBN	• Immunohistochemistry: HMB45[+], BAP1[+] • Normal melanoma FISH and cytogenetics
Atypical CBN	• Immunohistochemistry: HMB45[+], BAP1[+], increased Ki67 proliferation index • Normal melanoma FISH • Normal cytogenetics or loses or gains of single chromosomes or chromosomal segments
MBN	• Immunohistochemistry: may be HMB45[−], BAP1[−], high Ki67 proliferation index • Abnormal melanoma FISH • Abnormal cytogenetics: multiple losses or gains of chromosomal material involving multiple chromosomes • Mutations associated with melanoma progression such as TP53

prognosis in MBN Is at least as serious as in conventional melanoma. Lack of large series precludes definitive assessment of mortality, but most reported patients with MBN died because of widespread metastatic disease.[51,86–88] Treatment decisions regarding atypical CBN have to be made on a case-by-case basis. However, most are treated as CBN with more frequent follow-up.

REFERENCES

1. Adameyko I, Lallemend F, Aquino JB, et al. Schwann cell precursors from nerve innervation are a cellular origin of melanocytes in skin. Cell 2009;139(2):366–79.
2. Tieche M. Uber benigne Melanome (Chromatophorome) der Haut: blaue Naevi. Virchow Arch Pathol Anat 1906;186:212–29.
3. Bennaceur S, Fraitag S, Teillac-Hamel D, et al. Giant congenital blue nevus of the scalp. Ann Dermatol Venereol 1996;123(12):807–10 [in French].
4. Kawasaki T, Tsuboi R, Ueki R, et al. Congenital giant common blue nevus. J Am Acad Dermatol 1993;28(4):653–4.
5. Dorsey CS, Montgomery H. Blue nevus and its distinction from Mongolian spot and the nevus of Ota. Invest Dermatol 1954;22:225–36.
6. Rodriguez HA, Ackerman LV. Cellular blue nevus. Clinicopathologic study of forty-five cases. Cancer 1968;21(3):393–405.
7. Temple-Camp CR, Saxe N, King H. Benign and malignant cellular blue nevus. a clinicopathological study of 30 cases. Am J Dermatopathol 1988;10(4):289–96.
8. Buchner A, Leider AS, Merrell PW, et al. Melanocytic nevi of the oral mucosa: a clinicopathologic study of 130 cases from northern California. J Oral Pathol Med 1990;19(5):197–201.
9. Jiji V. Blue nevus of the endocervix. Review of the literature. Arch Pathol Lab Med 1971;92(3):203–5.
10. Mancini L, Gubinelli M, Fortunato C, et al. Blue nevus of the lymph node capsule. Report of a case. Pathologica 1992;84(1092):547–50.
11. Masci P, Ciardi A, Di Tondo U. Blue nevus of the lymph node capsule. J Dermatol Surg Oncol 1984;10(8):596–8.

12. Tannenbaum M. Differential diagnosis in uropathology. III. Melanotic lesions of prostate: blue nevus and prostatic epithelial melanosis. Urology 1974;4(5): 617–21.
13. Ferrara G, Argenziano G, Zgavec B, et al. "Compound blue nevus": a reappraisal of "superficial blue nevus with prominent intraepidermal dendritic melanocytes" with emphasis on dermoscopic and histopathologic features. J Am Acad Dermatol 2002;46(1):85–9.
14. Krause MH, Bonnekoh B, Weisshaar E, et al. Coincidence of multiple, disseminated, tardive-eruptive blue nevi with cutis marmorata teleangiectatica congenita [review] [23 refs]. Dermatology 2000;200(2):134–8.
15. Hendricks WM. Eruptive blue nevi. J Am Acad Dermatol 1981;4(1):50–3.
16. Walsh MY. Eruptive disseminated blue naevi of the scalp. Br J Dermatol 1999; 141(3):581–2.
17. Busam KJ, Woodruff JM, Erlandson RA, et al. Large plaque-type blue nevus with subcutaneous cellular nodules. Am J Surg Pathol 2000;24(1):92–9.
18. Wen SY. Plaque-type blue nevus. Review and an unusual case [review] [14 refs]. Acta Derm Venereol 1997;77(6):458–9.
19. Pittman JL, Fisher BK. Plaque-type blue nevus. Arch Dermatol 1976;112(8): 1127–8.
20. Betti R, Inselvini E, Palvarini M, et al. Agminate and plaque-type blue nevus combined with lentigo, associated with follicular cyst and eccrine changes: a variant of speckled lentiginous nevus. Dermatology 1997;195(4):387–90.
21. Ishibashi A, Kimura K, Kukita A. Plaque-type blue nevus combined with lentigo (nevus spilus). J Cutan Pathol 1990;17(4):241–5.
22. Bart BJ. Acquired linear blue nevi. J Am Acad Dermatol 1997;36(2 Pt 1):268–9.
23. Kang DS, Chung KY. Common blue naevus with satellite lesions: possible perivascular dissemination resulting in a clinical resemblance to malignant melanoma. Br J Dermatol 1999;141(5):922–5.
24. Balloy BC, Mallet V, Bassile G, et al. Disseminated blue nevus: abnormal nevoblast migration or proliferation? Arch Dermatol 1998;134(2):245–6.
25. Knoell KA, Nelson KC, Patterson JW. Familial multiple blue nevi [review] [17 refs]. J Am Acad Dermatol 1998;39(2 Pt 2):322–5.
26. Bondi EE, Elder D, Guerry D, et al. Target blue nevus. Arch Dermatol 1983; 119(11):919–20.
27. Sun CC, Lu YC, Lee EF, et al. Naevus fusco-caeruleus zygomaticus. Br J Dermatol 1987;117(5):545–53 [Erratum appears in Br J Dermatol 1988;118(2):314].
28. Zembowicz A, Mihm MC. Dermal dendritic melanocytic proliferations: an update [review] [94 refs]. Histopathology 2004;45(5):433–51.
29. Pulitzer DR, Martin PC, Cohen AP, et al. Histologic classification of the combined nevus. Analysis of the variable expression of melanocytic nevi. Am J Surg Pathol 1991;15(12):1111–22.
30. van Leeuwen RL, Vink J, Bergman W, et al. Agminate-type combined nevus consisting of a common blue nevus with a junctional Spitz nevus. Arch Dermatol 1994;130(8):1074–5.
31. Allen AC, Spitz S. Malignant melanoma. A clinicopathological analysis of criteria for diagnosis and prognosis. Cancer 1953;6:1–45.
32. Allen AC. A reorientation on the histogenesis and clinical significance of cutaneous nevi and melanomas. Cancer 1949;2:28–56.
33. Speakman JS, Phillips MJ. Cellular and malignant blue nevus complicating oculodermal melanosis (nevus of Ota syndrome). Can J Ophthalmol 1973;8(4): 539–47.

34. Micali G, Innocenzi D, Nasca MR. Cellular blue nevus of the scalp infiltrating the underlying bone: case report and review. Pediatr Dermatol 1997;14(3):199–203.
35. Michal M, Kerekes Z, Kinkor Z, et al. Desmoplastic cellular blue nevi. Am J Dermatopathol 1995;17(3):230–5.
36. Biernat W, Kordek R, Wozniak L. Cellular blue nevi with myxoid change–diagnostic difficulties and the review of the literature [review] [10 refs]. Pol J Pathol 1995;46(2):83–6.
37. Smith K, Germain M, Williams J, et al. CD34-positive cellular blue nevi. J Cutan Pathol 2001;28(3):145–50.
38. Carlson JA, Dickersin GR, Sober AJ, et al. Desmoplastic neurotropic melanoma. A clinicopathologic analysis of 28 cases. Cancer 1995;75(2):478–94.
39. Anstey A, Cerio R, Ramnarain N, et al. Desmoplastic malignant melanoma. An immunocytochemical study of 25 cases. Am J Dermatopathol 1994;16(1):14–22.
40. Longacre TA, Egbert BM, Rouse RV. Desmoplastic and spindle-cell malignant melanoma. An immunohistochemical study. Am J Surg Pathol 1996;20(12): 1489–500.
41. Skelton HG III, Smith KJ, Barrett TL, et al. HMB-45 staining in benign and malignant melanocytic lesions. A reflection of cellular activation. Am J Dermatopathol 1991;13(6):543–50.
42. Sun J, Morton TH Jr, Gown AM. Antibody HMB-45 identifies the cells of blue nevi. An immunohistochemical study on paraffin sections. Am J Surg Pathol 1990; 14(8):748–51.
43. Wood WS, Tron VA. Analysis of HMB-45 immunoreactivity in common and cellular blue nevi. J Cutan Pathol 1991;18(4):261–3.
44. Bhawan J, Cao SL. Amelanotic blue nevus: a variant of blue nevus. Am J Dermatopathol 1999;21(3):225–8.
45. Zembowicz A. Amelanotic cellular blue nevus: a hypopigmented variant of the cellular blue nevus: clinicopathologic analysis of 20 cases [article]. Am J Surg Pathol 2002;26(11):1493–500.
46. Carney JA, Ferreiro JA. The epithelioid blue nevus. A multicentric familial tumor with important associations, including cardiac myxoma and psammomatous melanotic schwannoma. Am J Surg Pathol 1996;20(3):259–72.
47. Zembowicz A, Carney JA, Mihm CM Jr. Pigmented epithelioid melanocytoma, a low grade melanoma indistinguishable from animal type melanoma and epithelioid blue nevus. Am J Surg Pathol 2004;28:31–40.
48. Yazdan P, Haghighat Z, Guitart J, et al. Epithelioid and fusiform blue nevus of chronically sun-damaged skin, an entity distinct from the epithelioid blue nevus of the Carney complex. Am J Surg Pathol 2013;37(1):81–8.
49. Cohen JN, Joseph NM, North JP, et al. Genomic analysis of pigmented epithelioid melanocytomas reveals recurrent alterations in PRKARIA and PRKCA genes. Am J Surg Pathol 2017, in press.
50. Connelly J, Smith JL. Malignant blue nevus. Cancer 1991;67(10):2653–7.
51. Goldenhersh MA, Savin RC, Barnhill RL, et al. Malignant blue nevus. Case report and literature review [review] [37 refs]. J Am Acad Dermatol 1988;19(4):712–22.
52. Mehregan DA, Gibson LE, Mehregan AH. Malignant blue nevus: a report of eight cases. J Dermatol Sci 1992;4(3):185–92.
53. Rubinstein N, Kopolovic J, Wexler MR, et al. Malignant blue nevus. J Dermatol Surg Oncol 1985;11(9):921–3.
54. Spatz A, Zimmermann U, Bachollet B, et al. Malignant blue nevus of the vulva with late ovarian metastasis. Am J Dermatopathol 1998;20(4):408–12.

55. Granter SR, McKee PH, Calonje E, et al. Melanoma associated with blue nevus and melanoma mimicking cellular blue nevus: a clinicopathologic study of 10 cases on the spectrum of so-called 'malignant blue nevus'. Am J Surg Pathol 2001;25(3):316–23.

56. Martin RC, Murali R, Scolyer RA, et al. So-called "malignant blue nevus": a clinicopathologic study of 23 patients. Cancer 2009;115(13):2949–55.

57. Pich A, Chiusa L, Margaria E, et al. Proliferative activity in the malignant cellular blue nevus. Hum Pathol 1993;24(12):1323–9.

58. Avidor I, Kessler E. 'Atypical' blue nevus–a benign variant of cellular blue nevus. Presentation of three cases. Dermatologica 1977;154(1):39–44.

59. Tran TA, Carlson JA, Basaca PC, et al. Cellular blue nevus with atypia (atypical cellular blue nevus): a clinicopathologic study of nine cases. J Cutan Pathol 1998;25(5):252–8.

60. Maize JC Jr, McCalmont TH, Carlson JA, et al. Genomic analysis of blue nevi and related dermal melanocytic proliferations. Am J Surg Pathol 2005;29(9):1214–20.

61. Zembowicz A, Carney JA, Mihm MC. Pigmented epithelioid melanocytoma: a low-grade melanocytic tumor with metastatic potential indistinguishable from animal-type melanoma and epithelioid blue nevus [article]. Am J Surg Pathol 2004;28(1):31–40.

62. Hung T, Argenyi Z, Erickson L, et al. Cellular blue nevomelanocytic lesions: analysis of clinical, histological, and outcome data in 37 cases. Am J Dermatopathol 2016;38(7):499–503.

63. Barnhill RL, Argenyi Z, Berwick M, et al. Atypical cellular blue nevi (cellular blue nevi with atypical features): lack of consensus for diagnosis and distinction from cellular blue nevi and malignant melanoma ("malignant blue nevus"). Am J Surg Pathol 2008;32(1):36–44.

64. Epstein JI, Erlandson RA, Rosen PP. Nodal blue nevi. A study of three cases. Am J Surg Pathol 1984;8(12):907–15.

65. Lamovec J. Blue nevus of the lymph node capsule. Report of a new case with review of the literature. Am J Clin Pathol 1984;81(3):367–72.

66. Sterchi JM, Muss HB, Weidner N. Cellular blue nevus simulating metastatic melanoma: report of an unusually large lesion associated with nevus-cell aggregates in regional lymph nodes. J Surg Oncol 1987;36(1):71–5.

67. Davies H, Bignell GR, Cox C, et al. Mutations of the BRAF gene in human cancer. Nature 2002;417(6892):949–54.

68. Pollock PM, Harper UL, Hansen KS, et al. High frequency of BRAF mutations in nevi. Nat Genet 2003;33(1):19–20.

69. Van Raamsdonk CD, Bezrookove V, Green G, et al. Frequent somatic mutations of GNAQ in uveal melanoma and blue naevi. Nature 2009;457(7229):599–602.

70. Saldanha G, Purnell D, Fletcher A, et al. High BRAF mutation frequency does not characterize all melanocytic tumor types. Int J Cancer 2004;111(5):705–10.

71. Emley A, Nguyen LP, Yang S, et al. Somatic mutations in GNAQ in amelanotic/hypomelanotic blue nevi. Hum Pathol 2011;42(1):136–40.

72. Van Raamsdonk CD, Griewank KG, Crosby MB, et al. Mutations in GNA11 in uveal melanoma. N Engl J Med 2010;363(23):2191–9.

73. Costa S, Byrne M, Pissaloux D, et al. Melanomas associated with blue nevi or mimicking cellular blue nevi: clinical, pathologic, and molecular study of 11 cases displaying a high frequency of GNA11 mutations, BAP1 expression loss, and a predilection for the scalp. Am J Surg Pathol 2016;40(3):368–77.

74. Held L, Eigentler TK, Metzler G, et al. Proliferative activity, chromosomal aberrations, and tumor-specific mutations in the differential diagnosis between blue nevi and melanoma. Am J Pathol 2013;182(3):640–5.
75. Vivancos A, Caratu G, Matito J, et al. Genetic evolution of nevus of Ota reveals clonal heterogeneity acquiring BAP1 and TP53 mutations. Pigment Cell Melanoma Res 2016;29(2):247–53.
76. Perez-Alea M, Vivancos A, Caratu G, et al. Genetic profile of GNAQ-mutated blue melanocytic neoplasms reveals mutations in genes linked to genomic instability and the PI3K pathway. Oncotarget 2016;7(19):28086–95.
77. Chan MP, Andea AA, Harms PW, et al. Genomic copy number analysis of a spectrum of blue nevi identifies recurrent aberrations of entire chromosomal arms in melanoma ex blue nevus. Mod Pathol 2016;29(3):227–39.
78. Gerami P, Pouryazdanparast P, Vemula S, et al. Molecular analysis of a case of nevus of ota showing progressive evolution to melanoma with intermediate stages resembling cellular blue nevus. Am J Dermatopathol 2010;32(3):301–5.
79. North JP, Yeh I, McCalmont TH, et al. Melanoma ex blue nevus: two cases resembling large plaque-type blue nevus with subcutaneous cellular nodules. J Cutan Pathol 2012;39(12):1094–9.
80. Harbour JW, Onken MD, Roberson ED, et al. Frequent mutation of BAP1 in metastasizing uveal melanomas. Science 2010;330(6009):1410–3.
81. Loghavi S, Curry JL, Torres-Cabala CA, et al. Melanoma arising in association with blue nevus: a clinical and pathologic study of 24 cases and comprehensive review of the literature. Mod Pathol 2014;27(11):1468–78.
82. Dai J, Tetzlaff MT, Schuchter LM, et al. Histopathologic and mutational analysis of a case of blue nevus-like melanoma. J Cutan Pathol 2016;43(9):776–80.
83. Gammon B, Beilfuss B, Guitart J, et al. Fluorescence in situ hybridization for distinguishing cellular blue nevi from blue nevus-like melanoma. J Cutan Pathol 2011;38(4):335–41.
84. Marano SR, Brooks RA, Spetzler RF, et al. Giant congenital cellular blue nevus of the scalp of a newborn with an underlying skull defect and invasion of the dura mater. Neurosurgery 1986;18:85–9.
85. Silverberg GD, Kadin ME, Dorfman RF, et al. Invasion of the brain by a cellular blue nevus of the scalp. A case report with light and electron microscopic studies. Cancer 1971;27(2):349–55.
86. Hernandez FJ. Malignant blue nevus. A light and electron microscopic study. Arch Dermatol 1973;107(5):741–4.
87. Kwittken J, Negri L. Malignant blue nevus. Case report of a Negro woman. Arch Dermatol 1966;94(1):64–9.
88. Mishima Y. Cellular blue nevus. Melanogenic activity and malignant transformation. Arch Dermatol 1970;101(1):104–10.

Sentinel Lymph Nodes in Cutaneous Melanoma

Victor G. Prieto, MD, PhD[a,b,]*

KEYWORDS

- Melanoma • Sentinel lymph node • Immunohistochemistry • Capsular nevus
- Tumor burden

KEY POINTS

- Sentinel lymph nodes provide very important prognostic information.
- Quantification of tumor burden correlates with prognosis.
- Immunohistochemistry is very helpful in the differential diagnosis among capsular nevus, macrophages, and melanoma.

INTRODUCTION

Cutaneous melanoma continues being a significant health problem. In addition to an increase in incidence for the last several decades, it has a relatively high mortality and affects relatively young patients, with the resulting social impact. Histologic examination of the melanoma lesion is still the gold standard to provide prognostic information, that is, Breslow thickness, ulceration, and mitotic figures; such information is compiled in the staging schema of the American Joint Committee on Cancer (AJCC) classification. However, there are still some patients with early stage (I or II) that progress to recur and metastasize. Therefore, in melanoma, as well as in other solid tumors, clinical research has focused on the detection of features that further refine the staging of these patients. Among them, examination of sentinel lymph node (SLN) has become probably the most popular method of early staging of these oncologic patients. SLN is defined as the lymph node that receives the lymphatic drainage from a particular anatomic area, and thus, it is the lymph node most likely to contain any metastatic deposits. Evaluation of SLN is used to help staging several malignancies, particularly

This is an update of the originally published article that appeared in *Clinics in Laboratory Medicine*, Volume 31, Issue 2, June 2011.

[a] Department of Pathology, University of Texas–MD Anderson Cancer Center, 1515 Holcombe Boulevard, Unit 85, Houston, TX 77030, USA; [b] Department of Dermatology, University of Texas–MD Anderson Cancer Center, 1515 Holcombe Boulevard, Unit 85, Houston, TX 77030, USA

* Department of Pathology, University of Texas–MD Anderson Cancer Center, 1515 Holcombe Boulevard, Unit 85, Houston, TX 77030.

E-mail address: vprieto@mdanderson.org

breast carcinoma and melanoma. SLN biopsy has a relatively low number/degree of side effects (when compared with complete lymphadenectomy). Another advantage is the restricted number of lymph nodes obtained (one or only few), thus allowing a more complete analysis in Pathology than in standard lymphadenectomy specimens (single, routine hematoxylin and eosin [H&E] section per paraffin block). Regarding its clinical significance, although it has been suggested that removal of SLN may improve overall survival, currently the main goal of examination of SLNs is to provide staging information, by more accurately defining the prognosis of these patients and providing more consistent grouping in clinical trials. This article discusses the main clinical, gross, histologic, and immunohistochemical features of SLN examination in patients with cutaneous melanoma.

GROSS FEATURES

Before starting the topic the processing of SLN, it is necessary to discuss the clinical criteria used to recommend SLN examination. Most protocols recommend SLN examination in patients with melanomas with Breslow thickness ≥1 mm or with ulceration. Formerly, many protocols also included Clark level IV, but since the publication of the 7th edition of the AJCC classification, most protocols instead consider the presence of any dermal mitotic figures in cases thinner than 1 mm (stage pT1b) as a criterion for possible SLN examination. It is important to highlight that the 8th edition of the AJCC modified the staging of thin melanomas (≤1 mm in thickness, pT1). In that 8th edition, melanomas ≤1 mm with ulceration, or between 0.8 and ≤1 mm (regardless ulceration), are staged as pT1b, again as a criterion for possible SLN examination.

At the author's institution, in addition, lesions with vascular invasion and satellitosis are also considered for SLN examination. It is unclear if the presence of regression correlates with higher rate of positive SLN,[1] so most protocols do not consider regression as a criterion for SLN analysis. Interestingly, a situation in which Breslow thickness does not appear to correlate with SLN positivity is in purely desmoplastic melanoma. When defining desmoplastic melanoma as such lesions having more than 90% of the invasive component with desmoplastic features (spindle cell dense collagenous stroma, relative hypocellularity composed of large spindle cells with hyperchromatic nuclei, clusters of lymphocytes), such lesions have a relatively low risk of distant metastasis, and it is generally not recommended to perform SLN examination.[2,3]

Regarding the surgical procedure, before the surgery, most institutions use lymphoscintigraphy to determine the drainage pattern of that particular area to then plan the surgical approach. As an example, a lesion on the foot will likely drain first to the popliteal lymph nodes and then to the groin; also, a lesion on the back may drain to either axillary or groin regions (cases have been seen of such lesions draining to 4 basins: right and left, axilla, and groin). After injection in the skin, the radioactive dye is transported by the lymphatic system to the associated lymphatic basin where it can be detected with a Geiger counter placed above the skin. Again, on the day of the surgery, the radioactive dye is injected in the area of the lesion and later, during the surgical procedure, a blue dye is also injected in the same area. With the Geiger counter, the surgeon determines the area in the basin(s) with the highest count and, after opening the skin, then locates the SLN(s) that are labeled with the blue dye.

Regarding the possible exposure to radioactivity in the department of Pathology, when the procedure is being developed as a new technique, it should be determined that the radioactive counts are within safe values by the time the specimen is to be processed in Pathology (with the standard procedures, it would be exceptional for an SLN not to have reached safe values by the time it is received in the Pathology department).

Frozen sections have been used in SLN to try to render an immediate diagnosis of metastatic melanoma during the surgical procedure. Those patients with positive SLN by frozen section would then undergo completion of the regional lymph nodes in the same surgical procedure. However, frozen sections provide a suboptimal morphology and may not contain the subcapsular region of the lymph node (likely area of early involvement by melanoma). Furthermore, because processing of the frozen tissue requires embedding and new sectioning of the paraffin block, it is possible that small, micrometastases are lost in the unexamined tissue.[4] Therefore, at least for SLN from melanoma patients, most investigators consider as gold standard the examination of routinely processed material (formalin-fixed, paraffin-embedded) and do not recommend frozen sections. An alternative is touch preparations/cytologic specimens[5,6]; however, it is not a widespread technique probably due to the sometimes difficult morphologic distinction between melanoma cells and pigmented macrophages.

Regarding grossing techniques, there is no complete agreement on how to process SLN.[7] However, it has become apparent that the classical processing used for non-SLNs, that is, bivalving of the node and examination of a single, routine H&E slide, is not sensitive enough. In an early study from the author's institution with 243 patients with SLN initially diagnosed negative when examining one H&E slide per block, 10 (4.3%) presented a recurrence in the same lymphatic basin. Of those 10 patients, when the original SLN was reexamined using new serial sections or immunohistochemistry, 8 (80%) were reclassified as positive.[8] In another study, 3 of 7 patients with recurrent disease had metastatic melanoma in the originally negative SLN after reexamination with serial sections and immunohistochemistry.[9] Based on these studies, most current protocols for examination of SLN require more than one H&E section or addition of immunohistochemistry.

The original protocol proposed by Cochran[10] called for bivalving the SLN through the hilum with the intent to allow examination of the lymphatic vessels of the lymph node. The original method bisects the lymph node along the long axis, through the lymph node hilum.[11] At the author's institution, breadloafing of the lymph node (perpendicular to the long axis) is recommended to allow examination of a large surface of the lymph node (**Fig. 1**), similar to other protocols,[12,13] and then one H&E slide is studied. If that H&E slide is positive, it is reported as such or else the block is submitted again to the laboratory to obtain a new H&E, deeper section slide (~200 μm deeper in the block), and 2 unstained slides. One of them is reacted with a panmelanocytic cocktail (combination of HMB45, anti-MART1, and anti-tyrosinase), and the other is left in case additional studies are needed (eg, HMB45, SOX10, and so forth) (**Fig. 2**).

An alternative processing of SLN, in the context of some clinical trials, calls for preserving a portion of the node for other studies (eg, polymerase chain reaction [PCR] analysis).

MICROSCOPIC FEATURES

Approximately 20% of patients with cutaneous melanoma show deposits of melanoma cells in the SLN. The amount of tumor in the SLN (tumor burden) ranges from solitary, rare cells, up to complete replacement of the lymph node. Most metastatic melanoma deposits are located within or close to the subcapsular sinus (**Fig. 3**). Less frequently, tumor cells are located within the parenchyma closer to the center

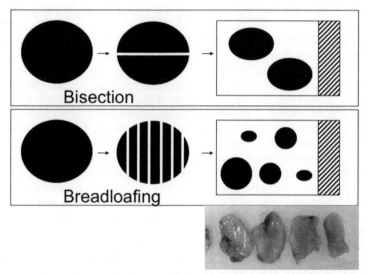

Fig. 1. Main techniques used to gross SLNs. MD Anderson Cancer Center protocols call for breadloafing and including as many fragments as possible within a single paraffin block.

of the lymph node (**Fig. 4**), and even rarely (less than 5% of cases), there is extracapsular extension into the perinodal fibroadipose tissues.

Metastatic melanoma cells may display a large variety of morphologies, although most commonly they resemble the cells in the primary lesion. Thus, at the time of examination of SLN, it is very important to study the original melanoma,

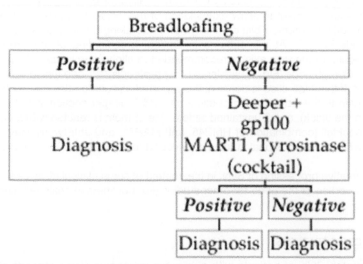

Fig. 2. Diagnostic algorithm used at MD Anderson Cancer Center. If the initial H&E is negative, the block is recut (after approximately 200 μm) in 3 sections. One is stained with H&E and another is stained with a panmelanocytic cocktail against gp100 (with HMB45), MART1, and tyrosinase. The third section is left for possible additional markers (eg, S100, SOX10).

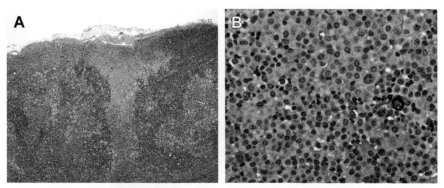

Fig. 3. (A) Cluster of metastatic melanoma involving the subcapsular region. (B) Note the large size, irregular nuclear contour, prominent nucleoli, and focal melanin pigment (H&E stain, original magnification (A) ×40, (B) ×200).

particularly to help distinguish metastatic melanoma cells from macrophages or nevus cells.

Immunohistochemical studies are very helpful when trying to detect small metastatic deposits and also at the time of differential diagnosis. Of the approximately 20% of patients that have metastasis to the SLN, 16% are detected in the initial H&E slide and the remaining 4% are detected with the serial sections or immunoperoxidase. Some investigators propose the use of anti-S100 protein.[14,15] However, in addition to melanoma cells, this marker also labels nevus cells and lymph node dendritic cells. The resulting high background labeling limits the practical utility of this immunohistochemical stain in this setting. Therefore, most investigators recommend the use of other markers.[16,17] Among the different options, the author agrees with the recommendation of using a panmelanocytic cocktail (HMB45, anti-MART1, and anti-tyrosinase) **(Fig. 5)** to increase the detection of tumor cells.[18] Occasionally, the author's institution uses HMB45 by itself or MiTF/SOX10 when trying to differentiate between macrophages and melanoma cells (see section Differential Diagnosis). The lack of expression of MART1 in a spindle cell melanocytic proliferation supports a diagnosis of

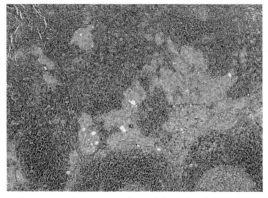

Fig. 4. Metastatic melanoma to intraparenchymal location (H&E stain, original magnification ×40).

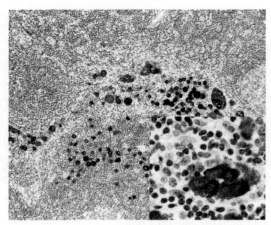

Fig. 5. Isolated, intraparenchymal tumor cells highlighted with a panmelanocytic cocktail, better seen at high magnification (*inset*, original magnification ×400) (panmelanocytic cocktail: HMB45, anti-MART1, and anti-tyrosinase; diaminobencidine and light hematoxylin, original magnification ×100).

melanoma[19]; in such cases of spindle cell melanoma lacking MART1 or gp100 (with HMB45) expression, the author may run antibodies against S100, SOX10, or MiTF (**Fig. 6**).

In most institutions, after detection of a positive SLN, the surgeon recommends completion lymphadenectomy of the affected basin, particularly in order to reduce the incidence to local recurrence in that basin. These lymphadenectomy specimens are examined histopathologically in a standard manner, identical to that used for other lymph nodes in the body. Briefly, the entire lymph node is processed and examined in H&E sections. Occasionally, immunohistochemical studies may be used if there are any cells suspicious for metastatic melanoma.

DIFFERENTIAL DIAGNOSIS

In general, it is relatively easy to detect melanoma cells in SLN. Such cells are usually large, with prominent nucleoli, focal cytoplasmic melanin pigment, and are arranged in clusters in the subcapsular region. However, and particularly in those cases in which there are isolated tumor cells, it may be difficult to distinguish them from macrophages or large lymphocytes. As mentioned, comparison with the original cutaneous melanoma may be helpful when trying to distinguish melanoma cells from macrophages or nevus cells. Also, immunohistochemical studies are helpful because the immense majority of metastatic melanoma cells to SLN will label for melanocytic markers. However, occasionally macrophages will label with anti-MART1[20]; therefore, if there are any doubts of isolated cells labeled with anti-MART1 actually being macrophages and not melanoma cells, the author recommends using HMB45 or anti-SOX10 by itself (in the author's experience, macrophages are rarely labeled with HMB45).[19]

The differential diagnosis also includes capsular nevi. These capsular nevi are clusters of benign melanocytes, most commonly present in the lymph node capsule. Up to 20% of lymphadenectomies from the axilla or groin contain such melanocytes.[21] The capsular location of these nevus deposits is different from the subcapsular

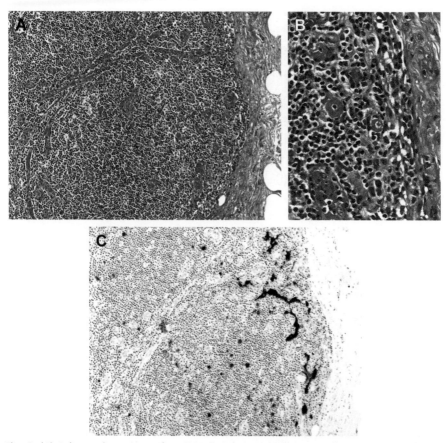

Fig. 6. (*A*) Subcapsular region of an SLN. No obvious melanoma cells, even at high power (H&E stain, original magnification ×100. (*B*) H&E stain, original magnification ×400. Note the large, elongated cells strongly positive for S100; these cells were completely negative with the panmelanocytic cocktail. (*C*) Anti-S100; diaminobencidine and light hematoxylin, original magnification ×100.

location of metastatic melanoma (**Fig. 7**). However, a potential problem is the presence of vascular metastasis detected in the intracapsular lymphatic vessels of the node. In such cases, use of anti-CD31, anti-CD34, or D2-40 may be helpful in detecting the rim of endothelial cells around the melanoma clusters, thus confirming the intravascular location. On the other hand, rarely, capsular nevi extend into the underlying node parenchyma. In general, those lymph nodes contain similar melanocytes in the capsular region, lack gp100 expression (with HMB45), and show very low Ki-67 expression.[22,23]

DIAGNOSIS

As mentioned before, if the original H&E slide is negative, the author's institution examines a deeper H&E slide as well as an immunoperoxidase slide labeled with the panmelanocytic cocktail. Then, the diagnosis includes the number of positive nodes and the total count. To avoid possible typographical errors, the author's

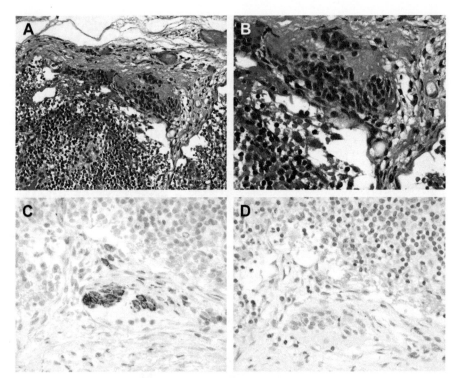

Fig. 7. (*A*) Nodal nevus. Notice the small melanocytes located in the capsule of the SLN (H&E stain, original magnification ×200). (*B*) At higher power, these cells show uniform nuclei with small nucleoli. Mitotic figures are not evident (H&E stain, original magnification ×400). (*C*) These cells express MART1 (anti-MART1; diaminobencidine and light hematoxylin as counterstain, original magnification ×100). (*D*) Nevus cells do not express gp100 (with HMB45; diaminobencidine and light hematoxylin as counterstain, original magnification ×400).

institution uses both the numbers and the spelling, for example, "one of two lymph nodes (1/2)." In addition, quantification of the amount of melanoma deposits in the SLN appears to provide prognostic information (see also next section on Prognosis). Based on the author's results,[24] the amount of melanoma cells seen in the SLN is measured as the size of the largest tumor deposit (in 2 dimensions, in millimeters), the location (subcapsular vs intraparenchymal/mixed subcapsular-intraparenchymal), and presence or absence of extracapsular extension (**Fig. 8**) (see also next section on Prognosis). For the purpose of measuring, when small aggregates are located in clusters in the same region of the SLN, they are measured overall as if they were a single nest (see **Fig. 8**). This practice of quantifying the amount of metastatic melanoma seems to be extending since a recent survey in Europe has shown that most participants report the size of the largest tumor deposit in the SLN[25] (see also Prognosis) (**Box 1**).

PROGNOSIS

Multiple studies have confirmed that SLN positivity is associated with impaired prognosis, along with Breslow thickness and ulceration.[26–29] In addition, the previous 7th edition of the AJCC included mitotic rate (>1 mitotic figure per squared

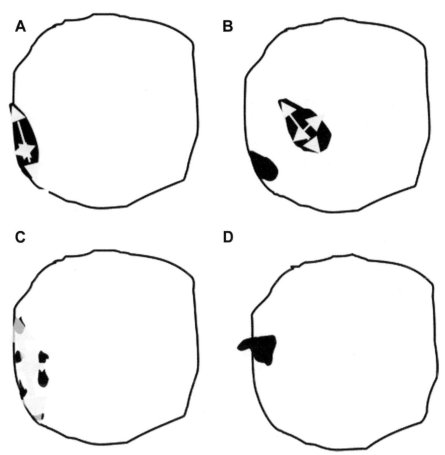

Fig. 8. (A) Measurement of a subcapsular nest. (B) Subcapsular and intraparenchymal nests. The larger is measured. (C) Cluster of small nests measured in aggregate. (D) Presence of extracapsular extension.

millimeter) as a component of stage pT1b, and thus a possible recommendation for SLN evaluation.[30] Although the current AJCC 8th edition does not consider mitotic count in thin melanomas (stage pT1, <1 mm),[31] mitotic rate still is an overall important prognostic factor in cutaneous melanoma.[32] There is still controversy about the clinical significance of SLN positivity in children, because it seems that, at least regarding spitzoid melanomas, there is a higher rate of SLN positivity compared

---

Box 1
Pitfalls

Macrophages can be labeled with anti-MART1

Capsular nevi can also (rarely) involve the node parenchyma

Spindle cell melanoma can be negative for gp100 (with HMB45) and MART1. Use as alternative an additional anti-S100 or anti-SOX10, or anti-MiTF in such cases.

with adults, and without equivalent worsening prognosis.[33,34] However, at least one recent study confirms correlation between positive SLN and impaired prognosis.[35]

Several studies have shown that quantification of the amount of melanoma in SLN correlates with subsequent involvement of non-SLNs (from the completion lymphadenectomy specimens)[36] and, furthermore, with prognosis.[24,37–42] The 2 main techniques suggested to perform this quantification are a modification of Breslow thickness (measurement of the distance between the capsule and the most deeply located deposit) and measurement of the size of the tumor deposits (in millimeters, in 1 or 2 dimensions).[43–45]

The author's preliminary data on 237 positive SLN out of 1417 patients[24] suggest a stratification in 3 groups with progressive worse prognosis:

1. Involvement of 1 or 2 SLN *AND* metastasis size ≤ 2 mm (in the largest nest) *AND* no ulceration (in the primary lesion)
2. Ulceration in the primary lesion *OR* metastasis size greater than 2 mm (in the largest nest)
3. Involvement of 3 or more SLN *OR* ulceration in the primary lesion *AND* metastasis size greater than 2 mm (in the largest nest).

Supporting these data, a large, recent study confirmed that maximum diameter of the SLN metastasis correlated with impaired prognosis in multivariate analysis.[46]

An important finding in the author's study was the lack of a cutoff in the metastasis size associated with no risk of subsequent metastasis (**Box 2**). The author has seen at least 2 cases in which only a single melanoma cell was identified in the SLN that recurred with multiple distant metastases within 4 years of diagnosis.

Quantification of vascularity within and around the melanoma metastasis in the SLN may help further refine the prognosis in such patients with positive SLN.[47] Some prior studies indicated that detection of melanocytic messenger RNA (mRNA) in SLN by PCR correlates with decreased survival,[48–50] but other investigators have not found significant differences.[51,52] A possible explanation for these differences may be the presence of nodal nevi in some SLN. Thus, even though it seems logical that detection of melanocytic mRNA in SLN should correlate with worse prognosis, it is likely that at least some of the SLN with positive PCR actually correspond to capsular nevi and not to metastatic melanoma deposits. Therefore, unless mRNA specific for melanoma cells becomes available for PCR studies, it seems that histologic examination will remain the gold standard in SLN for melanoma.

Another field of study is the determination of a gene signature that may help distinguish those patients with positive SLN with high or low risk for systemic disease.[53] Further studies are necessary to determine the clinical value of such signatures.

In summary, SLN is a technique widely used to stage patients with cutaneous melanoma. Ongoing studies are addressing the possible therapeutic effect secondary to the removal of positive SLN.

Box 2
Pathologic key features

Negative prognostic factors of metastasis to SLN:

Larger size (in mm)

Intraparenchymal location

Extracapsular extension

REFERENCES

1. Kaur C, Thomas RJ, Desai N, et al. The correlation of regression in primary melanoma with sentinel lymph node status. J Clin Pathol 2008;61(3):297–300.
2. Dunne JA, Wormald JC, Steele J, et al. Is sentinel lymph node biopsy warranted for desmoplastic melanoma? A systematic review. J Plast Reconstr Aesthet Surg 2017;70(2):274–80.
3. Pawlik TM, Ross MI, Prieto VG, et al. Assessment of the role of sentinel lymph node biopsy for primary cutaneous desmoplastic melanoma. Cancer 2006; 106(4):900–6.
4. Prieto VG. Use of frozen sections in the examination of sentinel lymph nodes in patients with melanoma. Semin Diagn Pathol 2008;25(2):112–5.
5. Messina JL, Glass LF, Cruse CW, et al. Pathologic examination of the sentinel lymph node in malignant melanoma. Am J Surg Pathol 1999;23(6):686–90.
6. Creager AJ, Shiver SA, Shen P, et al. Intraoperative evaluation of sentinel lymph nodes for metastatic melanoma by imprint cytology. Cancer 2002;94(11): 3016–22.
7. Cole CM, Ferringer T. Histopathologic evaluation of the sentinel lymph node for malignant melanoma: the unstandardized process. Am J Dermatopathol 2014; 36(1):80–7.
8. Gershenwald JE, Colome MI, Lee JE, et al. Patterns of recurrence following a negative sentinel lymph node biopsy in 243 patients with stage I or II melanoma. J Clin Oncol 1998;16(6):2253–60.
9. Clary BM, Brady MS, Lewis JJ, et al. Sentinel lymph node biopsy in the management of patients with primary cutaneous melanoma: review of a large single-institutional experience with an emphasis on recurrence. Ann Surg 2001; 233(2):250–8.
10. Cochran AJ. Surgical pathology remains pivotal in the evaluation of 'sentinel' lymph nodes. Am J Surg Pathol 1999;23(10):1169–72.
11. Morton DL, Wen DR, Wong JH, et al. Technical details of intraoperative lymphatic mapping for early stage melanoma. Arch Surg 1992;127(4):392–9.
12. Prieto VG, Clark SH. Processing of sentinel lymph nodes for detection of metastatic melanoma. Ann Diagn Pathol 2002;6(4):257–64.
13. Mitteldorf C, Bertsch HP, Zapf A, et al. Cutting a sentinel lymph node into slices is the optimal first step for examination of sentinel lymph nodes in melanoma patients. Mod Pathol 2009;22(12):1622–7.
14. Gibbs JF, Huang PP, Zhang PJ, et al. Accuracy of pathologic techniques for the diagnosis of metastatic melanoma in sentinel lymph nodes. Ann Surg Oncol 1999;6(7):699–704.
15. Yu LL, Flotte TJ, Tanabe KK, et al. Detection of microscopic melanoma metastases in sentinel lymph nodes. Cancer 1999;86(4):617–27.
16. Shidham VB, Qi DY, Acker S, et al. Evaluation of micrometastases in sentinel lymph nodes of cutaneous melanoma: higher diagnostic accuracy with Melan-A and MART-1 compared with S-100 protein and HMB-45. Am J Surg Pathol 2001;25(8):1039–46.
17. Abrahamsen HN, Hamilton-Dutoit SJ, Larsen J, et al. Sentinel lymph nodes in malignant melanoma: extended histopathologic evaluation improves diagnostic precision. Cancer 2004;100(8):1683–91.
18. Shidham VB, Qi D, Rao RN, et al. Improved immunohistochemical evaluation of micrometastases in sentinel lymph nodes of cutaneous melanoma with 'MCW

Melanoma Cocktail' - a mixture of monoclonal antibodies to MART-1, melan-A, and tyrosinase. BMC Cancer 2003;3(1):15.

19. Prieto VG, Shea CR. Use of immunohistochemistry in melanocytic lesions. J Cutan Pathol 2008;35(Suppl 2):1–10.

20. Trejo O, Reed JA, Prieto VG. Atypical cells in human cutaneous re-excision scars for melanoma express p75NGFR, C56/N-CAM and GAP-43: evidence of early Schwann cell differentiation. J Cutan Pathol 2002;29(7):397–406.

21. Carson KF, Wen DR, Li PX, et al. Nodal nevi and cutaneous melanomas. Am J Surg Pathol 1996;20(7):834–40.

22. Lohmann CM, Iversen K, Jungbluth AA, et al. Expression of melanocyte differentiation antigens and Ki-67 in nodal nevi and comparison of Ki-67 expression with metastatic melanoma. Am J Surg Pathol 2002;26(10):1351–7.

23. Biddle DA, Evans HL, Kemp BL, et al. Intraparenchymal nevus cell aggregates in lymph nodes: a possible diagnostic pitfall with malignant melanoma and carcinoma. Am J Surg Pathol 2003;27(5):673–81.

24. Prieto VG, Diwan AD, Lazar AFJ, et al. Histologic quantification of tumor size in sentinel lymph node metastases correlates with prognosis in patients with cutaneous malignant melanoma. Mod Pathol 2006;19:87A.

25. Batistatou A, Cook MG, Massi D. Histopathology report of cutaneous melanoma and sentinel lymph node in Europe: a web-based survey by the Dermatopathology Working Group of the European Society of Pathology. Virchows Arch 2009; 454(5):505–11.

26. Cascinelli N, Belli F, Santinami M, et al. Sentinel lymph node biopsy in cutaneous melanoma: the WHO Melanoma Program experience. Ann Surg Oncol 2000;7(6): 469–74.

27. Gershenwald JE, Thompson W, Mansfield PF, et al. Multi-institutional melanoma lymphatic mapping experience: the prognostic value of sentinel lymph node status in 612 stage I or II melanoma patients. J Clin Oncol 1999;17(3): 976–83.

28. Rousseau DL Jr, Ross MI, Johnson MM, et al. Revised American Joint Committee on Cancer staging criteria accurately predict sentinel lymph node positivity in clinically node-negative melanoma patients. Ann Surg Oncol 2003;10(5): 569–74.

29. Topping A, Dewar D, Rose V, et al. Five years of sentinel node biopsy for melanoma: the St George's Melanoma Unit experience. Br J Plast Surg 2004;57(2): 97–104.

30. Balch CM, Gershenwald JE, Soong SJ, et al. Final version of 2009 AJCC melanoma staging and classification. J Clin Oncol 2009;27(36):6199–206.

31. Amin MB, Greene FL, Edge SB, et al. The Eighth Edition AJCC Cancer Staging Manual: continuing to build a bridge from a population-based to a more "personalized" approach to cancer staging. CA Cancer J Clin 2017;67:93–9.

32. Mandala M, Galli F, Cattaneo L, et al. Mitotic rate correlates with sentinel lymph node status and outcome in cutaneous melanoma greater than 1 millimeter in thickness: a multi-institutional study of 1524 cases. J Am Acad Dermatol 2017; 76(2):264–73.e2.

33. Paradela S, Fonseca E, Pita-Fernandez S, et al. Spitzoid and non-spitzoid melanoma in children: a prognostic comparative study. J Eur Acad Dermatol Venereol 2013;27(10):1214–21.

34. Mills OL, Marzban S, Zager JS, et al. Sentinel node biopsy in atypical melanocytic neoplasms in childhood: a single institution experience in 24 patients. J Cutan Pathol 2012;39(3):331–6.
35. Kim J, Sun Z, Gulack BC, et al. Sentinel lymph node biopsy is a prognostic measure in pediatric melanoma. J Pediatr Surg 2016;51(6):986–90.
36. Gershenwald JE, Andtbacka RH, Prieto VG, et al. Microscopic tumor burden in sentinel lymph nodes predicts synchronous nonsentinel lymph node involvement in patients with melanoma. J Clin Oncol 2008;26(26):4296–303.
37. Debarbieux S, Duru G, Dalle S, et al. Sentinel lymph node biopsy in melanoma: a micromorphometric study relating to prognosis and completion lymph node dissection. Br J Dermatol 2007;157(1):58–67.
38. Rossi CR, De Salvo GL, Bonandini E, et al. Factors predictive of nonsentinel lymph node involvement and clinical outcome in melanoma patients with metastatic sentinel lymph node. Ann Surg Oncol 2008;15(4):1202–10.
39. van Akkooi AC, Bouwhuis MG, de Wilt JH, et al. Multivariable analysis comparing outcome after sentinel node biopsy or therapeutic lymph node dissection in patients with melanoma. Br J Surg 2007;94(10):1293–9.
40. Wright BE, Scheri RP, Ye X, et al. Importance of sentinel lymph node biopsy in patients with thin melanoma. Arch Surg 2008;143(9):892–9 [discussion: 899–900].
41. Guggenheim MM, Hug U, Jung FJ, et al. Morbidity and recurrence after completion lymph node dissection following sentinel lymph node biopsy in cutaneous malignant melanoma. Ann Surg 2008;247(4):687–93.
42. Satzger I, Völker B, Al Ghazal M, et al. Prognostic significance of histopathological parameters in sentinel nodes of melanoma patients. Histopathology 2007; 50(6):764–72.
43. Starz H, Balda BR, Kramer KU, et al. A micromorphometry-based concept for routine classification of sentinel lymph node metastases and its clinical relevance for patients with melanoma. Cancer 2001;91(11):2110–21.
44. Ranieri JM, Wagner JD, Azuaje R, et al. Prognostic importance of lymph node tumor burden in melanoma patients staged by sentinel node biopsy. Ann Surg Oncol 2002;9(10):975–81.
45. Scolyer RA, Li LX, McCarthy SW, et al. Micromorphometric features of positive sentinel lymph nodes predict involvement of nonsentinel nodes in patients with melanoma. Am J Clin Pathol 2004;122(4):532–9.
46. Egger ME, Bower MR, Czyszczon IA, et al. Comparison of sentinel lymph node micrometastatic tumor burden measurements in melanoma. J Am Coll Surg 2014;218(4):519–28.
47. Pastushenko I, Van den Eynden GG, Vicente-Arregui S, et al. Increased angiogenesis and lymphangiogenesis in metastatic sentinel lymph nodes is associated with nonsentinel lymph node involvement and distant metastasis in patients with melanoma. Am J Dermatopathol 2016;38(5):338–46.
48. Romanini A, Manca G, Pellegrino D, et al. Molecular staging of the sentinel lymph node in melanoma patients: correlation with clinical outcome. Ann Oncol 2005; 16(11):1832–40.
49. Gradilone A, Ribuffo D, Silvestri I, et al. Detection of melanoma cells in sentinel lymph nodes by reverse transcriptase-polymerase chain reaction: prognostic significance. Ann Surg Oncol 2004;11(11):983–7.

50. Mocellin S, Hoon DS, Pilati P, et al. Sentinel lymph node molecular ultrastaging in patients with melanoma: a systematic review and meta-analysis of prognosis. J Clin Oncol 2007;25(12):1588–95.
51. Scoggins CR, Ross MI, Reintgen DS, et al. Prospective multi-institutional study of reverse transcriptase polymerase chain reaction for molecular staging of melanoma. J Clin Oncol 2006;24(18):2849–57.
52. Hershko DD, Robb BW, Lowy AM, et al. Sentinel lymph node biopsy in thin melanoma patients. J Surg Oncol 2006;93(4):279–85.
53. Hao H, Xiao D, Pan J, et al. Sentinel lymph node genes to predict prognosis in node-positive melanoma patients. Ann Surg Oncol 2017;24(1):108–16.

Toward a Molecular-Genetic Classification of Spitzoid Neoplasms

Michael T. Tetzlaff, MD, PhD[a,b,*], Alexandre Reuben, PhD[c],
Steven D. Billings, MD[d], Victor G. Prieto, MD, PhD[a,e],
Jonathan L. Curry, MD[a,e]

KEYWORDS

- Spitz nevus • Atypical Spitz tumor • Spitzoid melanoma • *HRAS* • *BAP1*
- Comparative genomic hybridization • Fluorescence in situ hybridization
- Telomerase promoter

KEY POINTS

- The histopathologic spectrum of Spitzoid neoplasms includes Spitz nevi, atypical Spitz tumors, and Spitzoid melanomas; distinction among these lesions can be challenging.
- Recent studies have begun to elaborate a molecular–genetic framework by which to categorize Spitzoid neoplasms, predict their clinical behavior, and possibly inform therapeutic options.
- Spitzoid lesions with 11p amplification and/or *HRAS* mutations and Spitzoid lesions with *BAP1* loss and *BRAF* V600E mutation exhibit a typical morphology and predictably benign clinical behavior.
- Translocations involving different oncogenic kinase drivers occur across the spectrum of Spitzoid neoplasms and implicate critical oncogenic drivers that may be leveraged to inform therapeutic decisions.
- Spitzoid lesions with telomerase reverse transcriptase (*TERT*) promoter mutations exhibit a more aggressive clinical course; therefore, *TERT* promoter mutation may represent an additional marker of aggressive behavior.
- FISH identifies Spitzoid neoplasms with increased risk for metastasis and death including those with homozygous deletion of 9p21.

[a] Section of Dermatopathology, Department of Pathology, The University of Texas MD Anderson Cancer Center, 1515 Holcombe Boulevard, Unit 85, Houston, TX, USA; [b] Department of Translational and Molecular Pathology, The University of Texas MD Anderson Cancer Center, 1515 Holcombe Boulevard, Unit 85, Houston, TX, USA; [c] Department of Surgical Oncology, The University of Texas MD Anderson Cancer Center, 1515 Holcombe Boulevard, Houston, TX 77030, USA; [d] Department of Pathology, Cleveland Clinic, 9500 Euclid Avenue L25, Cleveland, OH, USA; [e] Department of Dermatology, The University of Texas MD Anderson Cancer Center, 1515 Holcombe Boulevard, Unit 85, Houston, TX, USA
* Corresponding author. Section of Dermatopathology, Department of Pathology, The University of Texas MD Anderson Cancer Center, 1515 Holcombe Boulevard, Unit 85, Houston, TX.
E-mail address: mtetzlaff@mdanderson.org

Clin Lab Med 37 (2017) 431–448
http://dx.doi.org/10.1016/j.cll.2017.05.003
0272-2712/17/© 2017 Elsevier Inc. All rights reserved.

INTRODUCTION

Spitz nevi were first described in 1948 by Sophie Spitz as "juvenile melanoma," a term intended to capture the important clinicopathologic differences between Spitz nevi, benign nevi in children, and malignant melanoma in adults.[1] A more descriptive term was subsequently proffered to capture the distinctive cytologic features Spitzoid lesions: "spindle and/or epithelioid cell nevi."[2,3] Traditionally, Spitzoid neoplasms comprise a challenging set of melanocytic lesions to diagnose because their morphology does not always reliably reflect their biological potential.[4–13] At one end of the spectrum, there are unequivocally benign Spitz nevi; at the other end, there are clearly malignant Spitzoid melanomas. These lesions exhibit sufficiently distinctive benign or malignant histopathologic features that support their diagnosis with reasonable certainty. However, there is a subset of so-called atypical Spitz tumors (ASTs) composed of spindled and/or epithelioid melanocytes with both incontrovertibly atypical and benign histopathologic features that preclude definitive classification as nevus or melanoma. An additional vexing consideration in the classification of ASTs is the well-recognized proclivity of a subset of these lesions to involve regional lymph nodes without further progression, prompting some to consider ASTs lesions of "intermediate malignancy,"[6,7,9,14–16] although not all authors agree with this concept, in part owing to the small fraction of ASTs with lethal clinical course despite their indeterminate morphology.[17] To date, no histopathologic criteria have been proffered that inform the diagnosis with confidence and reproducibly predict an aggressive clinical course for all Spitzoid neoplasms.[4–13] There is, therefore, a critical need to refine the existing diagnostic criteria for ASTs to facilitate accurate and reproducible diagnosis.

The past decade has witnessed an exponential expansion of our understanding of the molecular genetics underlying the development and progression of melanocytic tumors,[18–21] enabling more systematic and definitive classification of these lesions. This improvement in classification impacts both intelligent prognostication and more rational selection (and possibly earlier deployment) of systemic therapy. The application of comparative genomic hybridization (CGH) to melanocytic tumors demonstrated frequent genomic instability typical of melanomas, but not nevi.[22–27] This fundamental genetic disparity was leveraged in the development of the fluorescence in situ hybridization (FISH) assay, which interrogates a lesion for high-frequency copy number alterations to inform diagnosis and, more recently, prognosis.[28,29] In parallel, high-throughput sequencing analyses identified mutations prevalent in conventional melanomas and permitted molecular–genetic classification of melanomas according to driver mutations in *BRAF*, *RAS*, and *NF1*, or as "triple wild type."[19] Integration of histopathologic features with molecular–genetic changes underscores clinically actionable and/or prognostically relevant biomarkers associated with a particular lesion.[30]

As our understanding of these molecular–genetic features increases, knowledge of the molecular genetics unique to Spitzoid lesions has begun to be applied to their diagnosis, and the outlines of a molecular–genetic classification scheme for Spitzoid lesions are emerging. In addition to being classified on the basis of histomorphologic features, Spitzoid lesions can now be reasonably grouped according to molecular–genetic alterations driving tumor formation and/or possibly informing prognosis or therapy into a number of different subtypes, including Spitzoid lesions with (1) 11p amplification and/or *HRAS* mutations,[31,32] (2) homozygous deletion of 9p21,[33–35] (3) isolated loss of 6q23,[36,37] (4) BAP1 loss and *BRAFV600E* mutation,[38–41] (5) translocations involving different oncogenic kinase drivers, including *ROS1*, *ALK*, *NTRK1*, *NTRK3*, *MET*, *BRAF*, and *RET*,[42–44] and (6) mutations in the *TERT* promoter.[45]

SPITZ NEVI WITH 11P AMPLIFICATION AND/OR *HRAS* MUTATIONS

The first Spitzoid lesion recognized with specific molecular–genetic alterations that also correlated with both a relatively distinctive histomorphology and a benign clinical course[23,24] was identified by application of CGH applied to a series of Spitz nevi, revealing a small subset with isolated copy number gains of chromosome 11p. In addition, 67% of Spitz nevi carrying gains in 11p also had activating mutations in *HRAS*, compared with 5% of lesions without 11p gains.[23,24] Subsequent studies confirmed a low frequency (~15%) of *HRAS* mutations overall in Spitz nevi.[32,46]

Furthermore, Spitz nevi with 11p amplification (so-called 11p Spitz nevi) exhibit histopathologic features distinctive from those of lesions lacking this alteration. Specifically, 11p Spitz nevi are typically either compound or predominantly intradermal, and toward their base, exhibit an infiltrative single-cell pattern of growth amid a desmoplastic collagenous stroma with prominent nuclear pleomorphism in tumor cells (an example shown in **Fig. 1**). No morphologic differences existed between 11p Spitz nevi

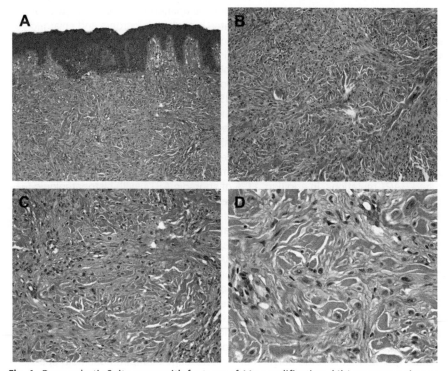

Fig. 1. Desmoplastic Spitz nevus with features of 11p amplification. (*A*) Low-power view reveals skin with an intradermal proliferation of melanocytes in a desmplastic stroma (stain: hematoxylin and eosin; original magnification, ×40). (*B*) Spindled and epithelioid melanocytes among thickened collagen bundles (stain: hematoxylin and eosin; original magnification, ×100). (*C*) Spindled and epithelioid melanocytes amid a fibrocollagenous stroma (stain: hematoxylin and eosin; original magnification, ×200). (*D*) Higher power examination reveals clusters of monotonous epithelioid melanocytes with increased pale eosinophilic cytoplasm and enlarged oval-irregular nuclei with conspicuous nucleoli amid a desmoplastic collagenous stroma (stain: hematoxylin and eosin; original magnification, ×400). (*Courtesy of* Dr Steven D. Billings, Cleveland Clinic.)

with *HRAS* mutations compared with wild-type *HRAS*,[23,24] and similar histopathologic features were described in *HRAS*-mutated Spitz nevi.[32]

Importantly, *HRAS* mutations have not yet been identified in unequivocal Spitzoid melanomas,[46–48] and 11p Spitzoid lesions with or without *HRAS* mutations have not been reported to produce metastases. Together, these findings thus defined the first set of lesions with Spitzoid morphology, a discrete molecular–genetic change (11p amplified and/or *HRAS* mutated), distinctive histopathologic/architectural features, and a predictable clinical course and, therefore, established the paradigm for subsequent studies aimed at defining other similarly morphologically, molecularly, and clinically distinctive subsets of Spitzoid lesions.

SPITZOID NEOPLASMS WITH BAP1 LOSS AND *BRAFV600E* MUTATION

A multiinstitutional study described 2 families whose offspring harbored numerous dome-shaped, well-circumscribed, tan to red papules and occasional affected offspring with of melanoma (uveal and cutaneous) with autosomal dominant inheritance.[39] Histopathologic examination of the papular lesions revealed a predominantly intradermal proliferation of variably sized atypical epithelioid melanocytes with abundant amphophilic cytoplasm, well-demarcated cytoplasmic borders and enlarged vesicular nuclei with prominent nucleoli (reminiscent of Spitz nevi) and an intimately associated lymphohistiocytic inflammatory infiltrate. Although these lesions resembled Spitz nevi, they were distinct from classic Spitz nevi in that they lacked the stereotypical (1) epidermal acanthosis and hypergranulosis, (2) cleft formation around junctional nests, and (3) Kamino bodies. In addition, 88% of the lesions harbored *BRAFV600E* mutations, which is not typical of Spitzoid lesions. Molecular–genetic studies identified inherited mutations in *BAP1* in the affected individuals with loss of heterozygosity confirmed in the majority of the papular lesions. Analysis of the contribution of *BAP1* to the development of sporadically acquired melanocytic lesions revealed a subset of uveal melanomas (40%) and cutaneous melanomas (7%) contained somatically acquired *BAP1* mutations. In addition, 11% of sporadic ASTs (with histopathologic features similar to those seen in the inherited lesions) lacked expression of nuclear *BAP1* and were positive for *BRAFV600E* mutations, further supporting a distinctive clinical and histopathologic phenotype associated with this genotype.[39]

The role of *BAP1* in the development of sporadic Spitzoid melanocytic tumors was formally assessed[41] and revealed loss of BAP1 protein expression in 28% of a series of sporadically occurring ASTs, which correlated with somatically acquired *BAP1* frameshift mutations. A *BRAFV600E* mutation was identified in most of these sporadic BAP1-negative tumors. More important, the sporadic BAP1-negative ASTs exhibited histopathologic features essentially identical to those seen in the familial cases.[41] Yeh and colleagues[40] also described histopathologically identical sporadically occurring *BAP1*-deficient Spitzoid melanocytic tumors by leveraging their CGH database to capture lesions with isolated deletion of variable lengths of chromosome 3 spanning the *BAP1* locus. Available clinical follow-up information revealed no evidence of recurrence in their series. Yeh and colleagues[40] were also the first to show BAP1 loss in a case of melanoma with features of a cellular blue nevus, suggesting an additional association between *BAP1* loss and blue nevus–like melanomas. Several subsequent studies have since confirmed this association.[49–52]

Two studies[38,53] described a series of sporadic compound *BAP1*-deficient Spitzoid nevi with *BRAFV600E* mutation. In contrast with the previous studies, the nevi described in these series exhibited a biphasic composition of small and large Spitzoid epithelioid melanocytes in a stereotypical dermal distribution: small nevoid melanocytes in the peripheral and deep aspects of the lesion blending together with larger Spitzoid epithelioid melanocytes situated in the center of the lesion. Whereas the epithelioid melanocytes lacked nuclear BAP1 expression, the banal nevoid melanocytes exhibited preserved nuclear BAP1 expression, and all the melanocytes were immunoreactive with antibodies for *BRAFV600E* (an example of such a lesion is shown in **Fig. 2**).[38,53] The overall indolent clinical behavior together with the longstanding

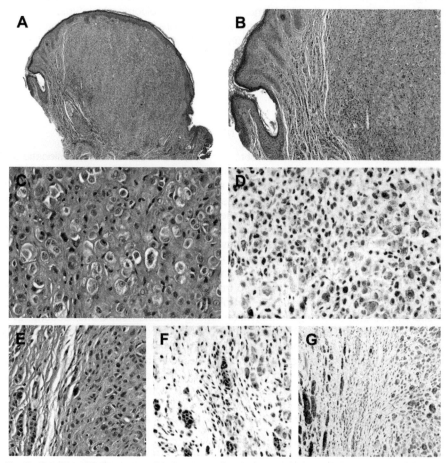

Fig. 2. Combined Spitz nevus with features of *BAP1* loss and *BRAFV600E* mutation. (*A*) Scanning magnification reveals papular architecture of predominantly intradermal proliferation of melanocytes (stain: hematoxylin and eosin; original magnification, ×20). (*B*) Biphasic proliferation of melanocytes with small banal melanocytes toward the periphery (*left*) and epithelioid melanocytes toward the center (stain: hematoxylin and eosin; original magnification, ×100). (*C*) Epithelioid melanocytes amid a fibrocollagenous stroma and variable lymphocytic infiltrate comprise the central portion of the lesion (stain: hematoxylin and eosin; original magnification, ×400), and (*D*) these lack nuclear expression of BAP1 (original magnification, ×400). (*E*) Juxtaposition of banal melanocytes (*left*) and epithelioid melanocytes (*right*; stain: hematoxylin and eosin; original magnification, ×200). (*F*) BAP1 immunohistochemistry reveals preserved nuclear expression of BAP1 protein in the nuclei of the banal melanocytes (*left*), but loss of nuclear BAP1 in the epithelioid forms (*right*; original magnification, ×200). (*G*) Immunohistochemical study for BRAFV600E (VE1) reveals *BRAFV600E* mutation in all cells of the lesion (original magnification, ×100).

presence of these lesions supported the benign diagnoses. In retrospect, this histo-pathologically distinct subset of Spitzoid tumors had been previously described, but without the connection to *BAP1*. Harvell and colleagues[54] described a series of Spit-zoid tumors exhibiting a combined morphology consisting of conventional banal nevoid melanocytes peripherally and centrally located epithelioid melanocytes with a distinctive lymphocytic "halo" response.

Together, these studies delineated a histopathologically distinct subset of Spitzoid neoplasms: predominantly intradermal proliferations of pleomorphic atypical epithe-lioid melanocytes (occasionally with an adjacent more banal nevoid proliferation of melanocytes) with an associated lymphohistiocytic inflammatory infiltrate and further defined by loss of nuclear BAP1 expression, often with coexisting *BRAFV600E* muta-tions,[41] and of particular significance, a predictably benign clinical course. The name "BAP1-inactivated Spitzoid nevi" is among the names proffered to describe such lesions.[55]

TRANSLOCATION-ASSOCIATED SPITZOID NEOPLASMS

Wiesner and colleagues[42] were the first to identify kinase fusion events (translocations) in Spitzoid lesions. Overall, kinase fusions were identified in 51% of lesions tested, including 55% of Spitz nevi, 56% of ASTs, and 39% of Spitzoid melanomas. Translo-cations involved the following kinase genes: *ROS1* (17%), *ALK* (10%), *NTRK1* (16%), *BRAF* (5%), and *RET* (3%). Activation of the aforementioned kinases by translocation events has also been described in numerous other cancer types.[56–70] The presence of one kinase fusion event was mutually exclusive with any other; each of the fusions was identified across the spectrum Spitzoid neoplasms; and each resulted in a fusion pro-tein with constitutive (ligand-independent) activation of the kinase.[42]

Many important conclusions emerged from this study. First, the high frequency of activating kinase fusion events (51% of Spitzoid lesions) suggests these represent a critical mechanism of oncogene activation among Spitzoid neoplasms. Second, the presence of these translocations across the histopathologic spectrum of Spitzoid le-sions argues that the translocation event is an early event in tumorigenesis. However, as of yet, no discrete translocation event by itself seemed to be sufficient for malignant transformation or to define a particular histopathologic or biological phenotype. Finally, given the tendency of ASTs and Spitzoid melanomas to produce metastases, the identification of recurring translocations activating kinases known to be clinically actionable reveals potentially susceptible targets for systemic therapy.[71–74]

Spitzoid Neoplasms with ALK Translocations

Distinctive clinical and/or pathologic features Spitzoid tumors containing *ALK* fusions have been described (**Table 1**).[75–78] *ALK*-rearranged Spitzoid lesions occur in adoles-cent patients without an apparent gender predilection most frequently on the extrem-ity (58%). The majority of *ALK*-rearranged Spitzoid lesions were classified as AST (62%); only 8% were classified as Spitzoid melanoma.[42,75–77] Immunohistochemistry (IHC) for ALK was positive in virtually all cases, and IHC is widely considered an accu-rate surrogate for *ALK* translocation.[42,75–77] The cases tested by melanoma FISH (6p25, 6q23, cep6, 11q13, cep9, and 9p21)[75,77] failed to meet criteria for malignancy.

ALK-rearranged Spitzoid tumors also exhibit distinctive histopathologic fea-tures.[75–78] Histopathologically, they are compound or predominantly intradermal, with an exophytic and/or wedge-shaped silhouette and plexiform growth pattern con-sisting of fusiform amelanotic melanocytes arranged in intersecting fascicles among dermal collagen bundles (an example shown in **Fig. 3**). Rare cases with metastases

Table 1
Summary of clinical characteristics of ALK-rearranged Spitzoid neoplasms

Author (Reference)	Busam et al,[75] 2014	Yeh et al,[76] 2015	Amin et al,[77] 2016	Totals
Gender				
Men	9	11	12	32
Women	8	21	5	34
Median age, y (range)	16 y (2–35 y)	12 y (5 mo–64 y)	13 y (1–38 y)	
Location				
Extremity (upper/lower)	8	18	11	37
Trunk/buttock	4	8	2	14
Head/neck	3	6	4	13
Diagnosis				
Spitz nevus	5	6	Not specified	11
Atypical Spitz tumor	12	22	Not specified	34
Spitzoid melanoma	0	4	0	4

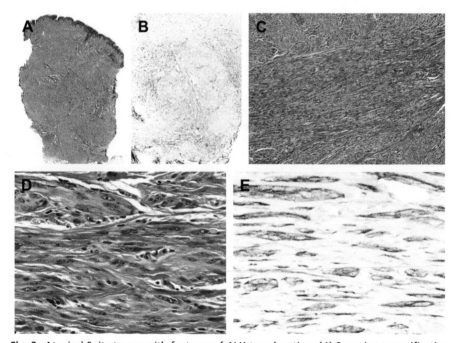

Fig. 3. Atypical Spitz tumor with features of ALK-translocation. (*A*) Scanning magnification reveals skin with a deeply infiltrative proliferation of melanocytes extending throughout the dermis (stain: hematoxylin and eosin; original magnification, ×20). (*B*) ALK immunohistochemistry highlight the pandermal proliferation of melanocytes (original magnification, ×20). (*C*) The lesion is composed of alternating fascicles of spindled melanocytes (stain: hematoxylin and eosin; original magnification, ×100). (*D*) Clusters of spindled melanocytes amid a dense fibrocollagenous stroma. (*E*) ALK immunohistochemical studies highlight the spindled melanocytes. (Courtesy of Dr Steven D. Billings, Cleveland Clinic.)

restricted to sentinel lymph nodes (SLNs) have been identified, but long-term follow-up has not identified further aggressive behavior. The 5' fusion partners with *ALK* vary; the most commonly reported are *TPM3* (tropomyosin 3) and *DCTN1* (dynactin subunit 1). To date, no discrete 5' fusion partner correlates with a distinctive clinical or histopathologic phenotype.[42,75–77]

Spitzoid Neoplasms with NTRK1 Translocations

The clinical and histopathologic characteristics of Spitzoid lesions with *NTRK1* translocations have also begun to coalesce.[34,42,77] Neither a gender predilection nor an anatomic preference has been described. Although most *NTRK1*-associated Spitzoid neoplasms reported to date were Spitz nevi or ASTs, a few were Spitzoid melanomas.[42,77] As for *ALK* rearranged Spitz lesions, IHC is a reliable surrogate for *NTRK1* rearrangement.[34,42,77] Some common histopathologic features of *NTRK1*-rearranged Spitzoid lesions have been reported[77] and include either an exophytic/verrucous (41%) or plaquelike (35%) configurations with frequent overlying epidermal hyperplasia (88%). Approximately one-half of *NTRK1*-rearranged Spitzoid lesions exhibit a wedge-shaped silhouette and contain Kamino bodies.[77] Although the tumor cells of *NTRK1*-rearranged Spitzoid lesions are most often small and spindled,[77] just fewer than one-half of cases have an epithelioid tumor cell morphology.[78] Among *NRTK1*-rearranged lesions tested using melanoma FISH (6p25, 6q23, cen6, 11q13, and 9p21), rare cases met criteria for malignancy (homozygous deletion of 9p21).[34,77]

Spitzoid Neoplasms with BRAF Translocations

Although activating *BRAF* mutations are vanishingly rare in Spitzoid neoplasms (except in *BAP1*-deficient tumors), activating *BRAF* translocations have recently been described.[34,42,72,77] To date, documented or suggested *BRAF* translocations have been reported in 28 Spitzoid lesions, including Spitz nevi, AST, and Spitzoid melanoma.[42,45,72,77] In the largest series of *BRAF*-rearranged Spitz lesions, one-half occurred on the extremities, with the remainder distributed on the head, neck, and trunk. Their architecture varied from plaquelike, nodular, or exophytic/verrucous. Most were compound with epidermal hyperplasia, but Kamino bodies were rare. *BRAF*-rearranged Spitz lesions essentially showed 1 of 2 histopathologic appearances: (1) a sheetlike or sclerosing growth pattern with medium to large epithelioid cells with prominent nuclear atypia and lacking prominent melanin pigmentation or (2) a plaquelike silhouette with the lesion exhibiting architectural features of dysplastic nevus and only moderate nuclear atypia.[77] Only 17% of *BRAF*-rearranged lesions tested exhibited melanoma FISH alterations: one with homozygous deletion of 9p21 and gains of 6p25, and a second case with gains of 6p25, although neither met histopathologic criteria for classification as Spitzoid melanoma.[77] In contrast with the other activating kinase fusions, IHC is not a discriminating marker for *BRAF*-rearranged lesions because the BRAF protein is endogenously expressed in melanocytes.

Spitzoid Neoplasms with NTRK3 and MET Translocations

Additional novel translocations in Spitzoid lesions were identified recently, including rearrangements activating *MET*[43] and *NTRK3*.[44] Each study drew from a collection of 1202 "difficult to classify melanocytic tumors" for which CGH was performed to inform diagnosis. Among these, 8 Spitzoid neoplasms with rearrangements in *NTRK3* and 6 Spitzoid neoplasms with rearrangements in *MET* were identified. Rearrangements in either *NTRK3* or *MET* were mutually exclusive with other translocations or with oncogenic mutations activating *BRAF*, *NRAS*, *HRAS*, *GNAQ*, and *GNA11*.

The majority of NTRK3-rearranged Spitzoid lesions occurred in females on the head and neck with a median age of 10 years. The lesions were classified as Spitz nevi or as ASTs. Mostly recurring 5' fusion partners were identified: ETV6 (n = 4), MYO5A (n = 3), and MYH9 (n = 1).[44] Histopathologically, most NTRK3-rearranged lesions exhibited a predominantly dermal location and had nonspecific Spitzoid morphology with frequent epidermal hyperplasia and clefting around junctional melanocytes. Patients with NTRK3-rearranged Spitzoid lesions had mostly negative follow-up (35 months to 4.5 years), although 1 NTRK3-rearranged AST produced metastases limited to the SLN but without evidence of recurrence after 3.5 years.[44]

All MET-rearranged Spitzoid tumors (n = 6) occurred in females, most commonly on the extremities, and with a median age at diagnosis of 20.5 years. Lesions were classified as Spitzoid melanomas or ASTs.[43] Histopathologically, MET-rearranged lesions exhibited a nonspecific Spitzoid morphology, and IHC for MET showed increased expression compared with non–MET-rearranged lesions. All patients with follow-up were free of disease. Many different 5' fusion partners were identified.[43]

CLINICAL BEHAVIOR IN SPITZOID NEOPLASMS AS PREDICTED BY MELANOMA FLUORESCENCE IN SITU HYBRIDIZATION ASSAY: SPITZOID LESIONS WITH HOMOZYGOUS DELETION OF 9P21 OR ISOLATED LOSS OF 6Q23
Fluorescence In Situ Hybridization in the Differentiation of Malignant From Benign Melanocytic Tumors

The melanoma FISH test emerged as a surrogate for the genomic instability described by CGH[22,23,25,26,79] and a potentially useful diagnostic test to delineate melanocytic lesions harboring chromosomal aberrations typical of melanoma.[28,80] The first study assessing the usefulness of melanoma FISH in a diagnostic setting demonstrated a sensitivity of 86.7% and a specificity of 95.4% in the distinction of unambiguous melanoma from nevus.[28] Subsequent confirmatory proof-of-principle studies validated the diagnostic usefulness of FISH in different (mostly unambiguous) diagnostic settings, reporting a similarly high sensitivity and specificity of FISH.[81–89] More recently, additional novel probe combinations improve the sensitivity and specificity of FISH in the distinction of benign from malignant.[29] In addition, FISH results correlate with clinical outcomes. Patients with FISH-positive melanomas more commonly develop metastases and have decreased disease-specific survival compared with patients with FISH-negative melanomas, and discrete FISH probes (8q24 and 11q13) show significant prognostic relevance among conventional melanomas.[33,90,91]

Prognostic Importance of Homozygous Deletion of 9p21 or Loss of 6q23 by Fluorescence In Situ Hybridization in Spitzoid Neoplasms

An important study assessing the prognostic relevance of FISH in a series of ASTs with annotated clinical follow-up showed that distinctive FISH alterations correlated with tumor aggressiveness.[36] FISH probes (including 6p25, cen6, 6q23, 11q13, 8q24, and 9p21)[28 29,92] were applied to 75 ASTs with carefully annotated clinical follow-up. All patients with tumor spread beyond the SLN ("high risk"), but only 23% of patients with limited disease (SLN positivity or less and benign follow-up of >5 years; "low risk") showed copy number alterations in at least 1 of the probes analyzed. Furthermore, among the "high-risk" patients, 82% (9 of 11) had homozygous deletion of 9p21 (including all who died of melanoma), whereas only 5% of the "low risk" patients (3 of 64) showed homozygous deletion of 9p21. Statistically significant indicators of the likelihood of tumor spread beyond a regional lymph node were (1) increased dermal mitotic rate and (2) homozygous loss of 9p21, and only homozygous deletion of 9p21 associated with increased risk of death from melanoma.[36]

The significance of the 9p21 locus to melanoma tumor biology relates to the *CDKN2A* gene (located at 9p21). *CDKN2A* encodes for 2 proteins: p16INK4a and p14ARF. p16INK4a inhibits cyclin D–mediated activation of CDK4 and CDK6, which inactivate Retinoblastoma to promote cell cycle entry. p14ARF inhibits MDM2-mediated destruction of p53. As such, homozygous *CDKN2A* deletion at 9p21 simultaneously abrogates Retinoblastoma-mediated control of cell cycle entry and p53-dependent cell cycle arrest, apoptosis, and DNA damage repair pathways.[30,93,94]

That FISH-positive ASTs represent a distinctive entity from FISH-positive conventional melanomas was explored by correlating FISH results with clinical outcomes among these lesions.[33] Similar to the previous findings, ASTs with metastatic disease beyond the SLN were enriched for homozygous deletion of 9p21 (78%, including 2 with brain metastases), whereas no clinical, histopathologic, or FISH feature correlated with outcome for the patients with conventional melanomas.[33] A study assessing the significance among ASTs of homozygous versus heterozygous deletion of 9p21[35] revealed that, whereas 41% of patients with homozygous deletion of 9p21 developed metastatic disease beyond the SLN, none with heterozygous deletion of 9p21 did. Finally, whereas 53% of conventional melanomas with biallelic loss of 9p21 also had *BRAFV600E*[35] (in line with prior reports[47]), only 2% of 9p21-deficient Spitzoid lesions were positive for BRAFV600E by IHC. Together, these findings underscore the prognostic significance of homozygous deletion of 9p21 among ASTs and confirm that Spitzoid melanomas are both histopathologically and genetically distinct from conventional melanomas in childhood.

Finally, FISH results were correlated with clinical behavior prospectively in a study of childhood Spitzoid lesions (n = 246).[34] FISH was positive in 13% cases overall. Among patients with disease spread beyond the SLN, 75% (3 of 4) harbored homozygous deletion of 9p21. FISH positivity correlated with recurrence and, more specifically, homozygous deletion of 9p21 strongly associated with likelihood of recurrence, although follow-up on at least some of the remaining cases with homozygous 9p21 deletion was not available.[34] As such, although these studies establish a strong association between homozygous deletion of 9p21 and an aggressive clinical course, this is not absolute because not all lesions with biallelic deletion of 9p21 exhibit an aggressive course. In fact, in an additional retrospective study of Spitzoid lesions, homozygous deletion of 9p21 did not associate with an aggressive clinical course. Only limited SLN involvement was identified in 50% of patients with homozygous 9p21 loss, but none showed evidence of distant recurrence.[95] In an additional retrospective study (described elsewhere in this article), homozygous deletion of 9p21 was detected in 24% of patients with a favorable clinical course and 50% with an unfavorable course.[45]

Taken together, homozygous deletion of 9p21 is an important (although not unequivocal) indicator of aggressive behavior and poor prognosis among Spitzoid neoplasms, and Spitzoid lesions carrying this alteration should be so designated ("Spitzoid melanoma/AST with homozygous deletion of 9p21"). Even among cases for which morphologic and immunophenotypic criteria are insufficient to permit a diagnosis of melanoma, the significance of this genomic alteration in the context of an AST and its correlation with a tendency for disease extension beyond the SLN should be emphasized somewhere in the diagnostic report.[34–36] A representative example is shown in **Fig. 4**.

In contrast, although homozygous deletion of 9p21 correlates with an aggressive phenotype, no AST with isolated loss of 6q23 developed advanced locoregional disease or distant metastasis and, accordingly, none died of disease with a follow-up of at least 5 years in the original study.[36] Isolated loss of 6q23 similarly predicted a benign clinical course in an additional retrospective review of 24 ASTs.[37] No patient in this series showed disease extension beyond the SLN (follow-up, 2–60 months), although 6 of

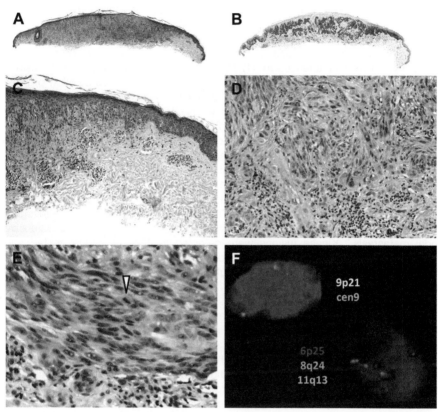

Fig. 4. Spitzoid melanoma with homozygous deletion of 9p21. (*A*) Scanning magnification reveals a mostly symmetric compound melanocytic proliferation (stain: hematoxylin and eosin; original magnification, ×20), which is highlighted by (*B*) Mart-1 immunohistochemistry (original magnification, ×20). (*C*) Toward the peripheral aspects of the lesion, the intraepidermal proliferation exhibits a single cell predominant pattern of growth (stain: hematoxylin and eosin; original magnification, ×100). (*D*) Atypical spindled and epithelioid melanocytes amid a variably dense lymphohistiocytic inflammatory infiltrate (stain: hematoxylin and eosin; original magnification, ×200). (*E*) Atypical spindled and epithelioid melanocytes with increased cytoplasm and enlarged oval-elongate nuclei. *Arrow* highlights a dermal mitotic figure (stain: hematoxylin and eosin; original magnification, ×400). (*F*) Fluorescence in situ hybridization reveals homozygous deletion of 9p21 with no copy number alterations identified at 6p25, 8q24, or 11q13.

11 patients in whom SLN biopsy was performed had a positive SLN. Of particular importance, however, the risk for developing disease beyond the SLN in ASTs with isolated loss of 6q23 was no different than that for ASTs without FISH-defined chromosomal abnormalities, supporting the assertion that patients whose Spitzoid lesions exhibit isolated loss of 6q23 typically have an overall benign clinical course.[37]

ATYPICAL SPITZ TUMORS WITH *TERT* PROMOTER MUTATIONS HAVE AN AGGRESSIVE PHENOTYPE

Recent studies implicated additional novel surrogates of clinically aggressive disease among ASTs.[45] Among 56 patients with an AST and available follow-up information,

52 patients who remained alive without disease ("favorable clinical course") and 4 died with widespread hematogenous metastases ("unfavorable clinical course"). Of note, one-half of the patients who underwent SLN biopsy in this series had at least 1 positive SLN, and 9 had "extensive nodal metastasis" (including the 4 who died of disease). These ASTs were characterized for (1) *TERT* promoter mutations, (2) kinase fusions (including *ROS1*, *NTRK1*, *ALK*, *BRAF*, and *RET*), (3) homozygous deletion of 9p21 by FISH, (4) *BRAF* and *NRAS* mutations, and (5) *PTEN* loss. *TERT* encodes the catalytic subunit for the telomerase complex, which maintains telomere length during DNA replication. In melanoma, mutations in the *TERT* promoter activate TERT expression, providing a pathway through which melanocytes bypass replicative senescence in the setting of activating oncogenic mutations (eg, in *BRAF*). Hot-spot *TERT* promoter mutations were identified in all 4 of the patients with an unfavorable clinical course who eventually died of disease, but in none with a favorable clinical course. As noted, homozygous deletion of 9p21 was detected in 14 of 53 patients tested, including 24% of patients with a favorable course but only 50% with an unfavorable course, although it was unclear whether any of the 12 with favorable course may have also had "extensive nodal metastasis." Kinase fusions were detected in 45% of tumors tested and included *ALK*, *ROS1*, *NTRK1*, *BRAF*, and *RET* fusions. Mutations in *BRAF* were detected in 3 ASTs (no correlation with outcome). Finally, biallelic deletion of *PTEN* was identified in 40% of samples tested with a favorable course and in none of the samples tested with an aggressive course.

Clinical and histopathologic features that correlated with extranodal disease and death included older age ($\geq$10 years), increased mitotic rate (>5/mm^2), and ulceration. Additionally, *TERT* promoter mutations significantly correlated with metastasis beyond the regional lymph nodes and with the risk of death. Homozygous deletion of 9p21 did not correlate with risk of extranodal metastasis or death. These findings suggest that Spitzoid lesions with *TERT* promoter mutations may represent an additional distinctive subtype with an aggressive clinical course; together with the caveats described, the findings of this study also question whether homozygous deletion of 9p21 absolutely predicts an aggressive clinical course among ASTs.[45]

A recent study, however, suggests that the clinical significance of *TERT* promoter mutations requires further investigation.[96] In this study, none of the Spitz/Reed nevi carried somatic mutations in the *TERT* promoter, whereas 2 of the ASTs/Spitzoid melanomas did. However, only 1 of the 2 patients with *TERT* promoter mutations developed subsequent metastases (isolated metastasis limited to the SLN), and both patients with *TERT* promoter mutations were free of disease at the last follow-up. Additional prospective studies are necessary to assess the absolute correlation of *TERT* promoter mutations with aggressive clinical behavior.[96]

SUMMARY

Together, these studies provide a framework to begin categorizing this morphologically ambiguous and biologically unpredictable group of lesions according to their histopathologic and genetic features. Morphologically atypical Spitzoid lesions with any of these changes might reasonably be predicted to have benign clinical follow-up: (1) mutations in *HRAS* and/or isolated gains in chromosome arm 11p, (2) loss of *BAP1* (3p21) and *BRAFV600E* mutations, and (3) isolated loss of 6q23. Some of these lesions—with *HRAS* mutations and/or gains of 11p or with BAP1 loss and *BRAFV600E* mutations—also exhibit stereotypical histopathologic features.

In contrast, ASTs with (1) homozygous deletion of 9p21 or (2) *TERT* promoter mutations might have a more aggressive clinical course. Although such lesions have not yet been shown to exhibit stereotypical histopathologic features, identification of these changes—in the context of otherwise Spitzoid morphology with atypical features—would provide sufficient justification for clinical management according to standard guidelines for melanoma.

Finally, there is a broad class of lesions with either (1) translocations resulting in constitutive activation of various oncogenic kinases: *ROS1, ALK, NTRK1, NTRK3, BRAF, MET,* or *RET* or (2) no genomic alterations. Still, the identification of recurrent kinase fusions as oncogenic driver events in Spitzoid neoplasms provides a molecular–genetic framework for pathologists and clinicians to conceptualize and potentially manage these tumors. Although no particular translocation correlates with a particular clinical course, these changes might eventually be leveraged to inform therapeutic decisions upon metastasis. Further evaluation of these molecular–genetic alterations in Spitzoid lesions will undoubtedly refine the biological significance of different genotypes as well as unveil morphologic clues regarding their presence.

REFERENCES

1. Spitz S. Melanomas of childhood. Am J Pathol 1948;24(3):591.
2. Echevarria R, Ackerman LV. Spindle and epitheloid cell nevi in the adult. Clinicopathologic report of 26 cases. Cancer 1967;20(2):175.
3. Kernen JA, Ackerman LV. Spindle cell nevi and epithelioid cell nevi (so-called juvenile melanomas) in children and adults: a clinicopathological study of 27 cases. Cancer 1960;13:612.
4. Barnhill RL. The Spitzoid lesion: the importance of atypical variants and risk assessment. Am J Dermatopathol 2006;28(1):75.
5. Barnhill RL. The Spitzoid lesion: rethinking Spitz tumors, atypical variants, 'Spitzoid melanoma' and risk assessment. Mod Pathol 2006;19(Suppl 2):S21.
6. Barnhill RL, Argenyi ZB, From L, et al. Atypical Spitz nevi/tumors: lack of consensus for diagnosis, discrimination from melanoma, and prediction of outcome. Hum Pathol 1999;30(5):513.
7. Cerroni L, Barnhill R, Elder D, et al. Melanocytic tumors of uncertain malignant potential: results of a tutorial held at the XXIX Symposium of the International Society of Dermatopathology in Graz, October 2008. Am J Surg Pathol 2010;34(3):314.
8. Gerami P, Busam K, Cochran A, et al. Histomorphologic assessment and interobserver diagnostic reproducibility of atypical Spitzoid melanocytic neoplasms with long-term follow-up. Am J Surg Pathol 2014;38(7):934.
9. Ludgate MW, Fullen DR, Lee J, et al. The atypical Spitz tumor of uncertain biologic potential: a series of 67 patients from a single institution. Cancer 2009; 115(3):631.
10. Mooi WJ, Krausz T. Spitz nevus versus Spitzoid melanoma: diagnostic difficulties, conceptual controversies. Adv Anat Pathol 2006;13(4):147.
11. Spatz A, Barnhill RL. The Spitz tumor 50 years later: revisiting a landmark contribution and unresolved controversy. J Am Acad Dermatol 1999;40(2 Pt 1):223.
12. Spatz A, Calonje E, Handfield-Jones S, et al. Spitz tumors in children: a grading system for risk stratification. Arch Dermatol 1999;135(3):282.
13. Walsh N, Crotty K, Palmer A, et al. Spitz nevus versus Spitzoid malignant melanoma: an evaluation of the current distinguishing histopathologic criteria. Hum Pathol 1998;29(10):1105.
14. Berk DR, Labuz E, Dadras SS, et al. Melanoma and melanocytic tumors of uncertain malignant potential in children, adolescents and young adults-the Stanford experience 1995-2008. Pediatr Dermatol 2010;27(3):244.

15. Hung T, Piris A, Lobo A, et al. Sentinel lymph node metastasis is not predictive of poor outcome in patients with problematic Spitzoid melanocytic tumors. Hum Pathol 2013;44(1):87.
16. Lallas A, Kyrgidis A, Ferrara G, et al. Atypical Spitz tumours and sentinel lymph node biopsy: a systematic review. Lancet Oncol 2014;15(4):e178.
17. Mones JM, Ackerman AB. "Atypical" Spitz's nevus, "malignant" Spitz's nevus, and "metastasizing" Spitz's nevus: critique in historical perspective of three concepts flawed fatally. Am J Dermatopathol 2004;26(4):310.
18. Bastian BC. The molecular pathology of melanoma: an integrated taxonomy of melanocytic neoplasia. Annu Rev Pathol 2014;9:239.
19. Cancer Genome Atlas Network. Genomic classification of cutaneous melanoma. Cell 2015;161(7):1681.
20. Shtivelman E, Davies MQ, Hwu P, et al. Pathways and therapeutic targets in melanoma. Oncotarget 2014;5(7):1701.
21. Woodman SE, Lazar AJ, Aldape KD, et al. New strategies in melanoma: molecular testing in advanced disease. Clin Cancer Res 2012;18(5):1195.
22. Bastian BC, LeBoit PE, Hamm H, et al. Chromosomal gains and losses in primary cutaneous melanomas detected by comparative genomic hybridization. Cancer Res 1998;58(10):2170.
23. Bastian BC, Olshen AB, LeBoit PE, et al. Classifying melanocytic tumors based on DNA copy number changes. Am J Pathol 2003;163(5):1765.
24. Bastian BC, Wesselmann U, Pinkel D, et al. Molecular cytogenetic analysis of Spitz nevi shows clear differences to melanoma. J Invest Dermatol 1999;113(6):1065.
25. Bauer J, Bastian BC. Distinguishing melanocytic nevi from melanoma by DNA copy number changes: comparative genomic hybridization as a research and diagnostic tool. Dermatol Ther 2006;19(1):40.
26. Curtin JA, Fridlyand J, Kageshita T, et al. Distinct sets of genetic alterations in melanoma. N Engl J Med 2005;353(20):2135.
27. Maize JC Jr, McCalmont TH, Carlson JA, et al. Genomic analysis of blue nevi and related dermal melanocytic proliferations. Am J Surg Pathol 2005;29(9):1214.
28. Gerami P, Jewell SS, Morrison LE, et al. Fluorescence in situ hybridization (FISH) as an ancillary diagnostic tool in the diagnosis of melanoma. Am J Surg Pathol 2009;33(8):1146.
29. Gerami P, Li G, Pouryazdanparast P, et al. A highly specific and discriminatory FISH assay for distinguishing between benign and malignant melanocytic neoplasms. Am J Surg Pathol 2012;36(6):808.
30. Wiesner T, Kutzner H, Cerroni L, et al. Genomic aberrations in Spitzoid melanocytic tumours and their implications for diagnosis, prognosis and therapy. Pathology 2016;48(2):113.
31. Bastian BC, LeBoit PE, Pinkel D. Mutations and copy number increase of HRAS in Spitz nevi with distinctive histopathological features. Am J Pathol 2000;157(3):967.
32. van Engen-van Grunsven AC, van Dijk MC, Ruiter DJ, et al. HRAS-mutated Spitz tumors: a subtype of Spitz tumors with distinct features. Am J Surg Pathol 2010;34(10):1436.
33. Gerami P, Cooper C, Bajaj S, et al. Outcomes of atypical Spitz tumors with chromosomal copy number aberrations and conventional melanomas in children. Am J Surg Pathol 2013;37(9):1387.
34. Lee CY, Sholl LM, Zhang B, et al. Atypical Spitzoid neoplasms in childhood: a molecular and outcome study. Am J Dermatopathol 2016;39:181–6.

35. Yazdan P, Cooper C, Sholl LM, et al. Comparative analysis of atypical Spitz tumors with heterozygous versus homozygous 9p21 deletions for clinical outcomes, histomorphology, BRAF mutation, and p16 expression. Am J Surg Pathol 2014;38(5):638.

36. Gerami P, Scolyer RA, Xu X, et al. Risk assessment for atypical Spitzoid melanocytic neoplasms using FISH to identify chromosomal copy number aberrations. Am J Surg Pathol 2013;37(5):676.

37. Shen L, Cooper C, Bajaj S, et al. Atypical Spitz tumors with 6q23 deletions: a clinical, histological, and molecular study. Am J Dermatopathol 2013;35(8):804.

38. Busam KJ, Sung J, Wiesner T, et al. Combined BRAF(V600E)-positive melanocytic lesions with large epithelioid cells lacking BAP1 expression and conventional nevomelanocytes. Am J Surg Pathol 2013;37(2):193.

39. Wiesner T, Obenauf AC, Murali R, et al. Germline mutations in BAP1 predispose to melanocytic tumors. Nat Genet 2011;43(10):1018.

40. Yeh I, Mully TW, Wiesner T, et al. Ambiguous melanocytic tumors with loss of 3p21. Am J Surg Pathol 2014;38(8):1088.

41. Wiesner T, Murali R, Fried I, et al. A distinct subset of atypical Spitz tumors is characterized by BRAF mutation and loss of BAP1 expression. Am J Surg Pathol 2012;36(6):818.

42. Wiesner T, He J, Yelensky R, et al. Kinase fusions are frequent in Spitz tumours and Spitzoid melanomas. Nat Commun 2014;5:3116.

43. Yeh I, Botton T, Talevich E, et al. Activating MET kinase rearrangements in melanoma and Spitz tumours. Nat Commun 2015;6:7174.

44. Yeh I, Tee MK, Botton T, et al. NTRK3 kinase fusions in Spitz tumours. J Pathol 2016;240(3):282.

45. Lee S, Barnhill RL, Dummer R, et al. TERT promoter mutations are predictive of aggressive clinical behavior in patients with Spitzoid melanocytic neoplasms. Sci Rep 2015;5:11200.

46. van Dijk MC, Bernsen MR, Ruiter DJ. Analysis of mutations in B-RAF, N-RAS, and H-RAS genes in the differential diagnosis of Spitz nevus and Spitzoid melanoma. Am J Surg Pathol 2005;29(9):1145.

47. Da Forno PD, Pringle JH, Fletcher A, et al. BRAF, NRAS and HRAS mutations in Spitzoid tumours and their possible pathogenetic significance. Br J Dermatol 2009;161(2):364.

48. Takata M, Lin J, Takayanagi S, et al. Genetic and epigenetic alterations in the differential diagnosis of malignant melanoma and Spitzoid lesion. Br J Dermatol 2007;156(6):1287.

49. Costa S, Byrne M, Pissaloux D, et al. Melanomas associated with blue nevi or Mimicking cellular blue nevi: clinical, pathologic, and molecular study of 11 cases Displaying a high frequency of GNA11 mutations, BAP1 expression loss, and a predilection for the scalp. Am J Surg Pathol 2016;40(3):368.

50. Dai J, Tetzlaff MT, Schuchter LM, et al. Histopathologic and mutational analysis of a case of blue nevus-like melanoma. J Cutan Pathol 2016;43(9):776.

51. Perez-Alea M, Vivancos A, Caratu G, et al. Genetic profile of GNAQ-mutated blue melanocytic neoplasms reveals mutations in genes linked to genomic instability and the PI3K pathway. Oncotarget 2016;7(19):28086.

52. Vivancos A, Caratu G, Matito J, et al. Genetic evolution of nevus of Ota reveals clonal heterogeneity acquiring BAP1 and TP53 mutations. Pigment Cell Melanoma Res 2016;29(2):247.

53. Busam KJ, Wanna M, Wiesner T. Multiple epithelioid Spitz nevi or tumors with loss of BAP1 expression: a clue to a hereditary tumor syndrome. JAMA Dermatol 2013;149(3):335.
54. Harvell JD, Meehan SA, LeBoit PE. Spitz's nevi with halo reaction: a histopathologic study of 17 cases. J Cutan Pathol 1997;24(10):611.
55. Vilain RE, McCarthy SW, Thompson JF, et al. BAP1-inactivated Spitzoid naevi. Am J Surg Pathol 2015;39(5):722.
56. Birchmeier C, Sharma S, Wigler M. Expression and rearrangement of the ROS1 gene in human glioblastoma cells. Proc Natl Acad Sci U S A 1987;84(24):9270.
57. Rikova K, Guo A, Zeng Q, et al. Global survey of phosphotyrosine signaling identifies oncogenic kinases in lung cancer. Cell 2007;131(6):1190.
58. Shaw AT, Costa D, Mino-Kenudson M, et al. Clinicopathologic features of EML4-ALK mutant lung cancer. J Clin Oncol 2009;27(15_suppl):11021.
59. Zhao Z, Verma V, Zhang M. Anaplastic lymphoma kinase: role in cancer and therapy perspective. Cancer Biol Ther 2015;16(12):1691.
60. Ciampi R, Knauf JA, Kerler R, et al. Oncogenic AKAP9-BRAF fusion is a novel mechanism of MAPK pathway activation in thyroid cancer. J Clin Invest 2005;115(1):94.
61. Ciampi R, Knauf JA, Rabes HM, et al. BRAF kinase activation via chromosomal rearrangement in radiation-induced and sporadic thyroid cancer. Cell Cycle 2005;4(4):547.
62. Cin H, Meyer C, Herr R, et al. Oncogenic FAM131B-BRAF fusion resulting from 7q34 deletion comprises an alternative mechanism of MAPK pathway activation in pilocytic astrocytoma. Acta Neuropathol 2011;121(6):763.
63. Palanisamy N, Ateeq B, Kalyana-Sundaram S, et al. Rearrangements of the RAF kinase pathway in prostate cancer, gastric cancer and melanoma. Nat Med 2010;16(7):793.
64. Haller F, Knopf J, Ackermann A, et al. Paediatric and adult soft tissue sarcomas with NTRK1 gene fusions: a subset of spindle cell sarcomas unified by a prominent myopericytic/haemangiopericytic pattern. J Pathol 2016;238(5):700.
65. Beimfohr C, Klugbauer S, Demidchik EP, et al. NTRK1 re-arrangement in papillary thyroid carcinomas of children after the Chernobyl reactor accident. Int J Cancer 1999;80(6):842.
66. Prasad ML, Vyas M, Horne MJ, et al. NTRK fusion oncogenes in pediatric papillary thyroid carcinoma in northeast United States. Cancer 2016;122(7):1097.
67. Vaishnavi A, Capelletti M, Le AT, et al. Oncogenic and drug-sensitive NTRK1 rearrangements in lung cancer. Nat Med 2013;19(11):1469.
68. Park do Y, Choi C, Shin E, et al. NTRK1 fusions for the therapeutic intervention of Korean patients with colon cancer. Oncotarget 2016;7(7):8399.
69. Pierotti MA. Chromosomal rearrangements in thyroid carcinomas: a recombination or death dilemma. Cancer Lett 2001;166(1):1.
70. Williams ED, Abrosimov A, Bogdanova T, et al. Thyroid carcinoma after Chernobyl latent period, morphology and aggressiveness. Br J Cancer 2004;90(11):2219.
71. Hutchinson KE, Lipson D, Stephens PJ, et al. BRAF fusions define a distinct molecular subset of melanomas with potential sensitivity to MEK inhibition. Clin Cancer Res 2013;19(24):6696.
72. Botton T, Yeh I, Nelson T, et al. Recurrent BRAF kinase fusions in melanocytic tumors offer an opportunity for targeted therapy. Pigment Cell Melanoma Res 2013;26(6):845.

73. Shaw AT, Ou SH, Bang YJ, et al. Crizotinib in ROS1-rearranged non-small-cell lung cancer. N Engl J Med 2014;371(21):1963.
74. Solomon B, Wilner KD, Shaw AT. Current status of targeted therapy for anaplastic lymphoma kinase-rearranged non-small cell lung cancer. Clin Pharmacol Ther 2014;95(1):15.
75. Busam KJ, Kutzner H, Cerroni L, et al. Clinical and pathologic findings of Spitz nevi and atypical Spitz tumors with ALK fusions. Am J Surg Pathol 2014;38(7): 925.
76. Yeh I, de la Fouchardiere A, Pissaloux D, et al. Clinical, histopathologic, and genomic features of Spitz tumors with ALK fusions. Am J Surg Pathol 2015; 39(5):581.
77. Amin SM, Haugh AM, Lee CY, et al. A Comparison of morphologic and molecular features of BRAF, ALK, and NTRK1 fusion Spitzoid neoplasms. Am J Surg Pathol 2016;41(4):491–8.
78. Kiuru M, Jungbluth A, Kutzner H, et al. Spitz tumors: comparison of histological features in relationship to immunohistochemical staining for ALK and NTRK1. Int J Surg Pathol 2016;24(3):200.
79. Bastian BC, Xiong J, Frieden IJ, et al. Genetic changes in neoplasms arising in congenital melanocytic nevi: differences between nodular proliferations and melanomas. Am J Pathol 2002;161(4):1163.
80. Morey AL, Murali R, McCarthy SW, et al. Diagnosis of cutaneous melanocytic tumours by four-colour fluorescence in situ hybridisation. Pathology 2009;41(4): 383.
81. Busam KJ, Fang Y, Jhanwar SC, et al. Distinction of conjunctival melanocytic nevi from melanomas by fluorescence in situ hybridization. J Cutan Pathol 2010;37(2): 196.
82. Dalton SR, Gerami P, Kolaitis NA, et al. Use of fluorescence in situ hybridization (FISH) to distinguish intranodal nevus from metastatic melanoma. Am J Surg Pathol 2010;34(2):231.
83. Gammon B, Beilfuss B, Guitart J, et al. Fluorescence in situ hybridization for distinguishing cellular blue nevi from blue nevus-like melanoma. J Cutan Pathol 2011;38(4):335.
84. Gerami P, Barnhill RL, Beilfuss BA, et al. Superficial melanocytic neoplasms with pagetoid melanocytosis: a study of interobserver concordance and correlation with FISH. Am J Surg Pathol 2010;34(6):816.
85. Gerami P, Wass A, Mafee M, et al. Fluorescence in situ hybridization for distinguishing nevoid melanomas from mitotically active nevi. Am J Surg Pathol 2009;33(12):1783.
86. Newman MD, Lertsburapa T, Mirzabeigi M, et al. Fluorescence in situ hybridization as a tool for microstaging in malignant melanoma. Mod Pathol 2009;22(8): 989.
87. Newman MD, Mirzabeigi M, Gerami P. Chromosomal copy number changes supporting the classification of lentiginous junctional melanoma of the elderly as a subtype of melanoma. Mod Pathol 2009;22(9):1258.
88. Pouryazdanparast P, Haghighat Z, Beilfuss BA, et al. Melanocytic nevi with an atypical epithelioid cell component: clinical, histopathologic, and fluorescence in situ hybridization findings. Am J Surg Pathol 2011;35(9):1405.
89. Pouryazdanparast P, Newman M, Mafee M, et al. Distinguishing epithelioid blue nevus from blue nevus-like cutaneous melanoma metastasis using fluorescence in situ hybridization. Am J Surg Pathol 2009;33(9):1396.

90. Gerami P, Jewell SS, Pouryazdanparast P, et al. Copy number gains in 11q13 and 8q24 [corrected] are highly linked to prognosis in cutaneous malignant melanoma. J Mol Diagn 2011;13(3):352.

91. North JP, Vetto JT, Murali R, et al. Assessment of copy number status of chromosomes 6 and 11 by FISH provides independent prognostic information in primary melanoma. Am J Surg Pathol 2011;35(8):1146.

92. Gammon B, Beilfuss B, Guitart J, et al. Enhanced detection of Spitzoid melanomas using fluorescence in situ hybridization with 9p21 as an adjunctive probe. Am J Surg Pathol 2012;36(1):81.

93. Serrano M, Lee H, Chin L, et al. Role of the INK4a locus in tumor suppression and cell mortality. Cell 1996;85(1):27.

94. Takata M, Saida T. Genetic alterations in melanocytic tumors. J Dermatol Sci 2006;43(1):1.

95. Massi D, Tomasini C, Senetta R, et al. Atypical Spitz tumors in patients younger than 18 years. J Am Acad Dermatol 2015;72(1):37.

96. Requena C, Heidenreich B, Kumar R, et al. TERT promoter mutations are not always associated with poor prognosis in atypical Spitzoid tumors. Pigment Cell Melanoma Res 2017;30(2):265.

The Immunology of Melanoma

Jennifer S. Ko, MD, PhD

KEYWORDS

- Tumor • Melanoma • Immunology • T cell • Type 1 • Checkpoint • Prognosis
- Immunotherapy

KEY POINTS

- Melanoma is thought to be the most immunogenic tumor due to its exceptionally high (UV-driven) mutational burden, which allows for the creation of neoantigens recognizable as "non-self" by host immunity.
- Immune editing refers to the process by which the host immune system modifies the quantity and quality of tumor growth, and by which the tumor adapts to grow under the selective pressure of the immune system. It occurs through 3 phases: immune surveillance/elimination, equilibrium, and escape.
- Brisk tumor-infiltrating lymphocytes are associated with improved survival in melanoma and imperfectly overlap with markers currently under investigation to predict responsiveness to immunotherapy.
- T-cell checkpoint inhibitor drugs break tumor-exploited mechanisms of peripheral tolerance at the T-cell priming phase (CTLA-4, ipilimumab) and the T-cell effector phase (PD-1, nivolumab, pembrolizumab) to produce unparalleled clinical responses in melanoma.
- Current research in melanoma is aimed at identifying (better) markers to predict response to immunotherapy, and at discovery of interventions to render immune-excluded tumors immunogenic and responsive to immunotherapy.

INTRODUCTION

Cutaneous melanoma is a relatively common, potentially lethal skin tumor of increasing incidence, with a propensity to affect relatively young patients, and a highly variable survival among patients with localized disease. It has a propensity for metastasis, with potential for visceral organ spread occurring remarkably early in its growth phase. Hence, melanoma has been the subject of intense research over the past several decades. Immunology is woven throughout the history of cancer, and the story of melanoma, in particular, with powerful prognostic and therapeutic influences.

Department of Anatomic Pathology, Cleveland Clinic, 9500 Euclid Avenue, L2-150, Cleveland, OH 44195, USA
E-mail address: koj2@ccf.org

Clin Lab Med 37 (2017) 449–471
http://dx.doi.org/10.1016/j.cll.2017.06.001
0272-2712/17/© 2017 Elsevier Inc. All rights reserved.

labmed.theclinics.com

Indeed, melanoma has paved the way for our understanding of immunotherapy, which now influences many other tumor types, including Merkel cell carcinoma, lung carcinoma, renal cell carcinoma, and many more. The interrelationship between the immune system and malignancy is best understood through the concept of cancer immunoediting, which exists in continuum from immunosurveillance to immune equilibrium to tumor escape. This review discusses the historical background, scientific basis, and clinical implications of melanoma's intricate relationship with host immunity, using the framework of immunoediting.

TUMOR IMMUNOLOGY: HISTORICAL PERSPECTIVE

The history of tumor immunology has been wrought with controversy. More than 100 years ago, Paul Ehrlich[1] initiated a century of contentious debate over immunologic control of neoplasia. He was a pathologist and chemist who won the Nobel Prize in 1908 mostly for his work with antibodies, antisera, and antitoxins. He observed that when tumors in mice were cultivated by sequential transplantation to other mice, their malignancy increased from generation to generation. He also noted that when a primary tumor was removed, the metastasis would precipitously increase. In an analogy to vaccination, he attempted to generate immunity to cancer by injecting weakened cancer cells. Based on his research, Ehrlich proposed in 1909 that tumor cells, due to altered patterns of protein expression, differ from their normal cellular counterparts, and that these differences allow them to be recognized and destroyed by immune cells via a process called immunosurveillance.[1] In 1957, Burnet and Thomas[2,3] formalized this proposal in their cancer immunosurveillance hypothesis, which predicted that the immune system recognizes and eliminates nascent transformed cells, based on "the emergence of a new and therefore foreign antigenic pattern" in cancer. In the same publication, they cited work by Black and colleagues,[4] which found a sharp correlation between the degree of lymphocytic inflammation in surgically removed tumors, and the likelihood of "cure" following surgery. The cancer immunosurveillance hypothesis also postulated that most tumors are eliminated before becoming clinically apparent, and that tumor development is usually suppressed. At the same time, landmark experiments by Old and colleagues[5] showed that inoculation with Bacillus Calmette-Guerin (BCG) was curative of bladder cancer in mice; and this observation has since led to the widespread clinical use of BCG as intravesicular immunotherapy for treating early-stage bladder cancer.[6]

In the following 2 decades, researchers sought to validate the immunosurveillance hypothesis by testing the incidence of spontaneous, chemically induced, or virally induced tumors in various populations of mice. Initial studies, done by Stutman and Rygaard and Povlsen,[7–9] showed that athymic nude mice failed to form more chemically induced or spontaneous tumors than their wild-type (WT) counterparts. Virally induced tumors occurred much more frequently in athymic nude mice, but this was thought to relate to increased viral replication.[10] Although it is now known that the negative results obtained by Stutman and Rygaard and Povlsen[7–9] were likely reflective of several important experimental caveats to their study design, including and not limited to the intact lymphocytes that still circulate in nude athymic mice, enthusiasm vanished for immunosurveillance by 1978, and researchers concluded that the cancer immunosurveillance hypothesis was dead.[11] Instead, the field of tumor immunology began to work on other areas, including defining the molecular nature of tumor antigens and the development of immunotherapeutic strategies for cancer. This abandonment is reflected in the Cell publication in 2000 by Hanahan and Weinberg,[12] in which they described the 6 crucial obstacles a cancer must overcome to become a clinical threat. Missing from this list was the requirement of a tumor to avoid host immune surveillance.

MODERN ACCEPTANCE OF TUMOR IMMUNOLOGY
Immunosurveillance

In the 1990s, several experiments pursuing similar hypotheses with alternative technical designs led to renewed interest in immunosurveillance. At that time, the functional CD4+ T-cell system was known to include at least 2 populations of helper cells, Th1 and Th2 (now at least 4 main populations, and other subpopulations, are known, **Fig. 1**), distinguished by the cytokines they produce following activation through the T-cell receptor (TCR). It was known that Th1 cells preferentially secrete interferon-gamma (IFN-γ) and Th2 cells-interleukin (IL)-4 and IL-5, and that Th1-biased responses direct cell-mediated immunity induced by intracellular pathogens, via stimulation of natural killer (NK) cells, cytotoxic CD8+ T-cell activation, and macrophage and dendritic cell (DC) activation. Meanwhile, Th2-biased responses lead to antibody production to target nematode infections.[13–16] Given this information, scientists used different mouse models to compare tumor growth under normal conditions in which endogenous IFN-γ was intact, compared with conditions in which IFN-γ was blocked. Along the same lines, tumor formation was compared in normal, WT mice with that in mice lacking perforin, a cytolytic agent used by cytotoxic T cells and NK cells.[16] In both types of experiments, mice lacking either IFN-γ or perforin were more likely to develop chemically induced tumors, grew more tumors, and grew larger tumors with a shorter latency time. In addition, untreated mice lacking IFN-γ[16–19] or perforin[19–23] were more likely to develop spontaneous lymphomas and

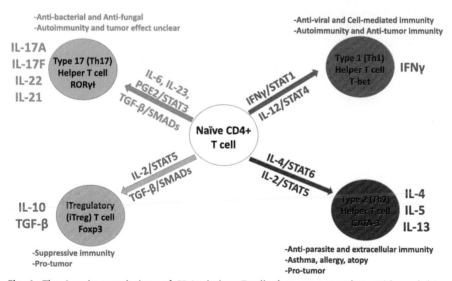

Fig. 1. The 4 main populations of CD4+ helper T cells that can expand to guide and drive the extent and type of immune response that ensues are depicted. The diagonal lines show the cytokines and the downstream transcription factors involved in programming each type of response. The circles also contain the master transcription factor regulator for each type of response. To the side are the main cytokines whose production defines each type of response. iTreg, inducible Tregulatory cell; ROR, retinoic acid receptor-related orphan receptor; TGF, transforming growth factor.

lung adenocarcinomas, a finding enhanced in mice lacking 1 of 2 *P53* tumor suppressor genes.

The creation of RAG knockout mice that completely lack NK T cells (NKT), T cells, and B cells, allowed for experiments that solidified proof of immunosurveillance.[24–26] These experiments showed that RAG-2−/− mice developed sarcomas more rapidly and frequently after exposure to the chemical methylcholanthrene (MCA), and developed more spontaneous epithelial tumors (lung, mammary, intestinal) than WT mice in a germ-free environment.[24–27] Following experiments observed increased tumor incidence and growth rate in mice missing isolated or combinations of defects in IFN-γ, RAG (all lymphocytes), αβT cells, NK cells, NKT cells, γδT cells, perforin, or IL-12 (which directs Th1 differentiation and IFN-γ production), hence showing that these tumor suppressor pathways are largely overlapping. As such, the Th1 type-1 driven cytotoxic response (IFN-γ) was accepted as the antitumor response, with the most robust tumor surveillance relying on combined functions of all T-cell and NK-cell subsets.[26–28]

Data to substantiate the clinical relevance of tumor immunosurveillance has been sought largely through epidemiologic studies. Early studies found that immunosuppressed patients with transplantation and patients with primary immunodeficiencies had a significantly higher relative risk for cancer development.[29–31] Over time, however, it has come to light that some of this risk was due to increased virally mediated tumors such as non-Hodgkin lymphoma (Epstein-Barr virus), Kaposi sarcoma (human herpesvirus 8), and anogenital/oropharyngeal carcinomas (human papilloma virus).[32,33] These data, although not negating the possibility that nonviral tumors are surveyed for by the immune system, make it harder to study the risk of nonvirally induced tumors, which develop more slowly. That said, greater relative risk ratios have been observed for a broad subset of tumors without known viral etiology. This includes an approximately fourfold increase in the incidence of de novo malignant melanoma development after organ transplantation.[34–36]

The modern era of gene sequencing, tumor atlases, and computational biology has led to exponential growth in the understanding of cancer genomics. Because of this, the hypothesis of early scientists that tumors express unique proteins compared with their normal counterparts, has been conclusively proven, and multiple tumor types shown to accumulate increasing somatic mutations during progression, due to inherent genetic instability.[37,38] In point, the so-called "driver" mutations, such as *BRAF*, *CKIT*, and *NRAS* in melanoma, which occur early in oncogenesis, are accompanied by numerous "passenger" mutations that do not necessarily contribute to pathogenicity, but that generate altered proteins serving as "neoantigens," which allow for immune cell recognition. Although the frequency of nonsynonymous mutations varies by more than 1000-fold across cancer types, it can exceed 100 per Mb in melanoma (range 0.1–100/Mb).[37] Indeed, melanoma is among the most mutated tumor types of all (along with lung adenocarcinoma). And so in summary, tumor mutations enable immune recognition early on, allowing for immune elimination in some circumstances, and also form the foundation for immunotherapy. The relatively high mutational burden in melanoma is one factor that is thought to contribute to its relatively high immunogenicity and responsiveness to immunotherapy, and because of this, melanoma has been the prototype tumor for immunotherapy of cancer.

Immune Equilibrium

Within the framework of immunoediting, cancers that are not recognized and eliminated during immunosurveillance go on to the second phase: immune equilibrium.

During this time, tumors enter a dynamic balance with the immune system wherein antitumor immunity contains, but does not fully eradicate, a heterogeneous population of tumor cells. Tumor cell genetic instability allows them to grow, under the selective pressure of the immune system, into edited, immune-selected variants that are largely capable of evading immune recognition or suppressing immune cell function through various mechanisms. Two landmark experiments that best demonstrate immune editing and immune equilibrium, respectively, are summarized in **Figs. 2** and **3**.

First, Shankaran and colleagues[25] compared carcinogen-induced tumors generated in and harvested from immunocompetent (WT) mice and immuno-deficient (RAG2−/−) mice to demonstrate *immune editing* (see **Fig. 2**). In these experiments, tumor cell lines were established from tumors arising in each group of mice, and these cells were then injected into immunodeficient (RAG2−/−) recipient mice or immunocompetent (WT) recipient mice. Tumors taken from WT mice formed progressively growing cancers when transferred to both WT and RAG2−/− mice 100% of the time. In contrast, although tumor cells from immunodeficient mice grew progressively

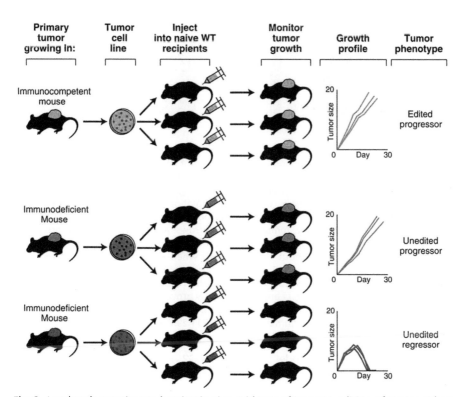

Fig. 2. Landmark experiment showing in vivo evidence of immuno editing of cancer. When tumors are grown in WT immune-competent mice (intact immune system edits tumor, *top*) they grow progressively 100% of the time whether they are transferred to WT (shown) or immunodeficient (not shown) mice. When tumors are grown in immunodeficient mice (no intact immune system to edit tumor, *bottom*) they only grow progressively 60% of the time when transferred to WT (shown) mice. They progress 100% of time in immunodeficient (not shown) mice. (*From* Schreiber RD, Old LJ, Smyth MJ. Cancer immunoediting: integrating immunity's roles in cancer suppression and promotion. Science 2011;331(6024):1566; with permission.)

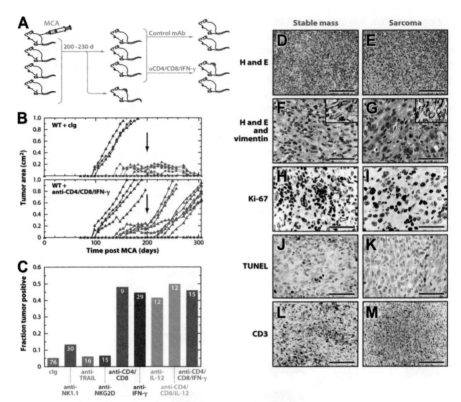

Fig. 3. Landmark experiment showing in vivo evidence of immune equilibrium in cancer. (*A*) Overall schema of experiment. After receiving a chemical to induce malignant transformation, a portion of mice develop progressively growing tumors (*red bump*). Within the portion of mice that are seemingly cancer free, depletion of various components of the type 1 immune response (listed in *C*) will lead to outgrowth of clinically dormant tumors that were held in equilibrium by immune cells (*B; arrows:* at day 200 antibodies are delivered to tumor-free mice; *violet triangles*: mice that develop tumors immediately; *blue triangles*: mice continue to live without tumor growth when control antibody is given; *red triangles*: mice grow tumors when T cells or other type 1–related factors are depleted with antibody). (*Right column*) Histologic comparison of stable nodules at tumor cell injection site, in equilibrium (*D, F, H, J, L*) and progressively growing tumors (*E, G, I, K, M*). H and E, hematoxylin-eosin. (*From* Vesely MD, Kershaw MH, Schreiber RD, et al. Natural innate and adaptive immunity to cancer. Annu Rev Immunol 2011;29:250; with permission.)

when transplanted into immunodeficient mice (RAG2−/−, 100%), only approximately half of these formed cancers in immunocompetent (WT) recipients, and the others were rejected. The results of this experiment show that tumors formed in mice that lack an intact immune system were, as a group, more immunogenic (hence classified as "unedited") than similar tumors generated in immunocompetent mice ("edited"). This increased immunogenicity is due to their growing without selective immune pressure to make competitive adaptations (ie, downregulation of recognized antigens). Importantly, these studies revealed that the immune system not only protects the host against tumor formation (controls tumor quantity via immune surveillance/immune elimination), but also shapes tumor immunogenicity (controls tumor quality), hence serving as the basis of the cancer immunoediting.[25]

The second landmark experiment, proving tumor *immune equilibrium*, used WT mice with intact immune systems (see **Fig. 3**). These mice were given a single low dose of chemical carcinogen (MCA) and monitored for progressive tumors over long periods of time (230 days). Mice that responded with progressively growing tumors were removed from the experiments (killed due to tumor size). The remaining mice, which appeared fine aside from small stable scarlike papules at the injection site, were then given either placebo control antibody or antibody/antibodies that deplete specific immunologic components. The results showed that approximately half of the mice who were seemingly cancer free grew progressive, lethal tumors when certain Type 1 (Th1) immune components were depleted. In these mice, depletion of either CD4 or CD8 T cells, IFN-γ, or IL-12p40 (critical for IFN-γ production) type 1 components, were equally effective in inducing tumor outgrowth.[28] Stable tumors examined histologically in equilibrium showed relatively increased tumor-infiltrating T cells (TILs), fibrosis, and low levels of Ki-67 + proliferating tumor cells. Meanwhile, progressively growing tumors showed minimal TIL and high fractions of Ki-67 + tumor cells. Importantly, those tumors, which were able to naturally become progressive out of equilibrium (without Th1 blockade), grew progressive masses whether transferred into WT or RAG2−/− mice. However, tumors in equilibrium that were able to grow only when Th1 immunity was blocked with antibodies, could not grow when transferred into WT mice (only RAG2−/− mice) because they remained immunogenic.[26–28] These experiments show that immune equilibrium is mechanistically distinguishable from elimination and escape, and that neoplastic cells in equilibrium are transformed, but proliferate poorly in vivo. They also show that tumor cells in equilibrium are unedited during the static phase, but are edited at the time of spontaneous tumor escape/clinical presentation.

Based on the previous results, one would hypothesize that the immune system can also restrain cancer growth for extended periods in patients with cancer. This time period, between definitive cancer treatment and cancer recurrence, or between cancer initiation and clinical presentation, is known as dormancy. Some tumors remain dormant forever with no apparent harm to patients. An example of this is seen in breast carcinoma, in which bone marrow aspiration with immunohistochemical and cytochemical detection of tumor cells was performed on thousands of patients at the time of surgery, as a prognostic factor and to assess for minimal residual disease. These studies show conclusively that the mere presence of micrometastatic tumor did not equate to recurrence or death of disease.[39–43] In the setting of melanoma in particular, numerous accounts exist of patients who were seemingly well clinically, but had died of other causes (eg, accidental, stroke) before donating organs to other patients in need. Organ recipients later went on to develop metastatic melanoma initiating within the transplanted organ. It was then discovered, that although there had been no history of cancer in the organ donor, said donor had essentially been living with occult metastatic melanoma that had been kept clinically dormant by the organ donor's immune system. Once transferred into the immunosuppressed microenvironment of the transplant recipients, the melanomas could grow unrestrained.[44–53] In rare cases, discontinuation of immunosuppressive medications along with allograft removal from organ recipients led to cancer cure. Finally, melanoma is also unique in its relative propensity for ultra-late recurrence, up to 41 years after primary tumor treatment.[54,55] These data highlight the very important nuance between living with cancer as a chronic disease and dying of progressive cancer. And, although all the factors that control tumor dormancy are not known, experimental evidence mostly points to the dominant role of the antitumor immune response and immune equilibrium.

Immune Escape

By the time a malignant tumor, including malignant melanoma, becomes clinically apparent, it has successfully escaped immune control as part of the third phase of immune editing (**Fig. 4**), immune escape. Despite this escape, a relatively small fraction (~3%–16%) of melanomas show brisk histologic infiltration by T-lymphocytes (**Fig. 5**): evidence of equilibrium at the time of pathologic evaluation. Other tumors show histologic regression (**Fig. 6**), which is likely the most histologically demonstrable evidence of escape that exists. As is discussed later, it is assumed that melanomas with brisk TIL perform relatively better based on their not having entirely completed tumor escape before treatment.

Cancers are known to accomplish *immune escape* via various mechanistic pathways of immune evasion and immune suppression previously outlined in great detail.[56–58] In general, the mechanisms used for tumor escape involve the exploitation of natural pathways of peripheral tolerance, as well as pathways designed to halt and contract the immune response following pathogen (microbial) clearance. The increasingly vast and detailed insight into these mechanisms have permitted the coming of age of immunotherapy in melanoma and other cancer types. In addition to this, malignancies can co-opt certain aspects of the immune system to promote their own growth and spread.[59] The mechanisms used typically involve the generation and recruitment of immune cells that inhibit cytotoxic T-lymphocytes, and, the promotion of angiogenesis, invasiveness, and distant tumor spread. The implicated pathways are

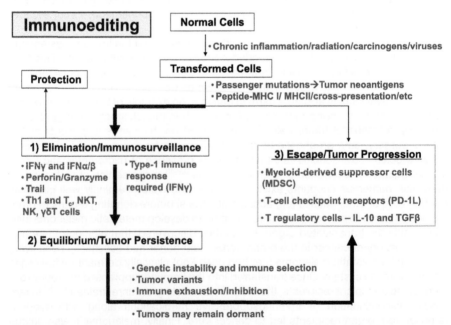

Fig. 4. Overview of immunoediting. It is not currently known whether all tumors pass through the processes of immunosurveillance/elimination, equilibrium, and escape, or whether some tumors progress directly through escape. Based on mouse experiments whereby 40% of tumors are rejected when transferred from an immunodeficient mouse to a WT mouse, and based on data regarding TIL prevalence and response rates to novel targeted immunotherapy, it is possible that approximately one-half of all tumors may avoid immunosurveillance and equilibrium and directly "escape" immune recognition.

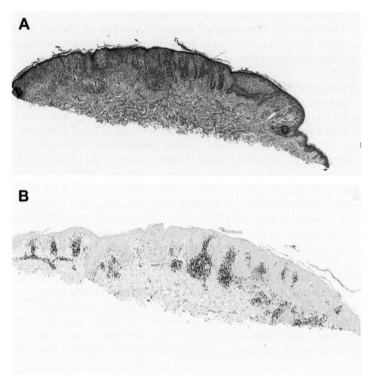

Fig. 5. Representative example of an early melanoma that is likely still in immune equilibrium. (*A*) Every focus of microinvasion is surrounded by a brisk lymphocytic infiltrate, H&E, 100× magnification. (*B*) The T-cell nature of the lymphocytic infiltrate is confirmed with CD3 immunohistochemical staining, original magnification ×100.

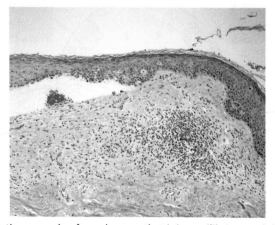

Fig. 6. Representative example of a melanoma that is in equilibrium and that shows at least partial regression. At the right aspect of the lesion, markedly atypical melanocytes are met with a brisk lymphocytic response. At the left aspect of the lesion, there is dermal fibrosis and angioplasia with rete ridge flattening, and without other features of trauma, consistent with regression H&E, original magnification ×200.

typically those involved in chronic innate immune stimulation. The recognition of this is reflected in Hanahan and Weinberg's[60] revised hallmarks of cancer, published in 2011, which cites avoidance of immune destruction and tumor-promoting inflammation as an emerging hallmark and an enabling characteristic (respectively) of all malignancies (**Fig. 7**).

Ko and colleagues[61–63] have well characterized myeloid-derived suppressor cells (MDSC) in patients with renal cell carcinoma (RCC) and melanoma, and in several mouse tumor models. MDSCs accumulate in tumor-bearing hosts and prevent T-cell–mediated tumor destruction via inhibition of type 1 T-cell functions. In mice, MDSCs are CD11b + Gr-1+ cells, which encompass monocytic (m-MDSC; CD11b + Ly6ChiLy6G−) and neutrophilic (n-MDSC; CD11b + Ly6CloLy6G+) subsets with varying degrees of maturity morphologically. In humans, MDSCs (all CD11b+) are identified in the mononuclear "buffy coat" fraction as n-MDSCs (CD14−CD33+HLADR−CD14−CD15+), m-MDSCs (HLA-DR−/loCD33 + CD14 + CD15−), and immature, lineage negative MDSC (Lin−HLA-DR−CD33 + CD14−CD15−) enriched for myeloid progenitors. Both n-MDSCs and m-MDSCs are known to be elevated in melanoma, and total MDSC percentages were recently correlated with overall survival in melanoma.[64,65] Although most studies indicate m-MDSCs predominate in melanoma tumors, we have observed an increase in circulating n-MDSCs in patients, and the literature suggests that establishment of the premetastatic niche is particular to the n-MDSC subset, possibly related to their proangiogenic properties.[66–72] We are currently investigating the relationship between n-MDSCs, angiogenesis, tumor-derived cytokines, and disease progression in melanoma. Other types of immune dysfunction observed in the setting of advanced melanoma have been extensively

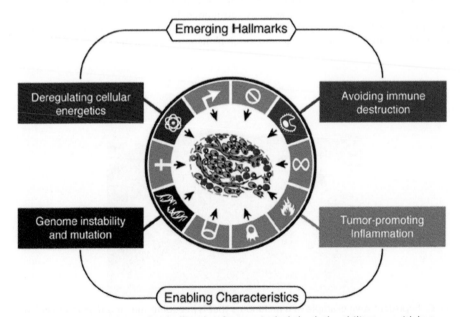

Fig. 7. Contemporary/emerging hallmarks of cancer include both the ability to avoid destruction by the host's immune system (*top right*), and the ability to use certain types of immune responses to promote tumor spread (*bottom right*). (*From* Hanahan D, Weinberg RA. Hallmarks of cancer: the next generation. Cell 2011;144(5):658; with permission.)

reported elsewhere, and include type 2 biased immune responses, elevated T regulatory (Treg) cells, and accumulation of non-mature DCs in lymph nodes.[73–77]

PROGNOSTIC VALUE OF TUMOR IMMUNE INFILTRATION

Although current American Joint Committee on Cancer staging criteria does not incorporate inflammation into melanoma (or any tumor) prognostication templates, the degree of tumor infiltration by lymphocytes (TIL) in melanoma has entered and exited the College of American Pathologists synoptic tumor reports, and is currently included. This reflects the controversial history of tumor immunology, and the extensive modern data showing that a brisk TIL response is associated with improved survival in melanoma. The conferred improved survival is presumed to be a reflection of TILs representing the histologic manifestation of immune equilibrium.

Tuthill and colleagues[78] published the first major report on the protective effect of TIL in melanoma. The investigators looked at 9 clinical and pathologic risk factors for disease progression in 259 patients with a median follow-up of 12.3 years. In this study, TIL was among Breslow thickness and tumor site as an independent predictor of survival ($P = .005$). TIL was characterized into 3 main categories: brisk, a bandlike lymphocytic infiltrate that surrounds the entire tumor front; nonbrisk, a defect in the banklike infiltrate that is 0.3 mm or greater; and absent, lymphocytes are in a perivascular distribution only, not interacting with tumor cells. Here, approximately 12% had brisk TIL, 37% had nonbrisk, and 51% had absent TIL.

Somewhat similar, but larger, studies were then completed by Taylor and colleagues[79] and Azimi and colleagues[80] in the more modern era of melanoma treatment, which included sentinel lymph node biopsy (SLNBx). First, Taylor and colleagues[79] studied prognostic factors in 875 patients who had undergone SLNBx, using the same TIL categorization criteria as Tuthill and colleagues.[78] Approximately 6% of cases showed brisk TIL, 75% were nonbrisk, and the remaining 20% had absent TIL. They found that absent TIL ($P = .0003$), Breslow thickness, ulceration, and male sex were all predictive of SLNBx positivity.[79] Importantly, the predictive value of TILs for SLNBx status was independent of tumor thickness. When disease-free survival (DFS) was examined, however, TILs were not found to predict DFS independently of sentinel lymph node (SLN) status. The investigators concluded that the protective effect of TIL in melanoma was related to impedance of SLN spread.[79] Finally, in 2012 Azimi and colleagues[80] used a 4-tiered TIL grading system based on both the density and distribution of lymphocytes, whereby they found that grades 3, 2, 1, and 0 TIL (more to less briskness) occurred in 3.2%, 16.3%, 45.1%, and 35.4% of patients, respectively. There was a significant, inverse association between TIL grade and SLNBx status ($P<.001$). Increasing TIL grade was independently associated with improved survival. It is interesting to note that the proportion of patients whose tumors show absent TILs throughout these studies somewhat approximates the percentage of patients with metastasis who do not benefit from treatment with modern immunotherapy, and this is discussed further.

The particular histologic finding of tumor regression is unique to melanoma and bares special mention. The prognostic significance of regression in primary melanoma has been debated for many years, with some large studies showing a protective effect and others showing a deleterious effect on survival. Because regression is understood to represent the end stage of immune equilibrium, and, by definition, a relatively effective immune response, it should be a positive prognostic factor. That said, some studies have previously found regression to be a poor prognostic factor. Gualano and colleagues[81] recently reviewed 183 articles of 1876 in a systematic review and meta-analysis to make final conclusions on the survival impact of regression in melanoma. Ten studies composed of 8557 patients were included. Overall, the investigators found that patients with histologic regression had a lower relative risk of death (0.772; 95% CI 0.612–0.973) than those without, and that regression is a protective factor for survival. One might surmise that those studies that previously showed an inverse relationship between survival and regression potentially did so due to an underestimation in tumor thicknesses (due to regression), although this cannot be known with certainty.

IMMUNOTHERAPY AND PREDICTIVE MARKERS IN MELANOMA

Metastatic melanoma is known for its resistance to traditional cancer treatments, including chemotherapy and radiotherapy, as well as its relative responsiveness to immunotherapy compared with other cancer types. Indeed, immunotherapy is the only treatment that can reproducibly result in cures in (albeit few) patients with metastatic melanoma. A timeline of melanoma treatments is shown in **Fig. 8** and summarized in several articles.[82–84] Briefly, before 1998, there were only 2 drugs approved by the Food and Drug Administration (FDA) for metastatic melanoma: dacarbazine (DTIC) and interleukin-2 (IL-2), with no additional treatments approved between 1998 and 2011. Adoptive T-cell therapy has achieved relative success over the years, but has remained experimental and is only offered at a few academic centers due to the intensive technical requirements involved.[85] In 1995, high-dose IFNα2b was FDA approved for stage III melanoma following completion lymph node dissection. Following decades of failed treatment attempts and negative clinical trials, explosive growth in the treatment of metastatic melanoma occurred between 2011 and 2014. This was initiated by FDA approval for the first of several generations of drugs in 2 main classes: (1) targeted kinase inhibitors and (2) T-cell checkpoint inhibitors, the propagation of which is ongoing. The potential synergy of kinase inhibitors with T-cell checkpoint inhibitors is under intense investigation because kinase inhibitors may enhance the immunogenicity of melanomas in vivo (reviewed in Luke and colleagues[83]). Several extensive articles have been published regarding targeted (kinase inhibitor) therapy for melanoma,[83,86,87] and discussion herein is limited to immunotherapy and its predictive markers. We are currently investigating peripheral blood T-cell polarization

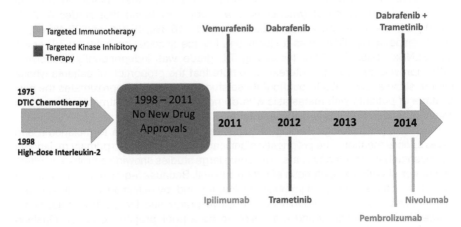

Fig. 8. Timeline of treatments for stage IV melanoma.

and activation responses in patients (stage 1–4), and their correlation with disease progression and response to therapy.

Interferon-α2b

INF-α is a multifunctional regulatory cytokine naturally produced in response to viral infection. It has pluripotent activities with immunomodulatory, antiangiogenic, prodifferentiation, antitumor/pro-apoptotic, and antiproliferative effects. It can promote tumor immunogenicity by enhancing DC maturation, antigen presentation, and antitumor responses, while directing T-cell differentiation preferentially from a Th2 toward a Th1 dominant antitumor response.[88–92] Adjuvant INF-α2b therapy in melanoma is somewhat controversial, albeit FDA approved, due to its toxicity and costs in comparison with its clinical benefit. Historically, high-dose IFN-α (HDI) has been the standard of care as adjuvant treatment for resected stage IIB/III melanoma, due to the findings from several randomized controlled phase III clinical trials (Eastern Cooperative Oncology Group (ECOG)/US Intergroup trials E1684, E1690, and E1694), which uniformly showed an improvement in relapse-free survival (RFS) compared with observation or vaccine. Improvement in overall survival (OS) was observed in only 2 of these 3 trials.[83,93–97]

As with all cancer therapies, there is a strong need to identify markers capable of predicting which patients will respond to a given type of immunotherapy. This need is particularly strong in the case of IFN-α, given its somewhat marginal clinical impact. Post hoc meta-analysis of several clinical trials including more than 2500 patients have indicated that primary tumor stage and ulceration are predictive factors of IFN efficacy, with the greatest risk reductions observed in patients with ulceration and stage IIb/III-N1. The efficacy was lower in patients with ulceration and stage III-N2 disease, and uniformly absent in patients without ulceration.[98,99]

The biologic basis for ulceration as a predictive marker for IFN-α efficacy has been studied by Busse and colleagues.[100] In multivariate analysis accommodating the deleterious impact of ulceration and increasing tumor thickness, higher expression of SOCS1 and SOCS3 (suppressor of cytokine signaling) mRNA at baseline was associated with worse RFS and distant metastasis-free survival (DMFS). IFN-α treatment decreased the mRNA expression of IFN-stimulated gene 15 (ISG15) overall, likely a feedback inhibitory mechanism. Nevertheless, higher decreases in ISG15 following IFN-α treatment were associated with worse RFS and DMFS compared to those with no or reduced decreases. In a somewhat similar study, patients who had a clinical response to high-dose IFN-α therapy showed lower peripheral blood lymphocyte interferon signaling capacity (measured via signal transducer and activator of transcription 1 [STAT1] activation) in T cells at baseline than nonresponders, and significant increases in STAT1 activation over the 4-week induction phase of IFN-α therapy. Interestingly, only patients who displayed modest signaling augmentation had good clinical outcome, whereas those with minimal or negative changes in phorylated STAT1 response, and also those who had "hyper" IFN-α signaling responses, had poor outcome.[101,102] Intratumoral predictors have not been described.

Interleukin-2

IL-2 is a cytokine that is produced by antigen-stimulated (primarily CD4+ helper) T cells, NK cells, and activated DCs. IL-2 primarily serves to induce T-cell expansion via its proliferative and antiapoptotic functions. It also augments effector T-cell function via downstream release of many proinflammatory cytokines (tumor necrosis factor-alpha [TNF-α], IL-beta/IL-1β, IL-6/IL-6, and IFN-γ).[103,104] On the downside, IL-2 is known to expand immunosuppressive CD4+CD25 + hiFOXP3+ Treg cells, and to promote activation-induced cell death of overactivated/exhausted T cells.[76,105] IL-2 is administered as a high-dose intravenous bolus and is plagued by flulike and other (hypotension, hypoxia) side effects, mandating hospitalization for treatment. Comparative analysis of several clinical trials, including 270 patients, showed an objective response rate of 16% in metastatic melanoma. The median duration of response was 8.9 months, and in those who responded, 28% (including 59% of those who achieved a complete response) were free of disease progression at 62 months of follow-up. Patients with ongoing responses at 30 months did not experience relapse. Because follow-up extended beyond 20 years, the potentially curative potential of IL-2 in a small subset of patients is well accepted in the medical community.[106,107]

IL-2 is offered only to a subset of (relatively healthy) patients with metastatic melanoma at a selective group of hospitals; and, because of this, data exploring pretreatment predictors of response are limited. Sabatino and colleagues[108] used multiplex array analysis of initially 111 proteins, largely composed of cytokines, chemokines, and proinflammatory and angiogenesis-related factors, in a training set of 10 patients and a validation set of 49 patients treated with high-dose IL-2, to identify serologic predictors of response. In these studies, high levels of vascular endothelial growth factor (>125 pg/mL) and fibronectin (>8 $\times$ 10^6 pg/mL) correlated with a lack of clinical response and worse OS. Other putative predictors of IL-2 response have been posttreatment-related variables, such as the height of rebound lymphocytosis, treatment-induced thrombocytopenia, development of autoimmune thyroiditis and vitiligo, and decreases in absolute number and frequency of peripheral Tregs.[109] Currently, there is at least 1 clinical trial under way that will use radiotherapy as an immunologic booster in patients with metastatic melanoma or RCC treated with high-dose IL-2. This study will evaluate the biomarkers of immunologic and therapeutic responses in the treatment cohort.[110]

Cytotoxic T-Lymphocyte–Associated Protein-4 Blockade/Ipilimumab

The "2-signal model" of T-cell activation refers to the fact that T-cell activation requires not only stimulation via the TCR through binding of the antigen/major histocompatibility complex (MHC) (signal 1), but also an additional costimulatory signal (signal 2). Engagement of CD28 on T cells by B7-1 (CD80) and B7-2 (CD86) on the antigen-presenting cell (APC) provides signal 2 (at least for naïve, antigen-inexperienced T cells). Without signal 2, stimulation through the TCR results in T-cell anergy. Overall, the tight regulation surrounding T-cell activation (costimulators and coinhibitors) is a critical component of peripheral tolerance, which prevents autoimmunity.[111]

Cytotoxic T-lymphocyte–associated protein-4 (CTLA-4) binds the same ligands as CD28 (signal 2 for T-cell activation), only with much higher avidity, and initiates a downstream inhibitory signal, therefore downregulating the immune response. It is constitutively expressed in Tregs in which context it serves as a key mediator of Treg effector T-cell suppressive capacity. CTLA-4 becomes upregulated in conventional T cells after activation. CTLA4 gene knockout in mice causes a lethal lymphoproliferative/autoimmune disorder. In humans, CTLA-4 gene variants are associated with an assortment of autoimmune diseases, and germline haploinsufficiency causes a rare immune disorder marked by lymphoproliferation, autoimmunity, hypogammaglobulinemia, recurrent infections, and slightly increased risk of lymphoma.[112]

The elucidation of T-cell checkpoint molecules, pioneered by CTLA-4 discovery, has led to the development of relatively more targeted forms of immunotherapy, the prototype of which is the anti–CTLA-4 antibody, ipilimumab.[113–115] Ipilimumab was the first T-cell checkpoint inhibitor to obtain FDA approval (2011) for metastatic melanoma (or any cancer). Although improvement in progression-free survival

(PFS) was not observed compared with standard DTIC chemotherapy, there was a highly significant increase in OS on ipilimumab (15.7 vs 9.1 months) with 38% of patients alive at 2 years on 10 mg/kg ipilimumab versus 17.9% on DTIC. The seemingly contradictory results between PFS and OS with immunotherapy is now known to reflect the atypical patterns of treatment responses seen, which have resulted in a formalized radiologic imaging criteria termed immune-related response criteria. A consistent observation is that a portion of patients have long-term survival independent of the extent of response. In a pooled analysis of all phase II and III clinical trials with ipilimumab, 22% of patients were alive at 3 years, and the plateau on the survival curve suggests that these patients are likely to survive long-term thereafter.

Interestingly, and pertinent to research regarding n-MDSC in melanoma, baseline neutrophils and the neutrophil-to-lymphocyte ratio (NLR) were recently shown to be associated with poor outcome in 720 patients with advanced melanoma receiving 3 mg/kg ipilimumab. In this study by Ferrucci and colleagues,[116] the optimal cutoff for NLR was 3. Baseline absolute neutrophil count (ANC) and NLR were significantly associated with disease progression and death ($P<.0001$), with prognosis worsening with each elevated variable. Patients with both ANC $\geq$7500 and NLR $\geq$3 had a significantly and independently increased risk of death and progression compared with patients with both lower ANC and dNLR. Patients with 1 of the 2 factors elevated had an intermediate risk of progression and death. The 1-year and 2-year survival rates were 2% and 0% for patients with ANC $\geq$7500 and dNLR $\geq$3, and 43% and 24% for patients with both lower ANC and dNLR. A similarly poor prognostic relevance has previously also been shown for neutrophils in patients with melanoma receiving biochemotherapy.[117]

Programmed Cell Death-1 Blockade

Programmed cell death-1 (PD-1, CD279) is an immune inhibitory receptor that is part of the CD28/CTLA-4 T-cell checkpoint receptor family. PD-1 plays an important role in (peripheral) self-tolerance by suppressing activated T-cell activity. Mechanisms of effector T-cell inhibition include reduced T-cell proliferation, reduced IFN-γ production, reduced cytotoxic molecule production, promotion of T-cell apoptosis in activated/effector T cells, and inhibition of apoptosis in Tregs. The PD-1 receptor becomes expressed within 24 hours of T-cell activation and declines with the clearance of antigen, reflecting the role of PD-1 in contracting the immune response at the appropriate time to prevent autoimmunity. Mice lacking PD-1 or its ligands do not automatically develop autoimmune disease; however, PD-1 deficiency or blockade can accelerate and exacerbate autoimmunity.

PD-1 has 2 ligands, programmed death-ligand 1 (PD-L1, CD274, B7-H1) and programmed death-ligand 2 (PD-L2, CD273, B7-DC), which are both expressed on APCs, as well as a host of other hematopoietic and nonhematopoietic cell types. PD-L1 is the most widely expressed ligand (including immune, epithelial, endothelial, and mesenchymal cells), where it is constitutively induced on exposure to proinflammatory cytokines (type 1 and 2 IFNs, especially IFN-γ, and TNF-α). PD-L2 is mostly limited to dendritic cells and macrophages, and is induced by many of the same cytokines as PD-L1. However, IL-4 and granulocyte-macrophage colony-stimulating factor are the most potent stimuli for PD-L2 expression. In the tumor microenvironment, tumor cells can express PD-L1 and/or PD-L2, as do many other cells (eg, fibroblasts, endothelial cells, immune cells). In addition to cytokines, PD-L1 and PD-L2 expression on tumor cells can rarely become upregulated by chromosomal copy gain (amplification of chromosome 9p24, which contains PD-L1 and PD-L2).[118]

PD-1 monoclonal antibodies, nivolumab and pembrolizumab, were FDA approved for the treatment of metastatic melanoma in 2014 based on highly significant tumor responses and improvements in OS (40%–44% response rate (RR) and median overall survival (OS) not reached at 1 and 2 years for nivolumab; 34% RR and median OS of 74% and 55% at 1 and 2 years for pembrolizumab). As would be intuitively expected, combination treatment with ipilimumab to stimulate T cells at the priming phase and nivolumab to stimulate them at the effector phase, resulted in improved clinical efficacy (58% RR and median OS at 1 and 2 years not reached).[83] Current understanding is that, although PD-L1 expression enriches for responders to PD-1 blockade treatment, responses can occur even when PD-1L expression in the tumor microenvironment is not observed. And, PD-1L expression is not needed for response to combined PD-1 and CTLA-4 therapy, which, although more effective, has a relatively higher toxicity compared with PD-1 blockade alone.[83,118–120]

Biomarkers of T-Cell Checkpoint Responsiveness

In general, mechanisms of resistance and biomarkers predictive of responsiveness to immunotherapy are ill-defined compared with kinase-targeted therapy. That said, it is currently understood that the "T-cell inflamed tumor microenvironment" characterized by (generally but not perfectly coexistent) increased CD8+ T-cell infiltration, some degree of PD1 and PD-1L expression, a relatively more clonal TCR repertoire, and expression of type 1 T-cell related cytokines and chemokines, is predictive of responsiveness to T-cell checkpoint inhibitor therapy.[121] These microenvironments are more likely to be found in tumors with a high mutational burden, although this relationship is not stringent because tumors with relatively fewer mutations occasionally produce the "right" mutation to generate a highly immunogenic neoantigen.[122–124] In general, the lack of an IFN-γ–associated gene-expression profile is highly correlated with a lack of clinical benefit from T-cell checkpoint inhibitors.[125] Preliminary evidence suggests that the so-called "T-cell excluded tumor microenvironment" may be more likely to occur in tumors with WNT/β-catenin signaling pathway activation, PTEN (phosphatase and tensin homolog) mutations, JAK (Janus kinase) 1 or 2 mutations, β2 microglobulin (an MHC class I subunit) mutations, or interferon regulatory factor 1 loss of expression. These tumors show deficits in autophagy, antigen presentation, and the type I interferon response.[126–129] As such, future drug development will likely focus on suppressing those pathways directing the T-cell excluded microenvironment and combining such drugs with immune-amplifying drugs, such as checkpoint inhibitors.

REFERENCES

1. Ehrlich P. Ueber den jetzigen stand der karzinomforschung. Ned Tijdschr Geneeskd 1909;5:73–290.
2. Burnet FM. Cancer, a biological approach. Br Med J 1957;1:841–7.
3. Thomas L. In: Lawrence HS, editor. Cellular and humoral aspects of the hypersensitive states. New York: Hoeber-Harper; 1959. p. 529–32.
4. Black MM, Opler SR, Speer FD. Microscopic structure of gastric carcinomas and their regional lymph nodes in relation to survival. Surg Gynecol Obstet 1954;98:725.
5. Old LJ, Clarke DA, Benacerraf B. Effect of bacillus Calmette-Guerin infection on transplanted tumours in the mouse. Nature 1959;184(Suppl 5):291–2.
6. Chou R, Selph S, Buckley DI, et al. Intravesical therapy for the treatment of nonmuscle invasive bladder cancer: a systematic review and meta-analysis [review]. J Urol 2017;197(5):1189–99.

7. Stutman O. Tumor development after 3-methylcholanthrene in immunologically deficient athymic-nude mice. Science 1974;183(4124):534–6.
8. Rygaard J, Povlsen CO. The mouse mutant nude does not develop spontaneous tumours. An argument against immunological surveillance. Acta Pathol Microbiol Scand B Microbiol Immunol 1974;82(1):99–106. No abstract available.
9. Stutman O. Chemical carcinogenesis in nude mice: comparison between nude mice from homozygous matings and heterozygous matings and effect of age and carcinogen dose. J Natl Cancer Inst 1979;62(2):353–8.
10. Stutman. Tumor development after polyoma infection in athymic nude mice. J Immunol 1975;114(4):1213–7.
11. Thomas L. On immunosurveillance in human cancer. Yale J Biol Med 1982; 55(3–4):329–33.
12. Hanahan D, Weinberg RA. The hallmarks of cancer. Cell 2000;100(1):57–70.
13. Schmitt N, Ueno H. Regulation of human helper T cell subset differentiation by cytokines. Curr Opin Immunol 2015;34:130–6.
14. Wynn TA. Type 2 cytokines: mechanisms and therapeutic strategies. Nat Rev Immunol 2015;15(5):271–82.
15. Boehm U, Klamp T, Groot M, et al. Cellular responses to interferon-gamma. Annu Rev Immunol 1997;15:749–95.
16. Russell JH, Ley TJ. Lymphocyte-mediated cytotoxicity [review]. Annu Rev Immunol 2002;20:323–70.
17. Dighe AS, Richards E, Old LJ, et al. Enhanced in vivo growth and resistance to rejection of tumor cells expressing dominant negative IFN gamma receptors. Immunity 1994;1(6):447–56.
18. Kaplan DH, Shankaran V, Dighe AS, et al. Demonstration of an interferon gamma-dependent tumor surveillance system in immunocompetent mice. Proc Natl Acad Sci U S A 1998;95(13):7556–61.
19. Street SE, Cretney E, Smyth MJ. Perforin and interferon-gamma activities independently control tumor initiation, growth, and metastasis. Blood 2001;97(1): 192–7.
20. Street SE, Trapani JA, MacGregor D, et al. Suppression of lymphoma and epithelial malignancies effected by interferon gamma. J Exp Med 2002; 196(1):129–34.
21. van den Broek ME, Kägi D, Ossendorp F, et al. Decreased tumor surveillance in perforin-deficient mice. J Exp Med 1996;184(5):1781–90.
22. Smyth MJ, Thia KY, Street SE, et al. Differential tumor surveillance by natural killer (NK) and NKT cells. J Exp Med 2000;191(4):661–8.
23. Smyth MJ, Thia KY, Street SE, et al. Perforin-mediated cytotoxicity is critical for surveillance of spontaneous lymphoma. J Exp Med 2000;192(5):755–60.
24. Shinkai Y, Rathbun G, Lam KP, et al. RAG-2-deficient mice lack mature lymphocytes owing to inability to initiate V(D)J rearrangement. Cell 1992;68(5):855–67.
25. Shankaran V, Ikeda H, Bruce AT, et al. IFNgamma and lymphocytes prevent primary tumour development and shape tumour immunogenicity. Nature 2001; 410(6832):1107–11.
26. Vesely MD, Kershaw MH, Schreiber RD, et al. Natural innate and adaptive immunity to cancer. Annu Rev Immunol 2011;29:235–71.
27. Schreiber RD, Old LJ, Smyth MJ. Cancer immunoediting: integrating immunity's roles in cancer suppression and promotion. Science 2011;331(6024):1565–70.
28. Koebel CM, Vermi W, Swann JB, et al. Adaptive immunity maintains occult cancer in an equilibrium state. Nature 2007;450(7171):903–7.

29. Starzl TE, Penn I, Halgrimson CG. Immunosuppression and malignant neo-plasms. N Engl J Med 1970;283(17):934.
30. Gatti RA, Good RA. Occurrence of malignancy in immunodeficiency diseases. A literature review [review]. Cancer 1971;28(1):89–98.
31. Penn I. Posttransplant malignancies. Transplant Proc 1999;31(1–2):1260–2.
32. Boshoff C, Weiss R. AIDS-related malignancies [review]. Nat Rev Cancer 2002; 2(5):373–82.
33. Saha A, Kaul R, Murakami M, et al. Tumor viruses and cancer biology: modulating signaling pathways for therapeutic intervention. Cancer Biol Ther 2010; 10(10):961–78.
34. Hoover RN. Origins of human cancer. In: Hiatt HH, Watson JD, Winsten JA, editors. The origins of human cancer. Cold Spring Harbor (NY): Cold Spring Harbor Laboratory Press; 1977. p. 369–79.
35. Sheil AG. Cancer after transplantation. World J Surg 1986;10(3):389–96.
36. Penn I. Malignant melanoma in organ allograft recipients. Transplantation 1996; 61(2):274–8.
37. Lawrence MS, Stojanov P, Polak P, et al. Mutational heterogeneity in cancer and the search for new cancer-associated genes. Nature 2013;499:214–8.
38. Schumacher TN, Schreiber RD. Neoantigens in cancer immunotherapy. Science 2015;348:69–74.
39. Diel IJ, Kaufmann M, Costa SD, et al. Micrometastatic breast cancer cells in bone marrow at primary surgery: prognostic value in comparison with nodal status. J Natl Cancer Inst 1996;88(22):1652–8.
40. Landys K, Persson S, Kovarik J, et al. Prognostic value of bone marrow biopsy in operable breast cancer patients at the time of initial diagnosis: results of a 20-year median follow-up. Breast Cancer Res Treat 1998;49:27–33.
41. Solomayer EF, Diel IJ, Krempien B, et al. Results of iliac crest biopsies taken from 1465 patients with primary breast cancer. J Cancer Res Clin Oncol 1998;124:44–8.
42. Mansi JL, Gogas H, Bliss JM, et al. Outcome of primary-breast-cancer patients with micrometastases: a long-term follow-up study. Lancet 1999;354:197–202.
43. Funke I. Meta-analyses of studies on bone marrow micrometastases: an independent prognostic impact remains to be substantiated. J Clin Oncol 1998; 16:557–66.
44. Loren AW, Desai S, Gorman RC, et al. Retransplantation of a cardiac allograft inadvertently harvested from a donor with metastatic melanoma. Transplantation 2003;76(4):741–3.
45. Stephens JK, Everson GT, Elliott CL, et al. Fatal transfer of malignant melanoma from multiorgan donor to four allograft recipients. Transplantation 2000;70(1): 232–6.
46. Milton CA, Barbara J, Cooper J, et al. Transmission of donor-derived malignant melanoma to a renal allograft recipient. Clin Transplant 2006;20(5):547–50.
47. Morris-Stiff G, Steel A, Savage P, et al, Welsh Transplantation Research Group. Transmission of donor melanoma to multiple organ transplant recipients. Am J Transplant 2004;4(3):444–6.
48. Bilal M, Eason JD, Das K, et al. Donor-derived metastatic melanoma in a liver transplant recipient established by DNA fingerprinting. Exp Clin Transplant 2013;11(5):458–63.
49. Buell JF, Beebe TM, Trofe J, et al. Donor transmitted malignancies. Ann Transplant 2004;9(1):53–6.

50. Kim JK, Carmody IC, Cohen AJ, et al. Donor transmission of malignant melanoma to a liver graft recipient: case report and literature review. Clin Transplant 2009;23(4):571–4.
51. Morath C, Schwenger V, Schmidt J, et al. Transmission of malignancy with solid organ transplants. Transplantation 2005;80(Suppl 1):S164–6.
52. Strauss DC, Thomas JM. Transmission of donor melanoma by organ transplantation. Lancet Oncol 2010;11(8):790–6.
53. Harvey L, Fox M. Transferral of malignancy as a complication of organ transplantation: an insuperable problem? J Clin Pathol 1981;34(2):116–22.
54. Tahery DP, Moy RL. Recurrent malignant melanoma following a 35-year disease-free interval. J Dermatol Surg Oncol 1993;19(2):161–3.
55. Terhorst D, Radke C, Trefzer U. Ultra-late recurrence of malignant melanoma after a disease-free interval of 41 years. Clin Exp Dermatol 2010;35(3):e20–1.
56. Mittal D, Gubin MM, Schreiber RD, et al. New insights into cancer immunoediting and its three component phases—elimination, equilibrium and escape. Curr Opin Immunol 2014;27:16–25.
57. Finn O. Cancer immunology. N Engl J Med 2008;358(25):2704–15.
58. Gabrilovich DI, Ostrand-Rosenberg S, Bronte V. Coordinated regulation of myeloid cells by tumours. Nat Rev Immunol 2012;12:253–68.
59. Nakamura K, Smyth MJ. Targeting cancer-related inflammation in the era of immunotherapy. Immunol Cell Biol 2017;95(4):325–32.
60. Hanahan D, Weinberg RA. Hallmarks of cancer: the next generation [review]. Cell 2011;144(5):646–74.
61. Ko J, Zea A, Rini B, et al. Sunitinib mediates reversal of myeloid-derived suppressor cell accumulation in renal cell carcinoma patients. Clin Cancer Res 2009;15(6):2148–57.
62. Ko J, Rayman P, Ireland J, et al. Direct and differential suppression of MDSC subsets by sunitinib is compartmentally constrained. Cancer Res 2010;70(9):3526–36.
63. Ko J, Bukowski R, Finke J. Myeloid-derived suppressor cells: a novel therapeutic target. Curr Oncol Rep 2009;11(2):87–93.
64. Stanojevic I, Miller K, Kandolf-Sekulovic L, et al. A subpopulation that may correspond to granulocytic myeloid-derived suppressor cells reflects the clinical stage and progression of cutaneous melanoma. Int Immunol 2016;28(2):87–97.
65. Chevolet I, Speeckaert R, Schreuer M, et al. Clinical significance of plasmacytoid dendritic cells and myeloid-derived suppressor cells in melanoma. J Transl Med 2015;13:9.
66. El Rayes T, Catena R, Lee S, et al. Lung inflammation promotes metastasis through neutrophil protease-mediated degradation of Tsp-1. Proc Natl Acad Sci U S A 2015;112(52):16000–5.
67. Ghajar CM, Peinado H, Mori H, et al. The perivascular niche regulates breast tumour dormancy. Nat Cell Biol 2013;15(7):807–17.
68. Shojaei F, Singh M, Thompson JD, et al. Role of Bv8 in neutrophil-dependent angiogenesis in a transgenic model of cancer progression. Proc Natl Acad Sci U S A 2008;105(7):2640–5.
69. Ardi VC, Kupriyanova TA, Deryugina EI, et al. Human neutrophils uniquely release TIMP-free MMP-9 to provide a potent catalytic stimulator of angiogenesis. Proc Natl Acad Sci U S A 2007;104(51):20262–7.
70. Shaked Y, McAllister S, Fainaru O, et al. Tumor dormancy and the angiogenic switch: possible implications of bone marrow-derived cells. Curr Pharm Des 2014;20(30):4920–33.

71. Bodogai M, Moritoh K, Lee-Chang C, et al. Immunosuppressive and prometa-static functions of myeloid-derived suppressive cells rely upon education from tumor-associated B cells. Cancer Res 2015;75(17):3456–65.

72. Wculek SK, Malanchi I. Neutrophils support lung colonization of metastasis-initiating breast cancer cells. Nature 2015;528(7582):413–7.

73. Tatsumi T, Kierstead LS, Ranieri E, et al. Disease-associated bias in T helper type 1 (Th1)/Th2 CD4(+) T cell responses against MAGE-6 in HLA-DRB10401(+) patients with renal cell carcinoma or melanoma. J Exp Med 2002;196(5):619–28.

74. Wesa AK, Mandic M, Taylor JL, et al. Circulating type-1 anti-tumor CD4(+) T cells are preferentially pro-apoptotic in cancer patients. Front Oncol 2014;4: 266, eCollection 2014.

75. Ascierto PA, Napolitano M, Celentano E, et al. Regulatory T cell frequency inpa-tients with melanoma with different disease stage and course, and modulating effects of high-dose interferon-alpha 2b treatment. J Transl Med 2010;8:76.

76. Cesana GC, DeRaffele G, Cohen S, et al. Characterization of CD4+ CD25+ reg-ulatory T cells in patients treated with high-dose interleukin-2 for metastatic mel-anoma or renal cell carcinoma. J Clin Oncol 2006;24(7):1169–77.

77. Elliott B, Scolyer RA, Suciu S, et al. Long-term protective effect of mature DC-LAMP+ dendritic cell accumulation in sentinel lymph nodes containing mi-crometastatic melanoma. Clin Cancer Res 2007;13(13):3825–30.

78. Tuthill RJ, Unger JM, Liu PY, et al, Southwest Oncology Group. Risk assessment in localized primary cutaneous melanoma: a Southwest Oncology Group study evaluating nine factors and a test of the Clark logistic regression prediction model. Am J Clin Pathol 2002;118(4):504–11.

79. Taylor RC, Patel A, Panageas KS, et al. Tumor-infiltrating lymphocytes predict sentinel lymph node positivity in patients with cutaneous melanoma. J Clin On-col 2007;25(7):869–75.

80. Azimi F, Scolyer RA, Rumcheva P, et al. Tumor-infiltrating lymphocyte grade is an independent predictor of sentinel lymph node status and survival in patients with cutaneous melanoma. J Clin Oncol 2012;30(21):2678–83.

81. Gualano MR, Osella-Abate S, Scaioli G, et al. Prognostic role of Histologic regression in primary cutaneous melanoma: a systematic review and meta-anal-ysis. Br J Dermatol 2017. http://dx.doi.org/10.1111/bjd.15552.

82. da Silveira Nogueira Lima JP, Georgieva M, Haaland B, et al. A systematic re-view and network meta-analysis of immunotherapy and targeted therapy for advanced melanoma. Cancer Med 2017;6(6):1143–53.

83. Luke JJ, Flaherty KT, Ribas A, et al. Targeted agents and immunotherapies: opti-mizing outcomes in melanoma. Nat Rev Clin Oncol 2017. http://dx.doi.org/10.1038/nrclinonc.2017.43.

84. Gorantla VC, Kirkwood JM. State of melanoma: an historic overview of a field in transition. Hematol Oncol Clin North Am 2014;28(3):415–35.

85. Yang JC, Rosenberg SA. Adoptive T-cell therapy for cancer [review]. Adv Immu-nol 2016;130:279–94.

86. Simeone E, Grimaldi AM, Festino L, et al. Combination treatment of patients with BRAF-mutant melanoma: a new standard of care [review]. BioDrugs 2017;31(1): 51–61.

87. Welsh SJ, Rizos H, Scolyer RA, et al. Resistance to combination BRAF and MEK inhibition in metastatic melanoma: where to next? [review]. Eur J Cancer 2016; 62:76–85.

88. Ferrantini M, Capone I, Belardelli F. Interferon-alpha and cancer: mechanisms of action and new perspectives of clinical use. Biochimie 2007;89(6–7):884–93.
89. Paquette RL. Interferon-alpha and granulocyte-macrophage colony-stimulating factor differentiate peripheral blood monocytes into potent antigen-presenting cells. J Leukoc Biol 1998;64:358–67.
90. Parlato S, Santini SM, Lapenta C, et al. Expression of CCR-7, MIP-3beta, and Th-1 chemokines in type I IFN-induced monocyte-derived dendritic cells: importance for the rapid acquisition of potent migratory and functional activities. Blood 2001;98:3022–9.
91. Brinkmann V, Geiger T, Alkan S, et al. Interferon alpha increases the frequency of interferon gamma-producing human CD4+ T cells. J Exp Med 1993;178:1655–63.
92. Wenner CA, Guler ML, Macatonia SE, et al. Roles of IFN-gamma and IFN-alpha in IL-12-induced T helper cell-1 development. J Immunol 1996;156:1442–7.
93. Kirkwood JM, Strawderman MH, Ernstoff MS, et al. Interferon alfa-2b adjuvant therapy of high-risk resected cutaneous melanoma: the Eastern Cooperative Oncology Group Trial EST 1684. J Clin Oncol 1996;14:7–17.
94. Kirkwood JM, Ibrahim JG, Sondak VK, et al. High- and low-dose interferon alfa-2b in high-risk melanoma: first analysis of intergroup trial E1690/S9111/C9190. J Clin Oncol 2000;18:2444–58.
95. Kirkwood JM, Richards T, Zarour HM, et al. Immunomodulatory effects of high-dose and low-dose interferon alpha2b in patients with high-risk resected melanoma: the E2690 laboratory corollary of intergroup adjuvant trial E1690. Cancer 2002;95:1101–12.
96. Eggermont AM, Suciu S, MacKie R, et al. Post surgery adjuvant therapy with intermediate doses of interferon alfa 2b versus observation in patients with stage IIb/III melanoma(EORTC 18952): randomised controlled trial. Lancet 2005; 366(9492):1189–96.
97. Kirkwood JM, Manola J, Ibrahim J, et al. A pooled analysis of Eastern Cooperative Oncology Group and intergroup trials of adjuvant high-dose interferon for melanoma. Clin Cancer Res 2004;10(5):1670–7.
98. Anaya DA, Xing Y, Feng L, et al. Adjuvant high-dose interferon for cutaneous melanoma is most beneficial for patients with early stage III disease. Cancer 2008;112(9):2030–7.
99. Eggermont AM, Suciu S, Testori A, et al. Ulceration and stage are predictive of interferon efficacy in melanoma: results of the phase III adjuvant trials EORTC 18952 and EORTC 18991. Eur J Cancer 2012;48(2):218–25.
100. Busse A, Rapion J, Fusi A, et al. Analysis of surrogate gene expression markers in peripheral blood of melanoma patients to predict treatment outcome of adjuvant pegylated interferon alpha 2b (EORTC 18991 side study). Cancer Immunol Immunother 2013;62:1223–33.
101. Wang W, Edington HD, Rao UN, et al. Modulation of signal transducers and activators of transcription 1 and 3 signaling in melanoma by high-dose IFNalpha2b. Clin Cancer Res 2007;13:1523–31.
102. Simons DL, Lee G, Kirkwood JM, et al. Interferon signaling patterns in peripheral blood lymphocytes may predict clinical outcome after high-dose interferon therapy in melanoma patients. J Transl Med 2011;5(9):52–60.
103. Tarhini AA, Agarwala SS. Interleukin-2 for the treatment of melanoma. Curr Opin Investig Drugs 2005;6:1234–9.
104. Boyman O, Sprent J. The role of interleukin-2 during homeostasis and activation of the immune system [review]. Nat Rev Immunol 2012;12(3):180–90.

105. Sim GC, Martin-Orozco N, Jin L, et al. IL-2 therapy promotes suppressive ICOS+ Treg expansion in melanoma patients. J Clin Invest 2014;124(1):99–110.
106. Fyfe G, Fisher RI, Rosenberg SA, et al. Results of treatment of 255 patients with metastatic renal cell carcinoma who received high-dose recombinant interleukin-2 therapy. J Clin Oncol 1995;13:688–96.
107. Atkins MB, Lotze MT, Dutcher JP, et al. High-dose recombinant interleukin 2 therapy for patients with metastatic melanoma: analysis of 270 patients treated between 1985 and 1993. J Clin Oncol 1999;17:2105–16.
108. Sabatino M, Kim-Schulze S, Panelli MC, et al. Serum vascular endothelial growth factor and fibronectin predict clinical response to high-dose interleukin-2 therapy. Clin Oncol 2009;27(16):2645–52.
109. Kirkwood JM, Tarhini AA. Biomarkers of therapeutic response in melanoma and renal cell carcinoma: potential inroads to improved immunotherapy. J Clin Oncol 2009;27(16):2583–5. No abstract available.
110. Ridolfi L, de Rosa F, Ridolfi R, et al. Radiotherapy as an immunological booster in patients with metastatic melanoma or renal cell carcinoma treated with high-dose Interleukin-2: evaluation of biomarkers of immunologic and therapeutic response. J Transl Med 2014;12:262.
111. Chen L, Flies DB. Molecular mechanisms of T-cell co-stimulation and co-inhibition [review]. Nat Rev Immunol 2013;13(4):227–42 [Erratum appears in Nat Rev Immunol 2013;13(7):542].
112. Walker LS, Sansom DM. The emerging role of CTLA4 as a cell-extrinsic regulator of T cell responses [review]. Nat Rev Immunol 2011;11(12):852–63.
113. Robert C, Thomas L, Bondarenko I, et al. Ipilimumab plus dacarbazine for previously untreated metastatic melanoma. N Engl J Med 2011;364:2517–26.
114. Hodi FS, O'Day SJ, McDermott DF, et al. Improved survival with ipilimumab in patients with metastatic melanoma. N Engl J Med 2010;363:711–23.
115. Ascierto PA, Del Vecchio M, Robert C, et al. Ipilimumab 10 mg/kg versus ipilimumab 3 mg/kg in patients with unresectable or metastatic melanoma: a randomised, double-blind, multicentre, phase 3 trial. Lancet Oncol 2017;18(5):611–22.
116. Ferrucci PF, Ascierto PA, Pigozzo J, et al. Baseline neutrophils and derived neutrophil-to-lymphocyte ratio: prognostic relevance in metastatic melanoma patients receiving ipilimumab. Ann Oncol 2016;27(4):732–8.
117. Schmidt H, Suciu S, Punt CJ, et al. Pretreatment levels of peripheral neutrophils and leukocytes as independent predictors of overall survival in patients with American Joint Committee on Cancer Stage IV Melanoma: results of the EORTC 18951 Biochemotherapy Trial. J Clin Oncol 2007;25(12):1562–9.
118. Baumeister SH, Freeman GJ, Dranoff G, et al. Coinhibitory pathways in immunotherapy for cancer. Annu Rev Immunol 2016;34:539–73.
119. Topalian SL, Hodi FS, Brahmer JR, et al. Safety, activity, and immune correlates of anti-PD-1 antibody in cancer. N Engl J Med 2012;366:2443–54.
120. Larkin J, Chiarion-Sileni V, Gonzalez R, et al. Combined nivolumab and ipilimumab or monotherapy in untreated melanoma. N Engl J Med 2015;373:23–34.
121. Tumeh PC, Harview CL, Yearley JH, et al. PD-1 blockade induces responses by inhibiting adaptive immune resistance. Nature 2014;515:568–71.
122. Gajewski TF, Louahed J, Brichard VG. Gene signature in melanoma associated with clinical activity: a potential clue to unlock cancer immunotherapy. Cancer J 2010;16:399–403.

123. Harlin H, Meng Y, Peterson AC, et al. Chemokine expression in melanoma metastases associated with CD8+ T-cell recruitment. Cancer Res 2009;69: 3077–85.

124. Ji RR, Chasalow SD, Wang L, et al. An immune-active tumor microenvironment favors clinical response to ipilimumab. Cancer Immunol Immunother 2011;61: 1019–31.

125. Ribas A, Robert C, Hodi S, et al. Association of response to programmed death receptor 1 (PD-1) blockade with pembrolizumab (MK-3475) with an interferon-inflammatory immune gene signature. J Clin Oncol 2015;33(Suppl) [abstract: 3001].

126. Spranger S, Bao R, Gajewski TF. Melanoma intrinsic β-catenin signalling prevents anti-tumour immunity. Nature 2015;523:231–5.

127. Peng W, Chen JQ, Liu C, et al. Loss of PTEN promotes resistance to T cell-mediated immunotherapy. Cancer Discov 2016;6:202–16.

128. Zaretsky JM, Garcia-Diaz A, Shin DS, et al. Mutations associated with acquired resistance to PD-1 blockade in melanoma. N Engl J Med 2016;375:819–29.

129. Shin DS, Zaretsky JM, Escuin-Ordinas H, et al. Primary resistance to PD-1 blockade mediated by JAK1/2 mutations. Cancer Discov 2017;7:188–201.

Molecular Melanoma Diagnosis Update

Gene Fusion, Genomic Hybridization, and Massively Parallel Short-Read Sequencing

Ursula E. Lang, MD, PhD[a,b], Iwei Yeh, MD, PhD[a,b],
Timothy H. McCalmont, MD[a,b],*

KEYWORDS

- Melanoma • Spitz nevus • BAP-1 inactivated spitzoid nevus • Kinase gene fusion
- Molecular • Comparative genomic hybridization

KEY POINTS

- Molecular evaluation of melanocytic tumors can be diagnostically useful to confirm malignancy or benignancy.
- Molecular tools are ancillary and supplemental to histopathologic evaluation and do not replace conventional microscopy.
- Immunohistochemistry, fluorescence in situ hybridization (FISH), array comparative genomic hybridization (aCGH), and massively parallel short-read sequencing, often referred to as next-generation sequencing (NGS), each provide varied (and often incomplete) additional information, and careful planning is necessary if tissue is limited.

Melanocytic tumor diagnosis remains a challenging area — if not the most challenging and controversial area — in dermatopathology, and analysis by conventional microscopy has limitations in defining entities precisely and in establishing biologic potential. Additionally, diagnostic criteria and diagnostic approaches vary considerably across the field, and because of fear of underdiagnosis, the diagnosis of melanoma is commonly, readily, and perhaps too easily rendered. Fortunately, molecular tools are available as ancillary techniques and hold the potential to provide some measure of diagnostic uniformity and insight in the evaluation of controversial tumors; additionally, these techniques provide the potential to unveil new oncogenic pathways that may disrupt existing morphology-based diagnostic conclusions and

[a] Department of Pathology, University of California, San Francisco, San Francisco, CA, USA;
[b] Department of Dermatology, University of California, San Francisco, San Francisco, CA, USA
* Corresponding author. UCSF Dermatopathology Service, University of California, San Francisco, 1701 Divisadero Street, Suite 280, San Francisco, CA 94105.
E-mail address: tim.mccalmont@ucsf.edu

Clin Lab Med 37 (2017) 473–484
http://dx.doi.org/10.1016/j.cll.2017.06.002
0272-2712/17/© 2017 Elsevier Inc. All rights reserved.

methods. There are various methods to probe the underlying genetic changes present in tumors, including immunohistochemistry, FISH,[1,2] aCGH,[3,4] and massively parallel short-read or NGS.[5] Each technique provides slightly different information with advantages and disadvantages. Herein, these techniques and how they can supplement conventional assessment are briefly described.

IMMUNOHISTOCHEMISTRY

The use of immunohistochemistry to evaluate the presence or absence of specific proteins constitutes a well established, widely available, nonmolecular approach, but selected stains can provide surrogate molecular information (**Table 1**). In conventional immunostaining, Melan-A, S100, and SOX-10 represent the most widely used reagents applied to melanocytic tumors in diagnostic dermatopathology. By contrast to traditional or mainstream approaches used to confirm lineage or define distribution, both p16 and BAP-1 are primarily used to provide a surrogate view of underlying molecular status.

At a cellular level, the importance of CDKN2A locus is its expression of tumor suppressors p16(Ink4a) and p19(Arf). A major function of p16 is through its suppression of cyclin-dependent kinase (CDK) 4 to inhibit cell cycle progression, while p19 functions through direct binding to the MDM2 protein, blocking degradation of p53.[6] Given its central importance in critical cellular pathways, p16 immunohistochemical expression has been extensively evaluated.[7–10] The underlying assumption is that initiating driver mutations that induce melanocyte proliferation (ie, mutation in BRAF) are maintained in a nonproliferative state by p16 activity. With CDKN2A loss or mutation, the affected melanocytes are then allowed to bypass this G1 checkpoint with an increased potential of malignancy. Although this is an oversimplification of the pathway, comprehensive studies examining the genomic alterations in advanced cutaneous melanoma have found up to 70% of cases having mutation, deletion, or methylation of CDKN2A.[11] Therefore, the complete

Table 1
Surrogate molecular information provided by selected immunostains

Determinant	Reactivity with Melanoma	Reactivity with Melanocytic Nevi	Comment
p16 (protein product of CDKN2A)	Potential loss (as a surrogate for CDKN2A loss)	Retained	High false-negative rate
BAP-1	Loss in blue nevus-like melanoma and ocular melanoma	Retained; loss in BAPoma	Expression loss corresponds to BAP-1 loss or chromosome 3p loss
ALK	• Positive if gene fusion present • Positive if ALK alternative transcription initiation present	Positive if gene fusion present	Kinase gene fusion common in a subset of Spitz nevi and Spitz tumors
NTRK1	• Strongly positive if NTRK1 gene fusion present • May cross-react with NTRK3 fusion	• Strongly positive if NTRK1 gene fusion present • May cross-react with NTRK3 fusion	Kinase gene fusion occurs in a subset of Spitz nevi and Spitz tumors

absence of staining for p16 in a melanocytic tumor is an obvious point of concern. The converse, however, is not true, because p16 expression can be maintained in a significant subset of melanomas.

Viewed simplistically, p16 immunostaining can be used as a rapid, readily available surrogate means to evaluate the genomic copy number status of *CDKN2A*. If complete loss of expression is observed, then there may be underlying mutation or homozygous loss in *CDKN2A*. Immunostaining results can be dramatic and diagnostically compelling in the context of biphasic tumor populations, such as melanoma arising in conjunction with a melanocytic nevus, in which a loss of p16 expression is observed in the component of melanoma and maintained expression is found in the component of precursor melanocytic nevus. Common use of the stain can be frustrating, however, because many tumors, whether presumed benign or malignant, exhibit partial labeling that is diagnostically inconclusive. Use of p16 immunohistochemistry as a screen for underlying genomic status is probably most effective when paired with FISH to evaluate *CDKN2A* copy number status. In effect, FISH can be applied to clarify copy number status when screening immunohistochemistry produces a diagnostically ambiguous result. Engaging in p16 immunohistochemistry on a daily basis in the absence of backup method, such as FISH, triggers the inclusion of many ambiguous statements in pathology reports.

BRCA-associated protein 1 (BAP-1) represents a tumor suppressor that is most widely known for its crucial role in the evolution of ocular melanoma.[12] In the ocular setting, subsequent to initiation through *GNAQ* or *GNA11* mutation, the addition of BAP-1 loss is sufficient to create a fully transformed (lethal) tumor. BAP-1 immunostaining results exhibit far greater correlation to underlying genetic status in comparison to p16.[13–15] If BAP-1 nuclear expression is lost, then either an interstitial deletion within chromosome 3p, chromosome 3p loss, or chromosome 3 loss can be presumed to be present (**Fig. 1**). Rarely, BAP-1 nuclear expression can be maintained in the face of BAP-1 deletion or genomic loss.

Sporadic BAPoma (also referred to as Wiesner nevus or BAP-1 inactivated spitzoid nevus) represents the most common cutaneous proliferation exhibiting BAP-1 genomic loss.[16] The full histopathologic spectrum associated with BAP-1 genomic loss continues to expand and also includes partially transformed tumors with a syncytial configuration as well as nevoid and conventional forms of melanoma (see **Fig. 1**). Sporadic BAPoma presents to the histopathologist most commonly as a combined melanocytic nevus, and these biphasic tumors were historically commonly interpreted as combined Spitz nevi. Because of the combination of large epithelioid and plasmacytoid (growth dysregulated) melanocytes — due to BAP-1 loss — with small conventional melanocytes, tumors in this spectrum may be overinterpreted as melanoma ex melanocytic nevus by the uninformed. With BAP-1 immunohistochemistry, both nonneoplastic background tissue and the component of conventional melanocytic nevus exhibit retained nuclear expression, whereas loss of nuclear BAP-1 expression is limited to enlarged melanocytes. In this context, the component of conventional melanocytic nevus is presumably triggered by *BRAF* mutation, and the addition of BAP-1 genomic loss or mutation permits a secondary population of enlarged melanocytes to emerge. The significance of BAP-1 inactivation or loss may vary depending on whether *BRAF* or *GNAQ/GNA11* mutation was the preceding initiating event.

Kinase gene fusion represents a not uncommon mechanism of induction associated with Spitz nevi, partially transformed Spitz tumors (atypical Spitz tumor), and spitzoid melanoma. Relevant genes include *ALK, BRAF, MET, NTRK1, NTRK3, RET,* and *ROS1.*[14,17–19] The fusion proteins produced are constitutively active as their kinase domains are uncoupled from the regulatory portion of the native kinase. In many

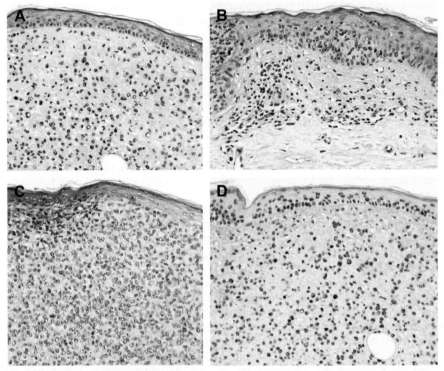

Fig. 1. Melanoma arising in conjunction with BAPoma. A focus of BAPoma shows large plasmacytoid and epithelioid melanocytes (*A*). To the side of this area, a component of melanoma in situ with a pagetoid distribution was noted (*B*). In a different focus, nevoid invasive melanoma with associated epidermal consumption was present (*C*). All 3 populations of melanocytes in this polymorphic tumor exhibited BAP-1 nuclear staining loss by immunohistochemistry (*D*). Note that the keratinocytes of the epidermis exhibit retained nuclear positivity as an internal control. *A–C*, H&E, original magnification ×100; *D*, BAP-1 immunostain, original magnification ×100.

cases, the fusion protein is also expressed at much higher levels than the native kinase. For example, ALK is not expressed in uninitiated melanocytes and is only expressed due to an ALK fusion (**Fig. 2**) or alternative transcription initiation.[20] The increase in expression of a portion of ALK can readily detected by immunohistochemistry. Currently, ALK immunohistochemistry is broadly available, and detection of the kinase domain of the ALK protein is highly predictive of the presence of an ALK fusion. Other fusion detection reagents (such as NTRK1 or ROS1) may be available in selected centers. Improvements that allow cogent evaluation for other kinase gene fusions may be forthcoming in the future.

Some Spitz tumors have gene fusion (alone) with no other detectable genomic changes and have historically been appropriately and safely interpreted as melanocytic nevi on histopathologic grounds. The determination as to whether additional genomic changes are present generally requires molecular assessment, although p16 immunohistochemistry can be used in conjunction with fusion transcript immunohistochemistry (such as ALK immunostaining) to screen for *CDKN2A* genomic loss, discussed previously. In the context of multiple genomic changes, including kinase gene fusion, current understanding suggests that diagnostic interpretation as a

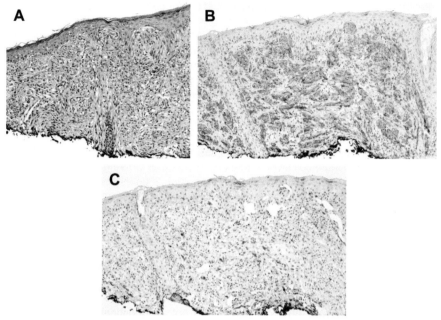

Fig. 2. Spitz nevus with ALK gene fusion. Conventional sections demonstrate a fascicular Spitz nevus with long dermal fascicles (*A*, H&E, original magnification ×100); particularly characteristic is a long vertical fascicle to the left of an eccrine duct. ALK immunohistochemistry shows diffuse positivity (*B*, ALK immunostain, original magnification ×100); dot cytoplasmic positivity can also be seen (not illustrated). Immunostaining for p16 demonstrated extensive expression loss (*C*, p16 immunostain, original magnification ×100) but targeted FISH using a CDKN2A probe showed no copy number loss, and thus the expression loss was interpreted as epigenetic in nature.

melanocytic nevus should be considered off the table. In this context, using current nosology, the differential diagnosis would instead be between partially transformation (atypical Spitz tumor) and frank spitzoid melanoma. Outcome studies are required, however, to explicitly define the significance of additional aberrations in the context of gene fusion.

ALK exhibits fusion promiscuity, meaning that multiple fusion partners have been defined. It seems possible that some fusion partners may lead to a molecular dead end — triggering a tumor that is, in effect, a melanocytic nevus — whereas other fusion partners may eventuate in additional transformation. This remains an area in need of both molecular and outcome studies.

FLUORESCENCE IN SITU HYBRIDIZATION

Both FISH and aCGH, discussed later, represent forms of genomic copy number analysis. Although both techniques are in some sense simplistic, because they do not provide specific information regarding mutation status and are simply a measure of genetic gain and/or loss, there is an established body of work that demonstrates that chromosomal copy number change represents a useful and readily detectable surrogate marker for underlying molecular events or molecular transformations that can be used to confirm or refute a diagnosis of melanoma.[3,4,21,22] As a case in point, copy number loss in chromosome 9 or 9p is taken as an indicator of *CDKN2A* loss or mutation. The identification of such loss should not (or cannot) necessarily be taken as providing full confirmation of a diagnosis of melanoma, but certainly the identification of chromosome 9 or 9p loss can be taken as excluding a conventional melanocytic nevus from the differential diagnosis. Copy number change cannot be viewed as a sine qua non of all malignancy, because oncogenic mechanisms, such as point mutation or balanced translocation, can produce profound genomic changes in the absence of genomic gain or loss, but the technique has proved highly effective in the context of melanocytic tumor diagnosis.

FISH as it applies to melanocytic tumors provides chromosomal copy number analysis at selected or targeted genomic loci.[1,2] Practical advantages to FISH include its wide availability, minimal tissue requirements, rapid turnaround time, and potential applicability to the single cell level. Although the operator working in a darkfield environment limits the full in situ qualities of the technique, if an established gain (or loss) was known to be present in a given tumor, FISH analysis could potentially be applied to highly specialized tasks, such as the evaluation of margin status.

FISH represents a targeted technique, because only selected loci are evaluated for copy number aberrations. A malignancy with an unconventional molecular profile could potentially have multiple copy number anomalies at nontested loci yet be FISH negative. In light of this, it is imperative that FISH be paired with thoughtful histopathologic evaluation by a skilled pathologist. To be completely explicit regarding the challenge of pairing FISH with microscopic evaluation, FISH-negative examples of melanoma are not rare, and, conversely indolent, diagnostically ambiguous, and potentially benign proliferations with a monoaberration, such as CDKN2A loss alone, can also be identified. In short, equating a normal or abnormal FISH result to a specific diagnosis in the absence of a histopathologic context could trigger misdiagnosis.

Commonly analyzed loci include 6p25 (RREB1), 6q23 (MYB), 8q24 (MYC), 9p21 (CDKN2A), and 11q13 (CCND1). Although a sensitivity of 94% and specificity of 98% were first reported for FISH in a validation cohort,[2] the application of FISH in the context of ambiguous melanocytic tumors has yielded varied results, suggesting that sensitivity of FISH may be lower in certain diagnostic situations. In routine diagnostic usage at the University of California, San Francisco, the differential diagnosis of Spitz versus melanoma constituted the most common testing scenario, and 88% received an enhanced classification as benign or malignant through the addition of molecular FISH evaluation.[1] Although positive FISH results ultimately led to a malignant diagnosis in 94% of these cases, FISH can also be used in dismissive fashion, with a lack of detectable copy number change eventuating in a diagnosis of melanocytic nevus. As an indication of the limitations of FISH, approximately 25% of cases with negative results eventuated, based on histopathologic findings, in either an equivocal (14%) or malignant (8%) diagnosis.[1] This reiterates the importance of using FISH results as supplemental tool. FISH does not replace careful histopathologic analysis by an experienced dermatopathologist.

In addition to copy number analysis, FISH can also be used to screen for or confirm the presence of gene fusion. This application is of the greatest benefit in the context of a rearrangement that is not readily or reliably detectable by immunohistochemistry. ALK fusion is predictably detectable by immunohistochemistry alone, but other fusions may require FISH analysis for consistent recognition.

ARRAY COMPARATIVE GENOMIC HYBRIDIZATION

In contrast to the targeted data provided by FISH, aCGH provides comprehensive chromosomal copy number status throughout the genome. Disadvantages to aCGH include its limited availability at selected centers, modest yet not insignificant tissue requirements (analysis may be impeded by low tumor volume), and lack of an in situ method of analysis. Any in situ information produced through the aCGH technique is derived from microdissection of unstained histopathologic sections based on the findings in paired stained sections.

The steps in aCGH analysis include careful stereoscopic microdissection to avoid tissue contamination, DNA extraction, DNA labeling, microarray hybridization, microarray scanning, and data analysis via software. The last 3 steps are typically completed using proprietary hardware and software. A summary graphic representation of all data points is generated from the scanned raw data (the aCGH graphs included in this article constitute examples of the summary data). An interpreting pathologist can also review the raw data in proprietary software, such as Nexus Copy Number (www.biodiscovery. com). Evaluation of the raw data is useful to confirm the precise location of small genomic changes, such as an interstitial deletion in chromosome 3p centered on *BAP-1* in the context of a BAPoma, or to confirm the precise genetic location of a chromosomal break in the context of subtotal genomic loss of a chromosomal arm. The raw aCGH data can also be used to screen for gene fusion and to identify the fusion partner, although typically this is most easily accomplished when the interpreting pathologist suspects, based on microscopic findings, that a particular gene fusion is present.

The principles used in the interpretation of aCGH tracings include the following:

1. Multiple chromosomal copy number gains or losses are construed as an indicator of genomic instability and support interpretation as melanoma (**Fig. 3**). This is especially true if the areas of genomic copy number change involve genomic loci of defined importance in the oncogenesis of melanoma, such as chromosomes 1, 6, 8, 9, and 11. Multiple copy number changes can provide diagnostic confirmation in diagnostically controversial, ambiguous, or uncomfortable tumors. In the context of a melanocytic tumor with multiple copy number aberrations, reasons to consider a diagnosis other than melanoma include microscopic findings incompatible with the diagnosis of melanoma or the identification of obscure or uncommon genomic changes not known to be relevant to the diagnosis of melanoma.

2. An absence of genomic gain or loss, or what could be termed a normal tracing, can be used to be dismissive of the diagnosis of malignancy. A normal aCGH result can be of tremendous value as a component of diagnostic reversal when an established diagnosis of melanoma becomes suspect and can also be helpful in refuting the possibility of melanoma in diagnostically challenging contexts, such as mitotically active melanocytic nevi.

3. A genomic monoaberration is not considered sufficient for a molecular diagnosis of melanoma. Many if not most monoaberrations are not of biologic significance, although the phenomenon does define a subset of partially transformed (or minimally transformed) tumors. Prototypical examples include HRAS-mutated desmoplastic Spitz nevus, in which a point mutation in HRAS correlates with chromosome 11p gain (**Fig. 4**), or BAPoma, in which BAP-1 genomic loss correlates with chromosome 3 loss (or, equivalently, chromosome 3p loss or an interstitial deletion in chromosome 3p).

4. Multiple whole chromosomal gains or losses can be identified in proliferative nodules that develop secondarily in congenital melanocytic nevi, typically large congenital melanocytic nevi, in infancy and early childhood (**Fig. 5**). Whole chromosomal gain or loss cannot be used as molecular support for a diagnosis of melanoma in this context. A diagnosis of atypical proliferative nodule — occurring in

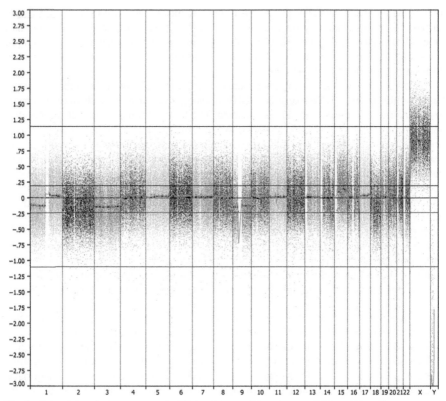

Fig. 3. Spitzoid melanoma occurring in a 70-year-old woman, aCGH tracing. Chromosomal copy number gain or loss involving chromosomes 1p, 1q, 3, 9, 15q, and 18 can be seen. Molecular analysis was pursued because although the diagnosis of desmoplastic Spitz nevus had been considered by the original pathologist, the age of the patient raised diagnostic doubt. The illustrated elevation in chromosome X represents a consequence of the use of male control genome and is not of diagnostic significance.

a nonpediatric context — should be viewed as suspect until it becomes established that the molecular oncogenesis is similar.

MASSIVELY PARALLEL SHORT-READ OR NEXT-GENERATION SEQUENCING

Massively parallel short-read sequencing determines the sequence of millions of fragments of DNA. After the sequences are determined they are mapped back to the reference genome sequence and the number of reads at each position and variations from the reference genome can be determined. This technology allows for the assessment of the entire genome of a sample in contrast to Sanger sequencing that assesses 1 polymerase chain reaction amplicon (exon) at a time and is not scalable to the entire genome. In addition to sequence variation, NGS can detect genome-wide copy number changes. NGS sequencing has been adopted by the oncology community for identification of targetable molecular alterations due to the growing number of actionable alterations. These assays target specific regions of the genome due to the substantial cost. The targeted regions are designed to include coding regions that are frequently mutated or amplified in cancer and may

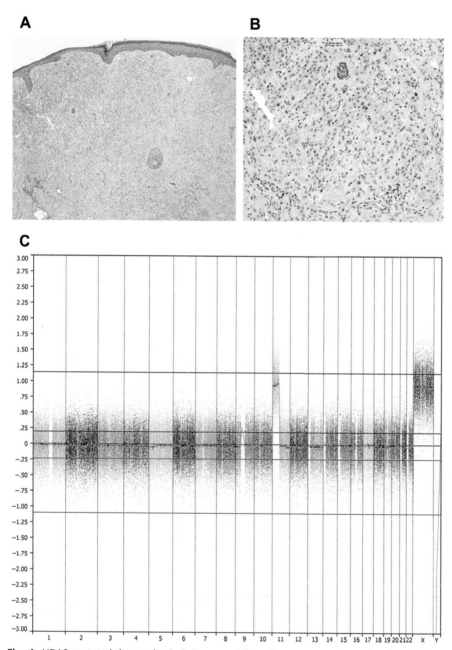

Fig. 4. HRAS-mutated desmoplastic Spitz nevus. There is a compound proliferation of large fusiform and epithelioid melanocytes without maturation (*A*, H&E, original magnification ×40). Often a broad horizontal axis of orientation is observed. The large dermal melanocytes are encompassed by sclerotic stroma (*B*, H&E, original magnification ×200) and may be found in mitosis, and thus the application of a traditional diagnostic paradigm (dermal melanocytes in mitosis, poor maturation) may trigger a false diagnosis of melanoma. aCGH analysis demonstrates gain in chromosome 11p, suggesting that HRAS mutation is present. No other copy number gains or losses are noted. The illustrated elevation in chromosome X represents a consequence of the use of male control genome and is not of diagnostic significance.

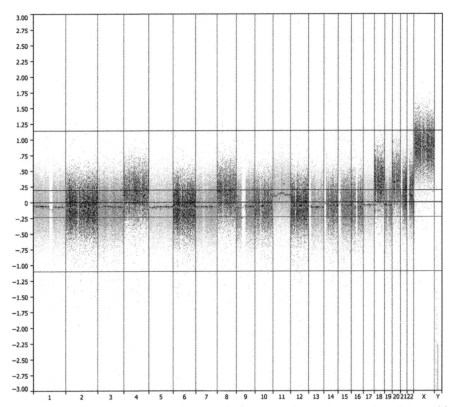

Fig. 5. Proliferative nodule occurring secondarily in a melanocytic nevus in a 3-year-old aCGH tracing. There are whole chromosomal gains in chromosomes 4, 8, 11, 18, and 20, and smaller gains in the acentric chromosomes 21 and 22 are also noted. Proliferative nodules represent an exception to the guideline that multiple aberrations should be construed as support for the diagnosis of melanoma. The illustrated elevation in chromosome X represents a consequence of the use of male control genome and is not of diagnostic significance.

include introns in which oncogenic rearrangements occur (ie, selected introns of *ALK*).

Nevi are characterized by a single initiating oncogene, such as $BRAF^{V600}$, $NRAS^{Q61}$, $GNAQ^{Q209}$, and $GNA11^{Q209}$ mutants or kinase fusions, and the initiating oncogene corresponds with the histopathologic subtype.[23–27] A recent study demonstrates that diagnostically challenging melanocytic tumors harbor a diverse array of oncogenic alterations that occur subsequent to acquisition of the initiating oncogene and lead to clonal outgrowth.[5] Alterations that follow the initiating oncogenic mutation in melanoma progression of are variable types in a broad range of genes, such as homozygous deletion of *CDKN2A*, mutations in the promoter of *TERT* resulting in elevated expression, and small or large deletions affecting the tumor suppressors *PTEN* and *NF1*. Genomic DNA-based NGS tests can detect all these alterations with varying sensitivity and specificity for types of variants and their genomic context and need to be designed to specifically target altered genomic regions. RNA-based NGS testing has higher sensitivity than DNA-based testing for detection of fusion genes due to limitations of short-read sequencing in determining alterations in repetitive regions, which are common in introns in which fusions occur. Adoption of these assays is well accepted for detecting single molecular alterations to predict drug sensitivity (ie, *BRAF* mutation or *ALK* fusion). Currently, these assays can be a helpful adjunct to histopathologic assessment because they provide similar information to aCGH with additional sequence information (ie, *TERT* promoter mutation). More studies are needed to determine how the results of this complex testing correspond with clinical outcomes and response to therapy.

REFERENCES

1. North JP, Garrido MC, Kolaitis NA, et al. Fluorescence in situ hybridization as an ancillary tool in the diagnosis of ambiguous melanocytic neoplasms: a review of 804 cases. Am J Surg Pathol 2014;38:824–31.

2. Gerami P, Jewell SS, Morrison LE, et al. Fluorescence in situ hybridization (FISH) as an ancillary diagnostic tool in the diagnosis of melanoma. Am J Surg Pathol 2009;33:1146–56.

3. Bastian BC, LeBoit PE, Hamm H, et al. Chromosomal gains and losses in primary cutaneous melanomas detected by comparative genomic hybridization. Cancer Res 1998;58:2170–5.

4. McCalmont TH, Vemula S, Sands P, et al. Molecular-microscopical correlation in dermatopathology. J Cutan Pathol 2011;38:324–6, 323.

5. Shain AH, Yeh I, Kovalyshyn I, et al. The genetic evolution of melanoma from precursor lesions. N Engl J Med 2015;373:1926–36.

6. Serrano M, Lee H, Chin L, et al. Role of the INK4a locus in tumor suppression and cell mortality. Cell 1996;85:27–37.

7. Mason A, Wititsuwannakul J, Klump VR, et al. Expression of p16 alone does not differentiate between Spitz nevi and Spitzoid melanoma. J Cutan Pathol 2012;39: 1062–74.

8. Lawrence NF, Hammond MR, Frederick DT, et al. Ki-67, p53, and p16 expression, and G691S RET polymorphism in desmoplastic melanoma (DM): a clinicopathologic analysis of predictors of outcome. J Am Acad Dermatol 2016;75:595–602.

9. DiSano K, Tschen JA, Cho-Vega JH. Intratumoral heterogeneity of chromosome 9 loss and CDKN2A (p16) protein expression in a morphologically challenging spitzoid melanoma. Am J Dermatopathol 2013;35:277–80.

10. Harms PW, Hocker TL, Zhao L, et al. Loss of p16 expression and copy number changes of CDKN2A in a spectrum of spitzoid melanocytic lesions. Hum Pathol 2016;58:152–60.

11. Cancer Genome Atlas Network. Genomic classification of cutaneous melanoma. Cell 2015;161:1681–96.

12. Harbour JW, Onken MD, Roberson ED, et al. Frequent mutation of BAP1 in metastasizing uveal melanomas. Science 2010;330:1410–3.

13. Wiesner T, Obenauf AC, Murali R, et al. Germline mutations in BAP1 predispose to melanocytic tumors. Nat Genet 2011;43:1018–21.

14. Botton T, Yeh I, Nelson T, et al. Recurrent BRAF kinase fusions in melanocytic tumors offer an opportunity for targeted therapy. Pigment Cell Melanoma Res 2013; 26:845–51.

15. Busam KJ, Sung J, Wiesner T, et al. Combined BRAF(V600E)-positive melanocytic lesions with large epithelioid cells lacking BAP1 expression and conventional nevomelanocytes. Am J Surg Pathol 2013;37:193–9.

16. Wiesner T, Murali R, Fried I, et al. A distinct subset of atypical spitz tumors is characterized by braf mutation and loss of BAP1 expression. Am J Surg Pathol 2012; 36:818–30.

17. Wiesner T, He J, Yelensky R, et al. Kinase fusions are frequent in Spitz tumours and spitzoid melanomas. Nat Commun 2014;5:3116.

18. Yeh I, Botton T, Talevich E, et al. Activating MET kinase rearrangements in melanoma and Spitz tumours. Nat Commun 2015;6:7174.

19. Yeh I, Tee MK, Botton T, et al. NTRK3 kinase fusions in Spitz tumours. J Pathol 2016;240:282–90.

20. Wiesner T, Lee W, Obenauf AC, et al. Alternative transcription initiation leads to expression of a novel ALK isoform in cancer. Nature 2015;526:453–7.

21. Mesbah Ardakani N, Thomas C, Robinson C, et al. Detection of copy number variations in melanocytic lesions utilising array based comparative genomic hybridisation. Pathology 2017;49:285–91.

22. Wang L, Rao M, Fang Y, et al. A genome-wide high-resolution array-CGH analysis of cutaneous melanoma and comparison of array-CGH to FISH in diagnostic evaluation. J Mol Diagn 2013;15:581–91.

23. Pollock PM, Harper UL, Hansen KS, et al. High frequency of BRAF mutations in nevi. Nat Genet 2003;33:19–20.

24. Yeh I, von Deimling A, Bastian BC. Clonal BRAF mutations in melanocytic nevi and initiating role of BRAF in melanocytic neoplasia. J Natl Cancer Inst 2013; 105:917–9.

25. Bastian BC, LeBoit PE, Pinkel D. Mutations and copy number increase of HRAS in Spitz nevi with distinctive histopathological features. Am J Pathol 2000;157: 967–72.

26. Van Raamsdonk CD, Bezrookove V, Green G, et al. Frequent somatic mutations of GNAQ in uveal melanoma and blue naevi. Nature 2009;457:599–602.

27. Van Raamsdonk CD, Griewank KG, Crosby MB, et al. Mutations in GNA11 in uveal melanoma. N Engl J Med 2010;363:2191–9.

Update on Merkel Cell Carcinoma

Paul W. Harms, MD, PhD[a,b,*]

KEYWORDS

- Merkel cell carcinoma • Merkel cell polyomavirus • T antigen
- Neuroendocrine carcinoma • Immunotherapy

KEY POINTS

- Merkel cell carcinoma (MCC) is a rare, highly aggressive cutaneous neuroendocrine malignancy.
- Most MCC tumors are associated with Merkel cell polyomavirus (MCPyV), which expresses viral oncoproteins including large T and small T antigens.
- A panel of immunohistochemical markers is necessary for the diagnosis of MCC and distinction from morphologically similar tumors involving the skin.
- MCCs do not consistently display activation of cellular oncogenes for which clinical inhibitors are available, therefore implementing targeted therapies for these tumors has been challenging.
- Viral antigens expressed by MCPyV-positive MCC, and mutation-associated neoantigens expressed by MCPyV-negative MCC, may render these tumors sensitive to immunotherapy.

INTRODUCTION

Primary cutaneous neuroendocrine carcinoma, or Merkel cell carcinoma (MCC), is a highly aggressive malignancy. Although rare, MCC represents the second most common cause of skin cancer death after melanoma.[1,2] MCC was originally described as "trabecular carcinoma" in 1972 by Toker.[3] Ultrastructural studies established similarity to Merkel cells (a type of cutaneous mechanoreceptor cell),[4] prompting the tumor to be renamed Merkel cell carcinoma. Most cases harbor the tumorigenic DNA virus Merkel cell polyomavirus (MCPyV) that expresses

---

No relevant conflicts of interest to disclose.
a Department of Pathology, University of Michigan Medical School, 3261 Medical Science I, 1301 Catherine Street, Ann Arbor, MI 48109-5602, USA; b Department of Dermatology, University of Michigan Medical School, 3261 Medical Science I, 1301 Catherine Street, Ann Arbor, MI 48109-5602, USA
* Department of Pathology, University of Michigan Medical School, 3261 Medical Science I, 1301 Catherine Street, Ann Arbor, MI 48109-5602.
E-mail address: paulharm@med.umich.edu

Clin Lab Med 37 (2017) 485–501
http://dx.doi.org/10.1016/j.cll.2017.05.004
0272-2712/17/© 2017 Elsevier Inc. All rights reserved.

oncogenic viral proteins including large T antigen (LTAg) and small T antigen (sTAg).[5] In contrast, MCC tumors lacking MCPyV demonstrate evidence of UV-associated genomic damage,[6–9] suggesting tumors may arise via viral-mediated or photodamage-mediated pathways.

EPIDEMIOLOGY

As of 2011, the annual incidence of MCC in the United States was 0.79 per 100,000, with slightly lower incidence in Europe and higher incidence in Australia.[1,10] There is higher incidence in fair-skinned populations.[1] The incidence of MCC has displayed a greater than three-fold increase in the past three decades, accompanied by increased mortality.[10]

MCC risk is influenced by patient factors including ethnicity, age, sex, and medical history. Greater than 95% of individuals with MCC are white.[11,12] There is male predominance.[11] The median age of incidence is approximately 76 years[11]; most patients are older than 50, and childhood cases are exceedingly rare.[12] UV exposure is a risk factor.[1] There is increased risk among patients with impaired immune function, including chronic lymphocytic leukemia, organ transplant, immunosuppressant medications, and human immunodeficiency virus.[1,12] Patients with MCC are at increased risk for a second malignancy, such as melanoma or hematologic malignancy.

CLINICAL PRESENTATION

MCC classically presents as a rapidly growing, firm, red or violaceous nodule on sun-exposed skin.[12] Clinical findings have been described by the AEIOU acronym (asymptomatic/lack of tenderness, expanding rapidly, immune suppression, older than 50 years, ultraviolet-exposed site on fair skin).[12] The clinical differential diagnosis often includes cyst, lipoma, or nonmelanoma skin cancer.[12,13]

PATHOLOGIC EVALUATION
Scanning Magnification Features

A basic approach for histopathologic evaluation of MCC is shown in **Box 1**. At low power, MCC typically forms a large nodule with infiltrative borders in the dermis or subcutis (**Fig. 1**A).[14] Circumscribed nodules or entirely infiltrative patterns (see **Fig. 1**B) may also be seen. Areas of cordlike or trabecular growth through thickened collagen are often present (see **Fig. 1**C). Some tumors display organoid patterning (see **Fig. 1**D, E). Tumor necrosis is common. Stromal changes may include mucin (see **Fig. 1**F), inflammation, and increased vascularity.[15]

High Magnification Features

At high magnification, tumors consist of small round cells with minimal cytoplasm and pale, finely stippled (salt and pepper) neuroendocrine chromatin (**Fig. 2**A). Hyperchromasia, molding, and crush artifact are often present (see **Fig. 2**B). Larger cells may form cords or trabeculae (see **Fig. 2**C). In some cases, small cells with hyperchromatic nuclei and minimal cytoplasm comprise part or all of the tumor (see **Fig. 2**D). Mitotic figures and apoptotic cells are usually numerous. Epidermal involvement with pagetoid scatter is present in a minority of cases (see **Fig. 2**E, F): entirely intraepidermal cases are rare.[15] Angiolymphatic invasion may be extensive. Rosettes may be observed (see **Fig. 2**G).[16] Rare morphologies include plasmacytoid, clear cell, or anaplastic.[16]

Box 1
Approach to histopathologic evaluation of MCC

Primary tumor
  Hematoxylin and eosin
- Confirm round cell neuroendocrine morphology.
- Measure tumor parameters as per College of American Pathologists or institutional template (including tumor thickness, mitotic rate, angiolymphatic invasion, distance to margins, tumor-infiltrating lymphocytes, presence of second malignancy, invasion of deep structures).

  Immunohistochemistry
- Basic immunohistochemical panel: broad-spectrum cytokeratin, cytokeratin 20 (CK20), neuroendocrine markers, thyroid transcription factor 1 (strongly recommended), possibly MCPyV.
- Paranuclear dotlike cytokeratin staining is helpful but not required.
- Expanded panel for cases lacking CK20 expression: cytokeratin 7, neurofilament, thyroid transcription factor 1; MCPyV may be of limited value.

  Comment section of report
- May note presence of divergent differentiation.
- There is no absolute distinguishing feature between primary and metastatic disease, therefore correlation with skin examination findings and any prior history of small cell carcinoma is necessary.
- If tumor is CK20$^+$, metastasis from an extracutaneous site is unlikely.

Sentinel lymph node biopsy
- Measure size of largest metastatic focus; note extracapsular extension.
- Immunohistochemical staining (broad-spectrum cytokeratin, CK20) to detect small metastatic deposits or scattered single cells.

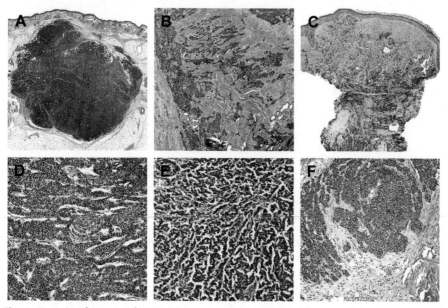

Fig. 1. Scanning features of MCC. (A) Large nodule with sheetlike growth (hematoxylin and eosin, original magnification ×5). (B) Diffusely infiltrative growth with small cell morphology (hematoxylin and eosin, original magnification ×40). (C) Trabecular/cord-like growth of tumor through thickened collagen (hematoxylin and eosin, original magnification ×40). (D) Organoid patterning (hematoxylin and eosin, original magnification ×100). (E) Serpiginous clefting (hematoxylin and eosin, original magnification ×100). (F) Stromal mucin may be prominent (hematoxylin and eosin, original magnification ×40).

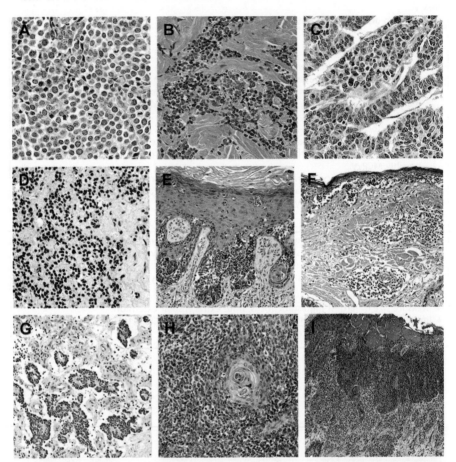

Fig. 2. Possible high magnification features of MCC. (*A*) Round blue cells with scant cytoplasm, neuroendocrine chromatin, and mitotic activity (hematoxylin and eosin, original magnification ×400). (*B*) Infiltrative cells with hyperchromasia and crush artifact (hematoxylin and eosin, original magnification ×400). (*C*) Trabeculae of larger cells (hematoxylin and eosin, original magnification ×400). (*D*) Small cell morphology characterized by tumor cells with small hyperchromatic nuclei (hematoxylin and eosin, original magnification ×400). (*E*) Intraepidermal scatter of MCC cells with distinctive neuroendocrine chromatin (hematoxylin and eosin, original magnification ×200). (*F*) Intraepidermal MCC with small cell morphology resembling lentigo maligna (hematoxylin and eosin, original magnification ×100). (*G*) Rosettes are a rare finding (hematoxylin and eosin, original magnification ×200). (*H*) Squamous differentiation (hematoxylin and eosin, original magnification ×200). (*I*) MCC with concurrent SCCIS (hematoxylin and eosin, original magnification ×40).

Divergent Differentiation in Merkel Cell Carcinoma

The most common form of divergent differentiation in MCC is squamous differentiation, typically manifesting as scattered clusters of atypical squamous cells that merge with the surrounding small blue cells (see **Fig. 2**H). The presence of squamous differentiation has been associated with molecular and immunophenotypic findings including absence of MCPyV.[13,17] Other forms of divergent differentiation include eccrine,[16] neuroblastic,[16] and sarcomatoid (including atypical fibroxanthoma, fibrosarcoma, leiomyosarcoma, or rhabdomyosarcoma).[15]

Coexisting Neoplasms

A second neoplastic process may be identified alongside MCC, most frequently squamous cell carcinoma (SCC), especially SCC in situ (SCCIS) (see **Fig. 2I**).[16] Other reported coexisting neoplasms include basal cell carcinoma (BCC), poroma, and trichoblastoma.[16,18–20]

Ancillary Studies

Immunohistochemistry

MCCs express keratins in a classic paranuclear dotlike pattern, cytoplasmic pattern, membranous pattern, or mixed pattern (**Fig. 3A, B**). Broad-spectrum cytokeratins (CAM5.2, AE1/AE3, and 34βE12) seem to be nearly 100% sensitive, although absence of cytokeratin expression has been reported.[21,22] Cytokeratin 20 (CK20) is a highly specific and sensitive marker for MCC (see **Fig. 3C**), especially when dotlike staining pattern is present. Most MCCs (reported range, 75%–100%) express CK20.[23–26]

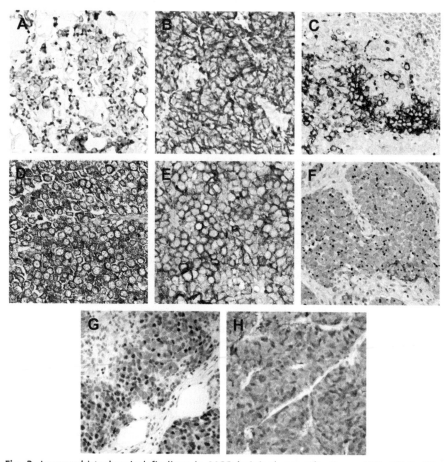

Fig. 3. Immunohistochemical findings in MCC (original magnification ×400). (A) Dotlike expression of broad-spectrum keratins. (B) MCC with mixed (dotlike and cytoplasmic) keratin pattern (by broad spectrum keratin). (C) Cytokeratin 20 expressed in a subset of cells. (D) Chromogranin A. (E) CD56. (F) Neurofilament (dotlike pattern). (G) MCPyV LTAg (nuclear pattern). (H) MCPyV LTAG (nuclear and cytoplasmic pattern).

CK20 expression may be diffuse or limited. Some tumors have only focal expression, requiring careful examination of the tumor in its entirety. A minority of MCCs completely lack CK20 expression, possibly because of partial loss of differentiation.[27] CK7 is expressed in a minority of MCC.[25,28]

MCCs express neuroendocrine markers including chromogranin A, neuron-specific enolase (NSE), and synaptophysin, as well as neural markers including neurofilament and CD56 (see **Fig. 3**D, E).[22,25,26,29,30] Chromogranin A, CD56, and synaptophysin are positive in most MCC cases, but no single marker is completely sensitive.[25,28] Neurofilament demonstrates a dotlike pattern (see **Fig. 3**F).[26]

Additional markers expressed in MCC, including TdT, PAX5, CD99, FLI1, CD117 (KIT), and p63,[22,25,30–32] are discussed in the differential diagnosis section.

Merkel cell polyomavirus detection

Detection of MCPyV (present in approximately 80% of MCC tumors) is entering clinical diagnostic use because of its high specificity for MCC, and may also have implications for prognosis and management.[33–35] MCPyV can be detected by approaches including immunohistochemical detection of viral T-antigen protein expression and polymerase chain reaction (PCR) detection of viral DNA sequences.

Immunohistochemistry studies report a MCPyV detection rate of approximately 70% (reported range, 18%–90%).[13,34,36,37] MCPyV LTAg may show cytoplasmic and/or nuclear distribution in tumor cells (see **Fig. 3**G, H). The most commonly used antibody, anti-LTAg clone CM2B4, is somewhat less sensitive than PCR for detection of MCPyV.[38–40] Other antibodies have been reported to have improved sensitivity for MCPyV,[39,40] but thus far the results have not been broadly replicated.

PCR for MCPyV T-antigen sequences is highly sensitive for detection of MCPyV. Both LTAg and sTAg must be targeted to achieve full sensitivity.[39] PCR may also detect background infection by wild-type MCPyV in the surrounding tissue.[41] Thresholds for distinguishing tumor-associated MCPyV from background wild-type MCPyV by quantitative PCR have not been established.

Differential Diagnosis

MCC may share features with other small cell and basaloid neoplasms of the skin, including BCC or other cutaneous carcinomas, small cell melanoma, lymphoma, Ewing sarcoma (ES), or metastasis from a noncutaneous small cell carcinoma (**Table 1**).[15]

Basal cell carcinoma

Most cases of BCC are easily distinguished from MCC. However, MCC and BCC share some morphologic features, leading to potential misdiagnosis in limited samples or cases with nonclassic morphology.

Both MCC and BCC may display stromal or intratumoral mucin, peripheral clefting around the edge of tumors (**Fig. 4**), and stromal amyloid.[16] However, BCCs are composed of cells with elongated nuclei with variable cytoplasm that display prominent peripheral palisading (see **Fig. 4**B), whereas MCCs are composed of round cells with neuroendocrine nuclei, minimal cytoplasm, and crush artifact, with focal or absent palisading (see **Fig. 4**C). Angiolymphatic invasion or intraepidermal spread occurs in a significant subset of MCCs, but is not expected in BCC.[15,16]

In challenging cases, immunohistochemistry is useful in distinction of MCC from BCC. CK20 and dotlike keratin expression are not seen in BCC. MCCs often express epithelial membrane antigen,[22] whereas BCCs lack epithelial membrane antigen expression except in squamous areas.[42] MCPyV LTAg is highly specific for MCC, with only rare reports in BCC.[36,37] Ber-EP4, BCL2, and neuroendocrine markers may be expressed in either tumor type.[15]

Other cutaneous carcinomas
Few other cutaneous carcinomas display true small round cell morphology. Small cell sweat gland carcinoma has morphologic overlap with MCC, but occurs in childhood and lacks expression of CK20 and neuroendocrine markers.[43] A case of nipple neuroendocrine adenocarcinoma mimicking MCC has also been reported; this case lacked CK20 expression.[44]

Melanoma
Small cell melanoma may enter the differential diagnosis for MCC. MCC may show pagetoid scatter and junctional nesting.[15] Immunohistochemistry for melanocytic and epithelial markers distinguishes melanoma from MCC,[29] with the caveat that S100 expression has been reported in some MCCs,[22,29] and melanomas may express keratins and NSE.[29]

Lymphoma
MCCs with brisk obscuring inflammation, or predominantly small cell morphology, may raise the differential diagnosis for lymphoma. MCCs express certain hematolymphoid markers, such as PAX5, TdT, and immunoglobulins,[30,31,45,46] but are negative for most other lymphoid markers including CD45, CD3, and CD20.[30]

Primary cutaneous Ewing sarcoma
Primary cutaneous ES is a rare small cell malignancy that may be mistaken for MCC.[15] A minority of ES express keratin. Both MCC and ES express CD99, FLI-1, and NSE.[15,22] There are no reports of CK20 expression or dotlike keratin expression in ES. Studies for *EWSR1* translocations may be useful in challenging cases, because these are absent in MCC.[7,15,47]

Metastatic Merkel cell carcinoma
MCC may develop in-transit or distant cutaneous metastases. Clinical correlation is required to distinguish primary from metastatic MCC, because no pathologic feature allows for absolute distinction. Epidermotropism in an MCC metastasis has been reported.[48] Regression or concurrent SCCIS favor a primary tumor.[15]

Metastatic small cell carcinoma from a noncutaneous site
In the absence of concurrent SCCIS, MCC is morphologically identical to metastatic small cell carcinoma from a noncutaneous site. CK20 is expressed in most MCC, but not in noncutaneous small cell carcinomas with the exception of parotid and cervical small cell carcinomas (**Table 2**).[21,23–25] Other markers expressed in MCC, but not small cell lung carcinoma, include neurofilament and MCPyV LTAg.[13,21,25] Most CK20-negative MCC are also MCPyV-negative, limiting the utility of MCPyV detection in this context.[6] Thyroid transcription factor 1 is commonly expressed in small cell lung carcinoma, and is negative in most MCCs[22,25,28,30] with the reported exception of MCCs combined with SCC or BCC.[49,50] As next generation sequencing enters widespread clinical use, the presence of UV signature mutations in MCPyV-negative MCC may be helpful in supporting a cutaneous origin in challenging cases.[27]

CLINICAL COURSE, STAGING, AND PROGNOSIS

MCC has a high rate of metastasis and mortality. A total of 26% of cases present with nodal metastatic disease, and 8% with distant metastatic disease.[11] In-transit and satellite cutaneous metastases can occur. Distant metastases may involve the skin,

Table 1
Differential diagnosis for MCC

| Diagnosis | Hematoxylin and eosin | | Immunohistochemistry | | Comments |
	Potentially Similar Findings	Distinguishing Findings	Potentially Overlapping Markers	Distinguishing Markers	
BCC	"Blue tumor" Nodular or infiltrative growth pattern Stromal mucin Inflammation Peripheral clefting Squamous foci Calcifications	MCC: small blue cells; angiolymphatic invasion; true palisading minimal/absent; tumor cells may disperse singly into stroma BCC: basaloid cells; extensive peripheral palisading with well-defined clefts	BCL2 Ber-EP4 Cytokeratins Neuroendocrine markers	MCC: dotlike keratin pattern; CK20, MCPyV, EMA	MCC and BCC coexist in rare cases
Melanoma (small cell)	Small cell morphology Intraepidermal pagetoid scatter	MCC: neuroendocrine chromatin; may have squamous foci Melanoma: may have coexisting pigmented lesion	S100 (reported in minority of MCC) NSE Cytokeratin	MCC: CK20, MCPyV Melanoma: HMB45, Melan-A, other melanocytic markers	Keratin in melanoma may show a globular staining pattern
Hematologic malignancy	Small hyperchromatic cells (for small cell MCC) Brisk inflammation may obscure MCC	MCC: neuroendocrine chromatin, may have squamous foci, rosettes, trabeculae B-cell lymphoma: aberrant lymphoid architecture as per lymphoma type	PAX5 Immunoglobulins TdT	MCC: keratins, CK20 Lymphoma: CD45, (also CD20, CD79a for B-cell lymphoma)	MCC and hematologic malignancy may coexist (especially chronic lymphocytic leukemia) Some MCC have clonal immunoglobulin rearrangements

Ewing sarcoma	Small blue cell morphology	MCC: concurrent SCCIS	CD99 FLI1 NSE Broad-spectrum keratin EMA	MCC: CK20, MCPyV	Molecular studies for t(11;22) translocation may be useful
Metastatic small cell lung carcinoma	Small cell neuroendocrine carcinoma	No reliable morphologic distinction	Neuroendocrine markers PAX5 CK7 (minority of MCC) Both may show dotlike keratin pattern	MCC: CK20, neurofilament, MCPyV, TdT Small cell lung carcinoma: TTF1, MASH1	
Parotid small cell carcinoma (vs metastatic MCC of unknown primary presenting in the parotid)	Small cell neuroendocrine carcinoma involving parotid	Metastatic MCC involves intraparotid lymph node	CK20 Neuroendocrine markers MCPyV	None	Definitive distinction may not be possible in some cases

Abbreviations: EMA, epithelial membrane antigen; SCCIS, squamous cell carcinoma in situ; TTF, thyroid transcription factor 1.

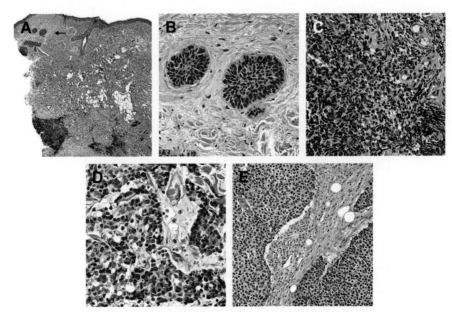

Fig. 4. (*A*) MCC (*yellow arrowheads*) with incidental BCC (*black arrow*) for comparison of low-power features. Both form blue tumors with stromal mucin (hematoxylin and eosin, original magnification ×40). (*B*) Elongated nuclei with distinctive palisading in BCC (hematoxylin and eosin, original magnification ×200). (*C*) Round cells with crush artifact in MCC (hematoxylin and eosin, original magnification ×200). (*D*) Intratumoral mucin in MCC (hematoxylin and eosin, original magnification ×200). (*E*) Cleft retraction in MCC (hematoxylin and eosin, original magnification ×400).

Table 2 Immunohistochemical distinction of MCC from SCLC			
Marker	**MCC**	**SCLC**	**Comment**
Broad-spectrum cytokeratins	Positive	Positive (majority)	Dotlike pattern may be seen in either SCLC or MCC
CK20	Positive in majority	Negative	CK20 also expressed in small cell carcinomas from the parotid and cervix, and large cell neuroendocrine carcinoma
CK7	Positive in minority (5%–20%)	Positive in majority	CK7⁺/CK20⁻ MCC has been reported
TTF1	Negative (>99%)	Positive in majority	Also positive in cervical small cell carcinomas; expression in rare cases of MCC (especially combined tumors)
Neurofilament	Positive (estimated 80%)	Negative	Dotlike pattern in MCC
MCPyV large T antigen	Positive (estimated 70%–80%)	Negative	Nuclear or nuclear and cytoplasmic
MASH1	Negative	Positive (83%)	
TdT	Positive (50%–70%)	Rarely positive (<10%)	

Abbreviations: CK, cytokeratin; SCLC, small cell lung carcinoma; TTF, thyroid transcription factor 1.

liver, bone, brain, or central nervous system. Reported mortality estimates vary. A recent study of 9387 patients reported 5-year overall survival rates of 51% for local disease, 35% for nodal disease, and 14% for distant disease.[11]

The strongest indicator of metastatic risk is primary tumor size. However, even small tumors are associated with a 10% to 20% risk of nodal metastasis.[51] Other primary tumor characteristics reported to influence prognosis include mitotic rate and infiltrative growth.[14,51]

Tumors with positive lymph nodes are associated with worse prognosis, and this effect increases with greater metastatic burden. Clinically detectable nodal disease is associated with worse outcome than clinically occult metastases.[11] Sheetlike nodal involvement by metastatic tumor[52] and increasing number of positive lymph nodes[53] have been associated with worse prognosis. However, metastases of any size are currently considered node-positive disease for staging purposes, and therefore immunohistochemical analysis of sentinel lymph nodes with broad-spectrum cytokeratin and CK20 is useful for identifying small metastatic deposits or isolated tumor cells.[54]

Based on the prognostic significance of primary tumor size, locoregional metastases, and distant metastases, these parameters have been incorporated into the American Joint Committee on Cancer consensus staging system for MCC.[11]

POTENTIAL PROGNOSTIC BIOMARKERS

Several potential prognostic biomarkers have been investigated for MCC.[1] Immune markers that may be informative include tumor PD-L1 expression and the presence of $CD8^+$ tumor-infiltrating lymphocytes.[55,56] Proangiogenic factor expression (vascular endothelial growth factor) and vascular density (by CD34) may be associated with worse outcome.[57,58] Other possible markers of poor prognosis include p63 and nuclear expression of survivin.[32,59]

Studies examining the prognostic significance of MCPyV in MCC have had mixed results.[33] Recently, Moshiri and colleagues[34] reported the largest prospective study to date on 282 MCC tumors, and found that MCPyV positivity was associated with significantly improved outcome relative to MCPyV-negative tumors.

Serologic studies for antibodies against MCPyV antigens may also be informative; patients with higher anti-VP1 titers have more favorable outcome,[60] whereas persistent or re-emergent anti-LTAg antibodies portend poor prognosis.[61]

CLINICAL MANAGEMENT

A multidisciplinary approach for the management of MCC is recommended. For local disease, wide local excision with 1- to 2-cm margins is a mainstay of therapy. Current guidelines recommend sentinel lymph node biopsy for all clinically node-negative patients.[62] Patients with positive sentinel lymph nodes generally receive lymph node dissection or radiotherapy to the nodal basin. Adjuvant or palliative radiotherapy is useful in some cases. Chemotherapy does not produce a durable response, and is generally reserved for palliation of stage IV disease.[1]

MOLECULAR FEATURES OF MERKEL CELL CARCINOMA AND IMPLICATIONS FOR NEW THERAPIES
Cell of Origin

MCCs resemble Merkel cells by immunophenotype and ultrastructure.[4,15] However, Merkel cells are postmitotic, and are not concentrated at the sites where most MCCs arise. MCCs express B-cell markers including PAX5 and immunoglobulins,[31,63] and may harbor clonal immunoglobulin rearrangements,[63] raising the possibility of a B-cell origin. More recently, epidermal progenitor cells have emerged as promising candidates for the origin of Merkel cells and possibly MCC.[64,65] Consistent with this notion, MCPyV sTAg is oncogenic in mouse epidermis.[66,67] More definitive mouse models may provide further evidence for the MCC cell of origin.

Mechanisms of Transformation by Merkel Cell Polyomavirus

MCPyV was first identified in MCC tumors by digital transcriptome subtraction.[5] Further studies found MCPyV infection to be highly prevalent in the healthy population.[33] Oncogenic (tumor-associated) MCPyV displays distinct features from wild type viral infection, including genomic integration and tumor-specific mutations.[68] Viral T antigens may drive tumorigenesis by several mechanisms. LTAg binds and inactivates the tumor suppressor RB1.[68] Possible roles for sTAg include regulation of oncoprotein stability and modulation of signaling pathways including AKT/mTOR and nuclear factor-κB.[40,48,69] A critical role for MCPyV is supported by the dependence of cultured MCC cells on MCPyV T-antigen expression.[40,70]

MCPyV-negative MCC display a high burden of UV signature mutations and TP53 and RB1 inactivation events,[7–9,71] implicating photodamage as a cause for MCPyV-negative MCC.

Oncogene Activation Events and Implications for Targeted Therapy

Direct activation of cellular oncogenes occurs in a minority of MCCs. Mutations of genes including PIK3CA and AKT1, may lead to phosphoinositide 3-kinase pathway activation.[7–9,27,72,73] Sensitivity to phosphoinositide 3-kinase inhibitors has been demonstrated in cultured MCC cells[72,73] and one clinical case of MCC.[74] The oncogene MYCL1 (L-Myc), amplified in 39% of MCC,[75] may be targetable by BET bromodomain inhibitors based on studies in other cell types.[76] Other hotspot oncogene mutations in MCC are infrequent, and most are not currently targetable with the exception of EZH2.[27] Highly recurrent amplifications or hotspot mutations of tyrosine kinases have not been described. Overexpressed oncogenes, such as BCL2 family members or survivin, may represent therapeutic targets.[35,77] Based on these observations, implementing targeted therapy in MCC may require precision medicine approaches to identify targets in a given tumor.[62]

Immunotherapy for Merkel Cell Carcinoma

The presence of viral antigens (MCPyV-positive MCC) and mutation-associated neoantigens (MCPyV-negative MCC) suggests potential susceptibility to immunotherapy.[9,78] One targetable mechanism of immune evasion by MCC is the PD-1/PD-L1 signaling axis, which inhibits antitumor immunity. A recent study demonstrated response to the anti-PD-L1 antibody avelumab in 28 of 88 patients with advanced MCC.[79] Others have reported successful use of antibodies targeting PD-1.[80–83] Another mechanism of immune evasion by MCC is suppression of HLA class I expression, which is reversed by several approaches.[84,85] Other immune-based therapies for MCC in clinical trials include interleukin-12, toll-like receptor 4 agonists, and ipilimumab.[1] Adoptive transfer of MCPyV-specific T cells was effective in one case.[85]

SUMMARY

As an aggressive malignancy with viral etiology and lack of targeted therapies, MCC represents an area of pressing clinical need, and a unique opportunity for tumor biology investigations. MCC must be distinguished from morphologically similar tumors including metastatic small cell carcinoma. Surgical management and radiotherapy are mainstays of current treatment of local and regional disease. Chemotherapy is currently the standard of care for stage IV disease, but promising new therapies including immunotherapy may provide more durable treatment responses.

REFERENCES

1. Schadendorf D, Lebbe C, Zur Hausen A, et al. Merkel cell carcinoma: epidemiology, prognosis, therapy and unmet medical needs. Eur J Cancer 2017;71: 53–69.
2. Agelli M, Clegg LX, Becker JC, et al. The etiology and epidemiology of Merkel cell carcinoma. Curr Probl Cancer 2010;34:14–37.
3. Toker C. Trabecular carcinoma of the skin. Arch Dermatol 1972;105:107–10.
4. Tang CK, Toker C. Trabecular carcinoma of the skin: an ultrastructural study. Cancer 1978;42:2311–21.
5. Feng H, Shuda M, Chang Y, et al. Clonal integration of a polyomavirus in human Merkel cell carcinoma. Science 2008;319:1096–100.
6. Miner AG, Patel RM, Wilson DA, et al. Cytokeratin 20-negative Merkel cell carcinoma is infrequently associated with the Merkel cell polyomavirus. Mod Pathol 2015;28:498–504.
7. Harms PW, Vats P, Verhaegen ME, et al. The distinctive mutational spectra of polyomavirus-negative Merkel cell carcinoma. Cancer Res 2015;75:3720–7.
8. Wong SQ, Waldeck K, Vergara IA, et al. UV-associated mutations underlie the etiology of MCV-negative Merkel cell carcinomas. Cancer Res 2015;75:5228–34.
9. Goh G, Walradt T, Markarov V, et al. Mutational landscape of MCPyV-positive and MCPyV-negative Merkel cell carcinomas with implications for immunotherapy. Oncotarget 2016;7:3403–15.
10. Fitzgerald TL, Dennis S, Kachare SD, et al. Dramatic increase in the incidence and mortality from Merkel cell carcinoma in the United States. Am Surg 2015; 81:802–6.
11. Harms KL, Healy MA, Nghiem P, et al. Analysis of prognostic factors from 9387 Merkel cell carcinoma cases forms the basis for the new 8th edition AJCC staging system. Ann Surg Oncol 2016;23:3564–71.
12. Heath M, Jaimes N, Lemos B, et al. Clinical characteristics of Merkel cell carcinoma at diagnosis in 195 patients: the AEIOU features. J Am Acad Dermatol 2008;58:375–81.
13. Busam KJ, Jungbluth AA, Rekthman N, et al. Merkel cell polyomavirus expression in Merkel cell carcinomas and its absence in combined tumors and pulmonary neuroendocrine carcinomas. Am J Surg Pathol 2009;33:1378–85.
14. Andea AA, Coit DG, Amin B, et al. Merkel cell carcinoma: histologic features and prognosis. Cancer 2008;113:2549–58.
15. Pulitzer MP, Amin BD, Busam KJ. Merkel cell carcinoma: review. Adv Anat Pathol 2009;16:135–44.
16. Plaza JA, Suster S. The toker tumor: spectrum of morphologic features in primary neuroendocrine carcinomas of the skin (Merkel cell carcinoma). Ann Diagn Pathol 2006;10:376–85.
17. Pulitzer MP, Brannon AR, Berger MF, et al. Cutaneous squamous and neuroendocrine carcinoma: genetically and immunohistochemically different from Merkel cell carcinoma. Mod Pathol 2015;28:1023–32.
18. Molina-Ruiz AM, Bernardez C, Requena L, et al. Merkel cell carcinoma arising within a poroma: report of two cases. J Cutan Pathol 2015;42:353–60.

Harms

19. Battistella M, Durand L, Jouary T, et al. Primary cutaneous neuroendocrine carcinoma within a cystic trichoblastoma: a nonfortuitous association? Am J Dermatopathol 2011;33:383–7.
20. Patel R, Adsay V, Andea A. Basal cell carcinoma with progression to metastatic neuroendocrine carcinoma. Rare Tumors 2010;2:e8.
21. Schmidt U, Muller U, Metz KA, et al. Cytokeratin and neurofilament protein staining in Merkel cell carcinoma of the small cell type and small cell carcinoma of the lung. Am J Dermatopathol 1998;20:346–51.
22. Llombart B, Monteagudo C, Lopez-Guerrero JA, et al. Clinicopathological and immunohistochemical analysis of 20 cases of Merkel cell carcinoma in search of prognostic markers. Histopathology 2005;46:622–34.
23. Chan JK, Suster S, Wenig BM, et al. Cytokeratin 20 immunoreactivity distinguishes Merkel cell (primary cutaneous neuroendocrine) carcinomas and salivary gland small cell carcinomas from small cell carcinomas of various sites. Am J Surg Pathol 1997;21:226–34.
24. Cheuk W, Kwan MY, Suster S, et al. Immunostaining for thyroid transcription factor 1 and cytokeratin 20 aids the distinction of small cell carcinoma from Merkel cell carcinoma, but not pulmonary from extrapulmonary small cell carcinomas. Arch Pathol Lab Med 2001;125:228–31.
25. Bobos M, Hytiroglou P, Kostopoulos I, et al. Immunohistochemical distinction between Merkel cell carcinoma and small cell carcinoma of the lung. Am J Dermatopathol 2006;28:99–104.
26. McCalmont TH. Paranuclear dots of neurofilament reliably identify Merkel cell carcinoma. J Cutan Pathol 2010;37:821–3.
27. Harms PW, Collie AM, Hovelson DH, et al. Next generation sequencing of cytokeratin 20-negative Merkel cell carcinoma reveals ultraviolet-signature mutations and recurrent TP53 and RB1 inactivation. Mod Pathol 2016;29:240–8.
28. Sidiropoulos M, Hanna W, Raphael SJ, et al. Expression of TdT in Merkel cell carcinoma and small cell lung carcinoma. Am J Clin Pathol 2011;135:831–8.
29. Kontochristopoulos GJ, Stavropoulos PG, Krasagakis K, et al. Differentiation between Merkel cell carcinoma and malignant melanoma: an immunohistochemical study. Dermatology 2000;201:123–6.
30. Sur M, AlArdati H, Ross C, et al. TdT expression in Merkel cell carcinoma: potential diagnostic pitfall with blastic hematological malignancies and expanded immunohistochemical analysis. Mod Pathol 2007;20:1113–20.
31. Dong HY, Liu W, Cohen P, et al. B-cell specific activation protein encoded by the PAX-5 gene is commonly expressed in Merkel cell carcinoma and small cell carcinomas. Am J Surg Pathol 2005;29:687–92.
32. Asioli S, Righi A, Volante M, et al. p63 expression as a new prognostic marker in Merkel cell carcinoma. Cancer 2007;110:640–7.
33. Coursaget P, Samimi M, Nicol JT, et al. Human Merkel cell polyomavirus: virological background and clinical implications. APMIS 2013;121:755–69.
34. Moshiri AS, Doumani R, Yelistratova L, et al. Polyomavirus-negative Merkel cell carcinoma: a more aggressive subtype based on analysis of 282 cases using multimodal tumor virus detection. J Invest Dermatol 2017;137(4):819–27.
35. Arora R, Shuda M, Guastafierro A, et al. Survivin is a therapeutic target in Merkel cell carcinoma. Sci Transl Med 2012;4:133ra156.
36. Mertz KD, Paasinen A, Arnold A, et al. Merkel cell polyomavirus large T antigen is detected in rare cases of nonmelanoma skin cancer. J Cutan Pathol 2013;40: 543–9.

37. Ota S, Ishikawa S, Takazawa Y, et al. Quantitative analysis of viral load per haploid genome revealed the different biological features of Merkel cell polyomavirus infection in skin tumor. PLoS One 2012;7:e39954.

38. Leroux-Kozal V, Leveque N, Brodard V, et al. Merkel cell carcinoma: histopathologic and prognostic features according to the immunohistochemical expression of Merkel cell polyomavirus large T antigen correlated with viral load. Hum Pathol 2015;46:443–53.

39. Rodig SJ, Cheng J, Wardzala J, et al. Improved detection suggests all Merkel cell carcinomas harbor Merkel polyomavirus. J Clin Invest 2012;122:4645–53.

40. Shuda M, Kwun HJ, Feng H, et al. Human Merkel cell polyomavirus small T antigen is an oncoprotein targeting the 4E-BP1 translation regulator. J Clin Invest 2011;121:3623–34.

41. Schowalter RM, Pastrana DV, Pumphrey KA, et al. Merkel cell polyomavirus and two previously unknown polyomaviruses are chronically shed from human skin. Cell Host Microbe 2010;7:509–15.

42. Heyderman E, Graham RM, Chapman DV, et al. Epithelial markers in primary skin cancer: an immunoperoxidase study of the distribution of epithelial membrane antigen (EMA) and carcinoembryonic antigen (CEA) in 65 primary skin carcinomas. Histopathology 1984;8:423–34.

43. Busam KJ, Gellis S, Shimamura A, et al. Small cell sweat gland carcinoma in childhood. Am J Surg Pathol 1998;22:215–20.

44. Mecca P, Busam K. Primary male neuroendocrine adenocarcinoma involving the nipple simulating Merkel cell carcinoma: a diagnostic pitfall. J Cutan Pathol 2008; 35:207–11.

45. Buresh CJ, Oliai BR, Miller RT. Reactivity with TdT in Merkel cell carcinoma: a potential diagnostic pitfall. Am J Clin Pathol 2008;129:894–8.

46. Kolhe R, Reid MD, Lee JR, et al. Immunohistochemical expression of PAX5 and TdT by Merkel cell carcinoma and pulmonary small cell carcinoma: a potential diagnostic pitfall but useful discriminatory marker. Int J Clin Exp Pathol 2013;6: 142–7.

47. Fernandez-Flores A, Suarez-Penaranda JM, Alonso S. Study of EWS/FLI-1 rearrangement in 18 cases of CK20+/CM2B4+ Merkel cell carcinoma using FISH and correlation to the differential diagnosis of Ewing sarcoma/peripheral neuroectodermal tumor. Appl Immunohistochem Mol Morphol 2013;21:379–85.

48. Griffiths DA, Abdul-Sada H, Knight LM, et al. Merkel cell polyomavirus small T antigen targets the NEMO adaptor protein to disrupt inflammatory signaling. J Virol 2013;87:13853–67.

49. Ishida M, Okabe H. Merkel cell carcinoma concurrent with Bowen's disease: two cases, one with an unusual immunophenotype. J Cutan Pathol 2013;40:839–43.

50. Koba S, Inoue T, Okawa T, et al. Merkel cell carcinoma with cytokeratin 20-negative and thyroid transcription factor-1-positive immunostaining admixed with squamous cell carcinoma. J Dermatol Sci 2011;64:77–9.

51. Schwartz JL, Griffith KA, Lowe L, et al. Features predicting sentinel lymph node positivity in Merkel cell carcinoma. J Clin Oncol 2011;29:1036–41.

52. Ko JS, Prieto VG, Elson PJ, et al. Histological pattern of Merkel cell carcinoma sentinel lymph node metastasis improves stratification of stage III patients. Mod Pathol 2016;29:122–30.

53. Iyer JG, Storer BE, Paulson KG, et al. Relationships among primary tumor size, number of involved nodes, and survival for 8044 cases of Merkel cell carcinoma. J Am Acad Dermatol 2014;70:637–43.

54. Su LD, Lowe L, Bradford CR, et al. Immunostaining for cytokeratin 20 improves detection of micrometastatic Merkel cell carcinoma in sentinel lymph nodes. J Am Acad Dermatol 2002;46:661–6.

55. Paulson KG, Iyer JG, Tegeder AR, et al. Transcriptome-wide studies of Merkel cell carcinoma and validation of intratumoral CD8+ lymphocyte invasion as an independent predictor of survival. J Clin Oncol 2011;29:1539–46.

56. Lipson EJ, Vincent JG, Loyo M, et al. PD-L1 expression in the Merkel cell carcinoma microenvironment: association with inflammation, Merkel cell polyomavirus and overall survival. Cancer Immunol Res 2013;1:54–63.

57. Ng L, Beer TW, Murray K. Vascular density has prognostic value in Merkel cell carcinoma. Am J Dermatopathol 2008;30:442–5.

58. Fernandez-Figueras MT, Puig L, Musulen E, et al. Expression profiles associated with aggressive behavior in Merkel cell carcinoma. Mod Pathol 2007;20:90–101.

59. Kim J, McNiff JM. Nuclear expression of survivin portends a poor prognosis in Merkel cell carcinoma. Mod Pathol 2008;21:764–9.

60. Touze A, Le Bidre E, Laude H, et al. High levels of antibodies against Merkel cell polyomavirus identify a subset of patients with Merkel cell carcinoma with better clinical outcome. J Clin Oncol 2011;29:1612–9.

61. Paulson KG, Carter JJ, Johnson LG, et al. Antibodies to Merkel cell polyomavirus T antigen oncoproteins reflect tumor burden in Merkel cell carcinoma patients. Cancer Res 2010;70:8388–97.

62. Cassler NM, Merrill D, Bichakjian CK, et al. Merkel cell carcinoma therapeutic update. Curr Treat Options Oncol 2016;17:36.

63. Zur Hausen A, Rennspiess D, Winnepenninckx V, et al. Early B-cell differentiation in Merkel cell carcinomas: clues to cellular ancestry. Cancer Res 2013;73:4982–7.

64. Van Keymeulen A, Mascre G, Youseff KK, et al. Epidermal progenitors give rise to Merkel cells during embryonic development and adult homeostasis. J Cell Biol 2009;187:91–100.

65. Morrison KM, Miesegaes GR, Lumpkin EA, et al. Mammalian Merkel cells are descended from the epidermal lineage. Dev Biol 2009;336:76–83.

66. Spurgeon ME, Cheng J, Bronson RT, et al. Tumorigenic activity of Merkel cell polyomavirus T antigens expressed in the stratified epithelium of mice. Cancer Res 2015;75:1068–79.

67. Verhaegen ME, Mangelberger D, Harms PW, et al. Merkel cell polyomavirus small T antigen is oncogenic in transgenic mice. J Invest Dermatol 2015;135:1415–24.

68. Shuda M, Feng H, Kwun HJ, et al. T antigen mutations are a human tumor-specific signature for Merkel cell polyomavirus. Proc Natl Acad Sci U S A 2008;105:16272–7.

69. Kwun HJ, Shuda M, Feng H, et al. Merkel cell polyomavirus small T antigen controls viral replication and oncoprotein expression by targeting the cellular ubiquitin ligase SCFFbw7. Cell Host Microbe 2013;14:125–35.

70. Houben R, Shuda M, Weinkam R, et al. Merkel cell polyomavirus-infected Merkel cell carcinoma cells require expression of viral T antigens. J Virol 2010;84:7064–72.

71. Cimino PJ, Robirds DH, Tripp SR, et al. Retinoblastoma gene mutations detected by whole exome sequencing of Merkel cell carcinoma. Mod Pathol 2014;27:1073–87.

72. Nardi V, Song Y, Santamaria-Barria JA, et al. Activation of PI3K signaling in Merkel cell carcinoma. Clin Cancer Res 2012;18:1227–36.

73. Hafner C, Houben R, Baeurle A, et al. Activation of the PI3K/AKT pathway in Merkel cell carcinoma. PLoS One 2012;7:e31255.
74. Shiver MB, Mahmoud F, Gao L. Response to idelalisib in a patient with stage IV Merkel-cell carcinoma. N Engl J Med 2015;373:1580–2.
75. Paulson KG, Lemos BD, Feng B, et al. Array-CGH reveals recurrent genomic changes in Merkel cell carcinoma including amplification of L-Myc. J Invest Dermatol 2009;129:1547–55.
76. Kato F, Fiorentino FP, Alibes A, et al. MYCL is a target of a BET bromodomain inhibitor, JQ1, on growth suppression efficacy in small cell lung cancer cells. Oncotarget 2016;7:77378–88.
77. Verhaegen ME, Mangelberger D, Weick JW, et al. Merkel cell carcinoma dependence on Bcl-2 family members for survival. J Invest Dermatol 2014;134:2241–50.
78. Carter JJ, Paulson KG, Wipf GC, et al. Association of Merkel cell polyomavirus-specific antibodies with Merkel cell carcinoma. J Natl Cancer Inst 2009;101:1510–22.
79. Kaufman HL, Russell J, Hamid O, et al. Avelumab in patients with chemotherapy-refractory metastatic Merkel cell carcinoma: a multicentre, single-group, open-label, phase 2 trial. Lancet Oncol 2016;17:1374–85.
80. Mantripragada K, Birnbaum A. Response to anti-PD-1 therapy in metastatic Merkel cell carcinoma metastatic to the heart and pancreas. Cureus 2015;7:e403.
81. Nghiem PT, Bhatia S, Lipson EJ, et al. PD-1 blockade with pembrolizumab in advanced Merkel-cell carcinoma. N Engl J Med 2016;374:2542–52.
82. Winkler JK, Bender C, Kratochwil C, et al. PD-1 blockade: a therapeutic option for treatment of metastatic Merkel cell carcinoma. Br J Dermatol 2017;176:216–9.
83. Walocko FM, Scheier BY, Harms PW, et al. Metastatic Merkel cell carcinoma response to nivolumab. J Immunother Cancer 2016;4:79.
84. Paulson KG, Tegeder A, Willmes C, et al. Downregulation of MHC-I expression is prevalent but reversible in Merkel cell carcinoma. Cancer Immunol Res 2014;2:1071–9.
85. Chapuis AG, Afanasiev OK, Iyer JG, et al. Regression of metastatic Merkel cell carcinoma following transfer of polyomavirus-specific T cells and therapies capable of re-inducing HLA class-I. Cancer Immunol Res 2014;2:27–36.

Cutaneous Squamous Cell Carcinoma

Vishwas Parekh, MD[a], John T. Seykora, MD, PhD[b],*

KEYWORDS

- Squamous cell carcinoma • Actinic keratosis • Keratoacanthoma
- Spindle cell squamous cell carcinoma • Desmoplastic squamous cell carcinoma
- Acantholytic squamous cell carcinoma • Pathogenesis

KEY POINTS

- There is a persistent trend for an increasing incidence of cutaneous squamous cell carcinoma (cSCC).
- It is crucial to differentiate cSCC from the benign and reactive squamoproliferative lesions and report the high-risk features associated with an aggressive tumor behavior.
- Understanding the molecular mechanisms that drive the development and progression of cSCC is necessary to develop diagnostic and prognostic assays and targeted therapies.

INTRODUCTION
Epidemiology

Nonmelanoma skin cancer is the most common malignancy worldwide. Historically, cutaneous squamous cell carcinoma (cSCC) has been thought to comprise about 20% of all nonmelanoma skin cancers, thus being the second most common malignancy after basal cell carcinoma (BCC), with a ratio of BCC to SCC estimated to be 4:1.[1,2] However, recent data indicate that there is a significant shift underway in the relative proportion of nonmelanoma skin cancer, with the ratio of BCC to SCC found to be 1.0 in the US Medicare population.[3] Several other studies bear out a trend for an increasing incidence of cSCC compared with BCC, particularly in the aging population.[4–8] An accurate incidence of cSCC is not known because it is not required to be reported to national cancer registries; however, a metaanalysis of population-based studies estimated that in 2012, 186,157 to 419,543 white individuals were diagnosed with cSCC in the United States alone. Note, these estimates do not include squamous cell carcinoma in situ (SCCIS), which likely occurs more frequently.[9]

[a] Department of Pathology, City of Hope Comprehensive Cancer Center, 1500 East Duarte Road, Duarte, CA, 91010, USA; [b] Department of Dermatology, Perelman School of Medicine, University of Pennsylvania, Room 1011 BRB II/III, 421 Curie Boulevard, Philadelphia, PA 19104, USA
* Corresponding author.
E-mail address: john.seykora@uphs.upenn.edu

Clin Lab Med 37 (2017) 503–525
http://dx.doi.org/10.1016/j.cll.2017.06.003
0272-2712/17/© 2017 Elsevier Inc. All rights reserved.

labmed.theclinics.com

Etiopathogenesis

Most cSCC arise in the sun-damaged skin of the elderly white individuals of European ancestry, in the background of preexisting lesions of actinic keratosis (AK).[1] Apart from ultraviolet (UV) radiation exposure, other predisposing factors include chronic immunosuppressed state (solid organ transplantation, human immunodeficiency virus infection),[10–13] chronic skin conditions (burn scars, hidradenitis suppurativa, chronic osteomyelitis, discoid lupus erythematosus, lichen plans, lichen slecrosus et atrophicus),[14–20] inherited genetic conditions (albinism, epidermolysis bullosa, xeroderma pigmentosum),[21–23] exposure to ionizing radiation,[24] chronic arsenic exposure,[25] human papillomavirus infection,[26,27] and treatment with BRAF inhibitors (vemurafenib and dabrafenib),[28] among others.

Clinical Features

AK and SCCIS are considered to be the precursor lesions of cSCC in most instances, and, frequently, patients present with cSCC in association with numerous precursor lesions. AK and SCCIS typically present as flesh-colored, pink, brown, often pigmented, scaly patches, papules, or plaques on an erythematous base. Lesions of cSCC manifest a range of clinical presentations, including papules, plaques, or indurated nodules with a smooth, scaly, verrucous, or ulcerative surface. Cutaneous SCC can be asymptomatic, pruritic, or tender. Local neuropathic symptoms such as numbness, burning, paresthesia, or paralysis are associated with perineural invasion.[29] Although cSCC typically arises on the sun-exposed areas of fair-skinned individuals and often on the sun-exposed areas of dark-skinned individuals, an involvement of the non–sun-exposed areas is more common in dark-skinned individuals.[30,31]

PRECURSOR LESIONS
Actinic Keratosis

Also known as solar keratosis, AK represents an early precursor lesion that can accumulate additional mutations and in some cases progress to SCCIS and invasive SCC.[32] Clinically, AKs often manifest spontaneous regression and approximately one-third of AKs exhibit regression in 1 year.[33]

Histologically, AK occurs as a proliferation of cytologically atypical keratinocytes that is confined to the lower levels of the epidermis. The lesional cells show loss of polarity, increased size, pleomorphic and hyperchromatic nuclei, and an increased number of mitoses. There is often an increased nuclear:cytoplasmic ratio within lesional cells. There is crowding of the basal portion of the epidermis with variable acanthosis and/or budding of the neoplastic keratinocytes in the papillary dermis, without breach of the basement membrane. By definition, the atypical proliferation does not occupy the full thickness of the epidermis. Hypogranulosis is often seen. The stratum corneum overlying the atypical keratinocytes typically shows hyperkeratosis with parakeratosis. Because the preneoplastic process usually spares the adnexal structures, this results in alternating areas of orthokeratosis and parakeratosis (flag sign). The underlying dermis almost invariably shows solar elastosis, which represents an important diagnostic clue. AKs exhibit a variety of histologic variants with a broad range of histologic patterns.[34,35]

Pigmented actinic keratosis

This variant shows hyperpigmentation of the lower epidermal layers owing to an increased amount of melanin in the basilar keratinocytes. Melanophages may be present in the superficial dermis. It is important to recognize this entity because it can be confused clinically, as well as histologically, with melanoma in situ, particularly in the presence of severe solar elastosis. There may be mild melanocytic hyperplasia of melanocytes typical of that seen in sun-damaged skin. Melanocytes in these lesions do not manifest cytologic atypia. Immunohistochemistry with melanocytic markers is useful in difficult cases.

Lichenoid actinic keratosis
This variant is characterized by a dense, bandlike lymphocytic infiltrate at the dermal–epidermal junction with focal vacuolar alteration and necrosis of the basal keratinocytes. This entity may be confused morphologically with benign lichenoid keratosis and lichenoid regression in melanoma.

Bowenoid actinic keratosis
In this variant, the atypical keratinocytes occupy almost the full thickness of epidermis and yet do not reach the level of SCCIS. There may be palisading in the basal layer. The adnexal sparing character of AK is often helpful in distinguishing this variant from SCCIS or Bowen's disease.

Proliferative actinic keratosis
In this variant, atypical keratinocytes extend fingerlike projections in the superficial dermis. Examination of multiple, deeper level sections is often helpful in allaying a concern for superficial invasion. This variant is associated with a more aggressive behavior.[36]

Hypertrophic actinic keratosis
This variant demonstrates epidermal hyperplasia with a prominent hyperparakeratotic stratum corneum. Often, the epidermal changes suggestive of a superimposed lichen simplex chronicus are also present.

Atrophic actinic keratosis
This variant shows atrophic changes in the form of thinned out epidermis and flattened rete ridges.

Acantholytic actinic keratosis
This variant is characterized by acantholysis of atypical keratinocytes resulting in detachment from each other and intraepidermal clefting. Dyskeratosis may be present. The differential diagnosis includes benign acantholytic disorders.

Squamous Cell Carcinoma In Situ

SCCIS occupies the intermediate step in the progression from AK to invasive SCC. Although some use SCCIS and Bowen's disease terminology interchangeably, Bowen's disease typically occurs in the anogenital region and is unrelated to UV-induced AK and more often associated with human papillomavirus infection, thus being more common in young adults.[37]

Histologically, SCCIS exhibits full-thickness atypia of the epidermis, sparing the adnexal structures. The hyperparakeratosis can be minimal or exuberant and can produce a cutaneous horn. The atypical keratinocytes show nuclear pleomorphism, hyperchromasia, frequent mitoses with atypical forms, and apoptosis. The loss of polarity imparts a "windblown" appearance. Frequently, the atypical keratinocytes spare the basal layer and produce a characteristic pattern called the "eyeliner sign," a useful diagnostic clue observable on a low-power examination. By definition, there is no dermal invasion. Similar to AK, several histomorphologic variants of SCCIS have been described, including hyperkeratotic, atrophic, verrucous, psoriasiform, acantholytic, clear cell, and pagetoid subtypes. It is important to histologically distinguish the pagetoid variant of SCCIS from extramammary Paget's disease and melanoma in situ. Immunohistochemical (IHC) markers such as CK7, CAM5.2, carcinoembryonic antigen, and epithelial membrane antigen (positive in extramammary Paget's disease, negative in SCCIS), p63 (positive in SCCIS, negative in extramammary Paget's disease), and MART1 (positive in melanoma in situ) are helpful in diagnosing difficult cases.[38,39]

INVASIVE CUTANEOUS SQUAMOUS CELL CARCINOMA

Cutaneous SCC can arise as the result of tumor progression in the sun-damaged skin or can occur de novo. It is characterized by invasion of the dermis by the neoplastic squamous epithelial cells. The invasive component can take the form of infiltrating cords, sheets, or single cells, or can present as well-circumscribed nodules, squamous islands, or cystic structures composed of malignant keratinocytes. Interestingly, in contrast with AK and SCCIS, the cytomorphology of malignant keratinocytes in cSCC can vary from a very banal appearance to a highly anaplastic one.[40,41]

Histologic Grading

Lesions of cSCC can be histologically divided into 3 grades based on their degree of differentiation: well, moderately, and poorly differentiated. The factors taken into consideration for this type of grading include the degree of keratinization, nuclear atypia, and the degree of architectural atypia (well circumscribed vs infiltrative).

A well-differentiated cSCC shows slightly enlarged keratinocytes with abundant, glassy-pink to eosinophilic cytoplasm. Intercellular bridges are generally visible. Keratinization is usually present and morphologically manifests as a central plug of keratinization within a nest of well-differentiated keratinocytes, commonly referred to as a "keratin pearl." Importantly, identifying the retention of keratinocyte nuclei (parakeratosis) within these keratin pearls is often useful in discriminating a well-differentiated cSCC from a benign squamoproliferative lesion in a superficial biopsy. Well-differentiated cSCC tends to be well-circumscribed with pushing margins and a lobulated appearance. In contrast, a poorly differentiated cSCC shows a highly infiltrative pattern and is composed of highly atypical keratinocytes with pleomorphic, hyperchromatic nuclei, numerous atypical mitotic figures, and shows little or no keratinization[40,42] **(Fig. 1)**.

Histologic Variants

Several histologic variants of cSCC have been described. Knowledge of these entities has diagnostic and prognostic significance.

Acantholytic squamous cell carcinoma

This variant is also known as adenoid SCC, adenoacanthoma of sweat glands, and pseudoglandular SCC. Rare subtypes such as small cell SCC, pseudovascular SCC, and pseudoangiosarcomatous SCC have been described. Histologically, the lesional cells show a variable degree of desmosomal disruption, resulting in rounded cells with centrally placed round nuclei. Acantholysis results in various morphologic patterns, such as pseudoglandular, pseudoalveolar, or pseudovascular spaces. Based on their involvement of the follicular epithelium alone or involvement of follicular epithelium and interfollicular epidermis, these tumors have also been further subdivided as the follicular type and follicular pattern, respectively[42–47] **(Fig. 2A)**.

The differential diagnoses for acantholytic SCC include adenoid BCC, eccrine carcinoma, metastatic adenocarcinoma, and, rarely, angiosarcoma. Identifying

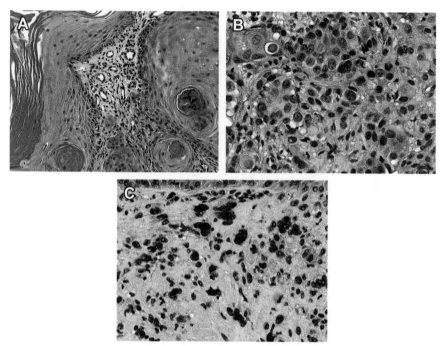

Fig. 1. Squamous cell carcinoma. (*A*) Well-differentiated. The tumor shows nests of mature keratinocytes with a low nuclear:cytoplasmic ratio and "keratin pearls" (original magnification, ×200), (*B*) Moderately differentiated. The tumor shows cellular pleomorphism, few, if any, keratin pearls and cells with more prominent cellular atypia (original magnification, ×400). (*C*) Poorly differentiated. The tumor shows infiltrative pattern and highly atypical keratinocytes with pleomorphic, hyperchromatic nuclei, and little to no keratinization (original magnification, ×400).

characteristic areas with basaloid cells, peripheral palisading, single cell necrosis, artifactual clefting, and stromal mucin would help to distinguish the adenoid BCC. Identifying ductal structures with a basal or myoepithelial layer that stains for smooth muscle actin, p63, calponin, or S100 protein, luminal borders that stain for carcinoembryonic antigen, and luminal secretions that stain with periodic acid–Schiff distase help to distinguish the eccrine carcinoma. Metastatic adenocarcinoma can be suspected from the clinical history, a multiplicity of lesions, and a lack of epidermal connection. Use of high- and low-molecular-weight cytokeratin antibodies and a battery of immunostains specific for adenocarcinomas from various sites of origin are essential in arriving at the correct diagnosis. Angiosarcoma can be suspected from blood-filled spaces and confirmed with various endothelial markers such as CD31, CD34, and ERG.

Adenosquamous carcinoma

This rare variant of cSCC is characterized by true glandular differentiation, in contrast with the pseudoglandular appearance seen in the acantholytic SCC. Histologically, the atypical squamoid cells are arranged as interconnecting nests, frequently forming keratocysts. Additionally, there are focal or diffuse areas of gland formation within the squamous nests. These glands are lined by cuboidal to low columnar epithelium that shows luminal positivity for carcinoembryonic antigen. The luminal secretions

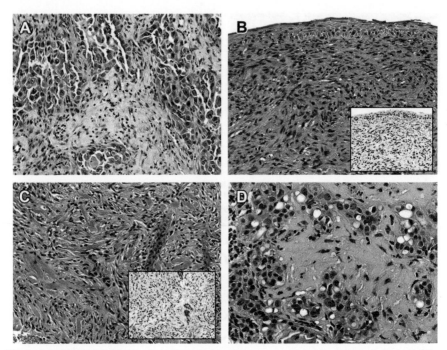

Fig. 2. Squamous cell carcinoma. (*A*) Acantholytic. Desmosomal disruption results in clefting and rounding of the tumor cells (original magnification, ×200). (*B*) Spindle cell. Haphazard growth of atypical spindle-shaped keratinocytes in the dermis. Inset: p63 immunostain confirms epithelial origin (original magnification, ×200). (*C*) Desmoplastic. Infiltrating cords of spindled tumor cells surrounded by a densely collagenous stroma. Inset: p63 immunostain (original magnification, ×200). (*D*) Signet ring cell. A variable number of tumor cells show clear cytoplasm that pushes the nucleus to the periphery imparting a signet ring appearance (original magnification, ×400).

stain with mucicarmine and Alcian blue at a pH of 2.5. The epidermal origin is evidenced by multifocal epidermal connections. The tumor commonly invades the deep dermis.[48–50]

The differential diagnosis for this variant includes primary cutaneous mucoepidermoid carcinoma and metastatic adenocarcinomas from various sites of origin. Primary cutaneous mucoepidermoid carcinoma is a controversial entity and, if it does exist, currently there is no reliable way to distinguish it from adenosquamous carcinoma.[51] Distinction from metastatic adenocarcinomas requires a thorough clinical history and imaging studies to identify a primary site, the presence of multiple lesions, histologic demonstration of a lack of epidermal connection, and, when necessary, judicious use of IHC markers.

Spindle cell squamous cell carcinoma

This variant is also known as sarcomatoid SCC. Histologically, this tumor is characterized by a haphazard growth of atypical spindle-shaped cells in the dermis. Connection with the epidermis is not always present. The atypical spindle cells may constitute all or part of the tumor, with none or a variable component of conventional SCC forming nests, cords, and keratin pearls. Occasionally, bizarre and pleomorphic giant cells and heterologous elements with numerous mitotic figures are seen. The tumor often infiltrates deep into the dermis, subcutis, fascia, muscle, and bone.[52–54] Importantly, there is not significant stromal desmoplasia (>30% of the tumor volume), because that would raise the diagnosis of the desmoplastic variant of cSCC[55] (see **Fig. 2**B).

The differential diagnosis for this variant, in the absence of an epidermal connection or an obvious evidence of keratinization, is an atypical spindle cell lesion of the dermis. This would include spindle cell/desmoplastic melanoma, leiomyosarcoma, and atypical fibroxanthoma or undifferentiated pleomorphic sarcoma, among other reactive and neoplastic dermal spindle cell proliferations. The use of the IHC markers is often required to derive a definitive diagnosis. Spindle cell SCC stains positively for p63, p40, and high-molecular-weight cytokeratins such as CK5/6.[56,57] Desmoplastic melanoma stains for S100 protein and SOX10, and leiomyosarcoma stains for smooth muscle actin and caldesmon.

Desmoplastic squamous cell carcinoma
Histologically, this variant is characterized by infiltrating cords of spindled–squamoid tumor cells surrounded by a densely collagenous (desmoplastic) stroma. In contrast with spindle cell SCC, the lesional squamous cells are oval to spindle shaped and can show single-cell keratinization. Keratin pearls are generally present, even in high-grade tumors, and the desmoplastic stromal component in this tumor should constitute greater than 30% of the tumor volume. Perineural invasion is frequent with this variant[55,58,59] (see **Fig. 2**C).

The differential diagnoses for this variant are entities that show sclerotic, desmoplastic stromal response with resultant infiltrative appearance. These include syringoma, desmoplastic trichoepithelioma, microcystic adnexal carcinoma, morpheaform BCC, and desmoplastic melanoma. The presence of epidermal squamous atypia and evidence of keratinization point to the diagnosis of desmoplastic SCC. Ductal differentiation points to the diagnoses of adnexal neoplasms. A diagnosis of morpheaform BCC would require identifying the typical findings of BCC, such as individual cell necrosis, mitotic figures and stromal retraction artifact in at least a focal manner. Additionally, the tumor cords in morpheaform BCC show sharp angulation that is quite characteristic. Desmoplastic melanoma is associated with the findings of in situ melanocytic lesion in the overlying epidermis and nodular lymphoid aggregates within the dermal component. Use of p63 (positive in SCC) and S100 and SOX10 (positive in desmoplastic melanoma) is helpful in difficult cases.

Clear cell squamous cell carcinoma
Also referred to as hydropic SCC or pale cell SCC, these rare tumors are subdivided into 3 categories: type I (keratinizing), type II (nonkeratinizing), and type III (pleomorphic). Type I tumors are characterized by sheets or islands of clear cells with peripherally displaced nuclei or central nuclei with bubbly cytoplasmic appearance, and focal areas of keratinization, even forming keratin pearls. Type II tumors are dermal masses without connection to the epidermis. Tumor cells show a cytoplasm with a finely reticulated clear appearance and are arranged in parallel or anastomosing cords separated by a fibrotic stroma with a heavy inflammatory infiltrate. There may be a central necrosis but, importantly, keratinization is absent. Type III tumors typically show extensive ulceration. Tumor cells are markedly pleomorphic with foci of acantholysis, dyskeratosis, keratinization, and perineural and lymphovascular invasion.[42,60]

The histologic differential diagnosis for clear cell SCC is broad: clear cell acanthoma, trichilemmoma, trichilemmal carcinoma, clear cell hidradenoma, hidradenocarcinoma, sebaceous tumors, clear cell BCC, balloon cell nevus, balloon cell melanoma, and metastatic renal cell carcinoma, among other entities with clear cell changes.[61] A high index of suspicion, a thorough analysis of all histologic sections, and a judicious use of IHC markers are necessary to arrive at this diagnosis.

Signet ring cell squamous cell carcinoma

This is an extremely rare variant. Histologically, this tumor is composed of a variable number of signet ring cells, where a clear cytoplasm pushes the nucleus to the periphery imparting a signet ring appearance. The cytoplasm is negative for mucin and shows focal PAS positivity with diastase sensitivity[62,63] (see **Fig. 2**D).

The differential diagnosis for this variant is extensive, because several primary cutaneous neoplasms such as BCC, melanoma, histiocytoid carcinoma of the eyelid, and lymphoproliferative diseases, as well as metastatic adenocarcinomas and soft tissue tumors can demonstrate signet ring cell changes. Once the signet ring cell changes are noted, identifying a focus of conventional SCC in the histologic sections in conjunction with IHC and special stains should promote derivation of the correct diagnosis.[64,65]

Pigmented squamous cell carcinoma

This variant is characterized by a colonization of the conventional SCC by benign, heavily pigmented dendritic melanocytes. Histologically, the tumor is composed of lobules, nests, and cords of atypical squamous cells showing evidence of keratinization. Intermixed within the tumor cells are numerous darkly pigmented dendritic melanocytes that stain for melanocytic markers such as MART1, HMB45, and S100 protein, although HMB45 can be negative in rare cases. Rare focal positivity of the squamoid tumor cells for melanocytic markers is likely secondary to antigen transfer.[66–68]

The histologic differential diagnosis for this variant includes other pigmented entities such as seborrheic keratosis, melanoacanthoma, pigmented trichoblastoma, pigmented pilomatricoma, pigmented BCC, melanoma with pseudoepitheliomatous hyperplasia, and an exceedingly rare dermal squamomelanocytic tumor.[69] Of these, the one tumor that is easy to be confused with pigmented SCC with potentially serious consequences is melanoma with pseudoepitheliomatous hyperplasia, where the malignant and benign components are transposed. A careful examination and identification of atypical melanocytes is essential to avoid this pitfall.

Verrucous carcinoma

This variant has a very distinctive silhouette owing to its endo-exophytic growth, and prominent acanthosis, papillomatosis, and hyperkeratosis. One key histologic feature is the blunt, broad, squamous epithelial projections that push into the dermis, rather than infiltrate the dermis. The tumor cells show a bland cytomorphology and the human papillomavirus-related cytopathic changes are not obvious. Rabbit burrow-like sinuses and keratocysts, and a dense inflammatory infiltrate are typically seen in carcinoma cuniculatum, a subtype of verrucous carcinoma localized to the plantar surface[42,70,71] (**Fig. 3**A).

The histologic differential diagnosis for this variant includes condyloma acuminatum, verruca vulgaris, keratoacanthoma, prurigo nodularis, and pseudoepitheliomatous hyperplasia. Clinicopathologic correlation and the availability of adequate biopsy material that includes the base of the tumor are essential for arriving at the correct diagnosis.

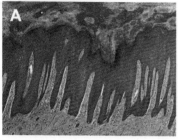 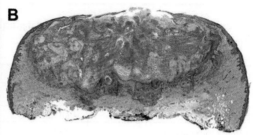

Fig. 3. (*A*) Verrucous carcinoma. Blunt, broad-based, squamous epithelial projections that push, rather than infiltrate, into the dermis (original magnification, ×20). (*B*) Keratoacanthoma. Dome-shaped nodule with a central keratin-filled crater (original magnification, ×20).

Keratoacanthoma

KA commonly presents as a rapidly growing, solitary, dome-shaped nodule with a central keratin-filled crater. The fact that it undergoes spontaneous resolution has led to a decades-long debate and uncertainty over the classification of this lesion with views ranging from KA being a benign squamoproliferative lesion, a continuum between benign and malignant proliferation, to an outright cSCC that has the biological capacity to regress. We have incorporated this entity here to enable its recognition from conventional SCC. Several clinical variants of KA are recognized including giant KA, mucosal KA, subungual KA, keratoacanthoma centrifugum marginatum, and multiple KAs associated with Ferguson-Smith disease, generalized eruptive keratoacanthomas of Grzybowski, multiple familial keratoacanthoma of Witten and Zak, Muir-Torre syndrome, and subungual tumors associated with incontinentia pigmenti[42,72–74] (see **Fig. 3**B).

Histologically, KAs are composed of mature-appearing keratinocytes that form a large, symmetric, exo-endophytic mass with a central crateriform invagination filled with a keratin plug. Typically, there is buttressing of the surrounding normal epidermis around the mass. The tumor cells have a characteristic pink, glassy cytoplasm and lack the pleomorphism and atypia seen in conventional SCC. Most KAs show scattered neutrophils and eosinophils, occasionally forming microabscesses. Perforating elastic fibers are a characteristic finding.[75] Mixed inflammatory infiltrate and small islands of tumor cells may be present in the underlying dermis, and the lesions lack infiltrative features. The histologic differential diagnosis for KA includes well-differentiated conventional SCC and pseudoepitheliomatous hyperplasia found in association with inflammatory or reactive conditions.

High-Risk Features

Although the vast majority of cSCCs are cured with complete excision, a subset of cSCCs with certain histologic and clinical features exhibits a significantly increased risk of local recurrence and metastasis, and resultant poorer prognosis.[76–78] The incidence of regional or distant metastases is estimated to be as high as 2% to 6% in such cases.[79,80] Several staging systems have been proposed to stratify the cSCC prognosis based on a number of known risk factors. These include the 2002 TNM staging system proposed by the American Joint Committee on Cancer,[81] the revised American Joint Committee on Cancer and International Union Against Cancer staging systems,[77,82] Brigham and Women's Hospital tumor staging system,[83] National Comprehensive Cancer Network guidelines[84] (**Table 1**), and European Organization for Research and Treatment of Cancer guidelines[85] (**Table 2**).

Table 1
National Comprehensive Cancer Network clinical practice guidelines, version I.2017: risk factors for local recurrence or metastasis

History and Physical Examination	Low Risk	High Risk
Location/size[a]	Area L <20 mm Area M <10 mm[d]	Area L ≥20 mm Area M ≥10 mm Area H[e]
Borders	Well defined	Poorly defined
Primary vs recurrent	Primary	Recurrent
Immunosuppression	(−)	(+)
Site of prior RT or chronic inflammatory process	(−)	(+)
Rapidly growing tumor	(−)	(+)
Neurologic symptoms	(−)	(+)
Pathology	**Low Risk**	**High Risk**
Degree of differentiation	Well or moderately differentiated	Poorly differentiated
Adenoid (acantholytic), adenosquamous (showing mucin production), desmoplastic, or metaplastic (carcinosarcomatous) subtypes	(−)	(+)
Depth[b,c]: Thickness or Clark level	<2 mm or I, II, III	≥2 mm or IV, V
Perineural, lymphatic, or vascular involvement	(−)	(+)

Area H = "mask areas" of face (central face, eyelids, eyebrows, periorbital, nose, lips [cutaneous and vermilion], chin, mandible, preauricular and postauricular skin/sulci, temple, ear), genitalia, hands, and feet. Area M = cheeks, forehead, scalp, neck, and pretibia. Area L = trunk and extremities (excluding pretibia, hands, feet, nail units, and ankles).
[a] Must include peripheral rim of erythema.
[b] If clinical evaluation of incisional biopsy suggests that microstaging is inadequate, consider narrow margin excisional biopsy.
[c] A modified Breslow measurement should exclude parakeratosis or scale crust, and should be made from base of ulcer if present.
[d] Location independent of size may constitute high risk.
[e] Area H constitutes high risk based on location, independent of size. Narrow excision margins owing to anatomic and functional constraints are associated with increased recurrence rates with standard histologic processing. Complete margin assessment, such as with Mohs micrographic surgery, is recommended for optimal tumor clearance and maximal tissue conservation. For tumors less than 6 mm in size, without other high-risk features, other treatment modalities may be considered if at least 4-mm clinically tumor-free margins can be obtained without significant anatomic or functional distortions.
From Bichakjian CK, Farma JM, Schmults CD, et al. NCCN Clinical Practice Guidelines in Oncology (NCCN Guidelines) Squamous Cell Skin Cancer. Fort Washington (PA): National Comprehensive Cancer Network, Inc; 2016; with permission.

Clinical high-risk features
Tumor location Tumors arising in head and neck locations (eg, forehead, temporal region, scalp, lips, ears) show increased rates of local recurrence and metastasis.[79,86,87] A recent metaanalysis showed that the anatomic locations of lips, ears, and temple are independent predictors of metastasis, although, in this analysis, tumor location on lips or ears did not independently predict local recurrence.[88] Additionally, tumors developing in chronic wounds or scars or at the site of prior burns or radiation therapy

Table 2
European Organization for Research and Treatment of Cancer Guidelines: prognostic risk factors in primary cutaneous squamous cell carcinoma

	Tumor Diameter	Location	Depth/Level of Invasion	Histologic Features	Surgical Margins	Immune Status
Low risk	<2 cm	Sun exposed sites (except ear/lip)	<6 mm/invasion above subcutaneous fat	Well-differentiated common variant or verrucous	Clear	Immunocompetent
High risk	>2 cm	Ear/lip Non–sun-exposed sites (sole of foot) SCC arising in radiation sites, scars, burns or chronic inflammatory conditions Recurrent SCCs	>6 mm/invasion beyond subcutaneous fat	Moderately or poorly differentiated grade Acantholytic, spindle, or desmoplastic subtype Perineural invasion	Incomplete excision	Immunosuppressed (organ transplant recipients, chronic immunosuppressive disease or treatment)

Abbreviation: SCC, squamous cell carcinoma.
From Stratigos A, Garbe C, Lebbe C, et al. Diagnosis and treatment of invasive squamous cell carcinoma of the skin: European consensus-based interdisciplinary guideline. Eur J Cancer 2015;51(14):1989–2007; with permission.

are more likely to behave aggressively in terms of local recurrence and increased rate of metastasis.[89–91]

Recurrence status Not surprisingly, tumor recurrence itself is a high-risk feature.[88] Recurrent tumors tend to be larger, are more likely to manifest perineural invasion, lymphovascular invasion, subcutaneous invasion, and lymph node metastasis, and are associated with poorer disease-specific survival.[86,87,92,93]

Number of tumors Multiple cSCC are associated with an increased risk of local recurrence and lymph node metastasis. In 1 study, having more than 1 tumor increased the risk of local recurrence and nodal metastasis by 2- to 4-fold and 3- to 4-fold, respectively.[94]

Immunosuppression Solid organ transplant recipients on immunosuppressive therapy develop aggressive tumors at an increased frequency. This increased incidence is estimated to be as high as 65- to 250-fold as compared with the general population.[11,95] These tumors also exhibit rapid growth, an increased rate of local recurrence, and metastasis.[96,97] Thus, the immunosuppressed state is an independent predictor of poor outcomes.[98]

Histopathologic high-risk features
Tumor size Cutaneous SCC tumors with a 2.0-cm or greater maximum diameter are more likely to metastasize.[79,86] A metaanalysis has shown that a tumor diameter of 2.0 cm or greater is independently predictive of recurrence and metastasis.[88] The increased recurrence and metastasis rates for an SCC 2.0 cm or greater in size arising on lips and skin were 2-fold and 3.3-fold, respectively, when compared with tumors less than 2.0 cm in size.[87]

Tumor thickness and depth of invasion Tumor thickness and depth of invasion are independent predictors of both local recurrence and metastasis.[79,88] The American Joint Committee on Cancer and National Comprehensive Cancer Network guidelines consider an invasion depth of 2.0 mm or greater or Clark level IV or higher as the high-risk factor.[77,84] A corollary of the prognostic significance of the depth of invasion could be that cSCC tumors of identical thickness may show different clinical behavior based on their body location, owing to the varying thickness of dermis and subcutaneous tissue.

Margin status Margin-positive reexcision is recently identified as an independent risk factor for locoregional recurrence, whereas margin-negative reexcision is associated with a low-risk prognosis (29% vs 5% local recurrence). Hence, while evaluating a reexcision specimen, patients with a positive margin should be considered at high risk for recurrence.[85,99]

Histologic grade Tumor differentiation grade is an independent predictor of recurrence, metastasis, and patient survival.[79,86,88] Indeed, in 1 study, well-differentiated cSCC showed a local recurrence rate of 13.6%, and a 5-year cure rate of 94.6%, whereas the poorly differentiated cSCC showed a recurrence rate of 28.6% and 5-year cure rate of 61.5%.[87] A more recent metaanalysis showed that the 5-year metastasis-free and overall survival rates were significantly higher in well-differentiated tumors (70%) as compared with moderately differentiated (51%) and poorly differentiated (26%) tumors.[88]

Histologic subtype Although it is customary to think of several cSCC histologic subtypes as being associated with an aggressive tumor behavior, for the most part, there are insufficient data in this regard. For example, acantholytic SCC is thought to be highly aggressive, but this is not convincingly supported by published literature.[47,100] In contrast, desmoplastic SCC or tumors with infiltrative and desmoplastic growth patterns are associated with aggressive behavior in terms of local recurrence and metastasis.[59,101] The 2016 National Comprehensive Cancer Network Clinical Practice Guidelines for cSCC designates acantholytic, adenosquamous, and desmoplastic SCC subtypes as high-risk factors.[84] The current European Organization for Research and Treatment of Cancer guidelines list acantholytic, spindle, and desmoplastic subtypes as the high-risk prognostic factors.[85] KA, when identified with certainty based on clinical and histologic features, is not regarded as a subtype of cSCC and that is borne out by a recent metaanalysis of 445 cases of KA with reported follow-up; none of these cases resulted in death or distant metastases.[102]

Perineural invasion Perineural invasion independently predicts increased rate of local recurrence and metastasis. In particular, perineural invasion of large-caliber nerves ($\geq$0.1 mm) is associated with an increased likelihood of lymph node metastasis and higher mortality rate.[92,103,104] In cSCC of the head and neck region, 1 study found perineural invasion in 14% of all cases, which was associated with increased incidence of cervical lymphadenopathy, distant metastasis, and a significantly reduced survival.[105]

Lymphovascular invasion Lymphovascular invasion is an independent predictor of lymph node metastasis[106,107] and disease-specific death.[103]

Our recommendations for pathology reporting

Based on this discussion of the current evidence and guidelines, we recommend that a pathology report includes a comment on the following features:

- *Tumor size* - particularly when approaching or more than 2 cm
- *Tumor thickness* - particularly when approaching or more than 2 mm
- *Tumor depth* - particularly when approaching or more than Clark level IV
- *Margin status* - particularly in the reexcision specimens
- *Histologic grade* - particularly when poorly differentiated
- *Histologic subtype* - particularly when acantholytic, adenosquamous, spindle cell, or desmoplastic
- *Perineural invasion* - particularly when involving a nerve approaching or greater than 0.1 mm in diameter
- *Lymphovascular invasion*

MOLECULAR PATHOGENESIS
Importance

The high burden of cSCC produces significant morbidity and mortality around the world; therefore, diagnosing and treating cSCC early in its development is crucial and will minimize morbidity and conserve health care resources. Unfortunately, owing to their cosmetic or functional consequences, dermatologic biopsies are often small and superficial, and hence the entire lesion is frequently not available for examination. This often leads to 1 of 3 undesirable consequences: (1) repeat biopsy, which increases health care costs, (2) overdiagnosis, which leads to an unnecessary reexcision, increased morbidity, and an increased health care costs, or (3) underdiagnosis, which results in a missed opportunity to diagnose cSCC early and may result in increased morbidity and mortality. Therefore, identifying the unique molecular alterations associated with cSCC development, and developing assays that use these molecular alterations as markers of malignancy is of paramount importance. Ideally, such assays would significantly increase the diagnostic yield even with a limited biopsy specimen. Moreover, in regard to cSCC treatment, there is no standard of care beyond complete surgical excision of the lesion, and the therapeutic options for locally advanced and metastatic disease are limited. Consequently, identifying molecular targets and pathways that drive cSCC development is imperative. We provide a brief overview of the current state of knowledge.

Chromosomal Aberrations, Instability, and Epigenetic Changes

Cytogenetic studies in cSCC have revealed a large number of complex allelic alternations such as deletions, insertions, and translocations.[108] The chromosomes most commonly affected include chromosomes 1, 11, 8, 9, 5, 3, and 7. The most frequently rearranged chromosomal sites are pericentromeric, such as 8q10-q11, 1p10-q12, 5p10-q11, 11p15, and 9p10-q10. Recurrent anomalies such as i(1q), i(8q), i(5p), i(1p), i(9p), and i(9q); losses of part of or the entire chromosomes 2, 4, 8, 9, 11, 13, 14, 18, 21, X and Y, and overrepresentation of 1q, chromosome 7, and 8q have been identified as most frequent cytogenetic aberrations.[109] A large-scale genome-wide association study of cSCC has identified 10 single nucleotide polymorphism (SNP) loci, 6 of which encompass pigmentation genes associated with skin cancer risk. These include nonsynonymous SNPs in SLC45A2 gene on chromosome 5p13 and in TYR gene on chromosome 11q14, as well as a functional intronic SNP in IRF4 gene on chromosome 6p25. Three more previously unreported SCC-associated SNPs were identified in HERC2/OCA2 genes at 15q13, DEF8 gene at 16q24, and RALY gene at 20q11.[110]

A genome-wide SNP microarray analysis showed that well-differentiated cSCCs are a genetically distinct subpopulation among all cSCCs. Extensive loss of heterozygosity were seen at 3p and 9p. Loss of 9p could result in inactivation of protein tyrosine phosphatase delta, proposed as a candidate tumor suppressor gene in cSCC. Protein tyrosine phosphatase delta microdeletions were also demonstrated in a subset of cSCCs. Fragile histidine triad, a recognized tumor suppressor gene on 3p14.2 was proposed as another candidate gene that undergoes inactivation.[111] Another study demonstrated that there were 2 distinct telomere phenotypes in cSCCs (and AKs), suggesting 2 modes of initiation of chromosomal instability in cSCCs. One of the telomere phenotypes was associated with a higher degree of aberrant p53 and cyclin D1 expression as well as a more complex karyotype.[112]

Specific Gene Mutations

A unique aspect of the skin biology is the presence of a high number of cancer driver gene mutations in the histologically normal sun-exposed skin. It has been shown that there are thousands of evolving cellular clones in the aged, sun-exposed, physiologically normal skin with more than one-quarter of cells carrying cancer-causing mutations in genes such as TP53, NOTCH1, NOTCH2, and FAT1.[113] Although this intriguing observation has the potential to provide insights into the early stages of squamous carcinogenesis, it also points to a potential impediment in being able to use these genes as diagnostic or prognostic biomarkers, or therapeutic targets. Another study, despite the high mutational background caused by UV exposure, has identified 23 candidate driver genes in aggressive cSCC that include TP53, CDKN2A, NOTCH1, NOTCH2, AJUBA, HRAS, CASP8, FAT1, KMT2C (MLL3), PARD3, and RASA1.[114] We discuss in detail some of the genes frequently found to be mutated in cSCC.

TP53

It has been well-established that a large proportion of cSCC and precursor lesions harbor UV radiation–induced TP53 mutations. These UV signature mutations are found in up to 90% of all cSCC. The fact that TP53 mutations have been found in precursor lesions suggests that this might be an early event in squamous carcinogenesis.[115–117] However, the increased expression levels of mutant p53 also predict aggressive tumor behavior. One study showed that the IHC scores of p53 protein expression had a strong association with histologic grades and TNM stages of cSCC, with tumors expressing high score of p53 being more aggressive as compared with tumors having low score of p53.[118]

CDKN2A

Tumor suppressor genes p16INK4a and p14ARF are the alternative reading frames of CDKN2A locus on 9p21, which is frequently deleted in cSCC. Deletion of p16INK4a is thought to correlate with progression from AK to cSCC.[119,120]

NOTCH

NOTCH is a direct target of p53 that plays a role in the differentiation of epidermal keratinocytes. NOTCH1 is expressed in full thickness of the epidermis, whereas NOTCH2 expression is localized mainly to the basal layer of epidermis. Loss of function NOTCH1 and NOTCH2 mutations are identified in more than 75% of cSCC. NOTCH1 mutation is considered an early event in squamous carcinogenesis of the skin and has been demonstrated to lead to a patchy loss of expression in the normal epidermis.[117–121] Precise exomic sequencing of UV-exposed epidermis and SCCIS also implicates NOTCH1, NOTCH2 and multiple nulceoporins in the early stages of UV-induced carcinogenesis (Seykora and colleagues, unpublished data, 2017).

RAS

The dysregulation of the RAS protooncogene has been implicated in the cSCC initiation in mouse models of chemical carcinogenesis. Recent studies have shown activating mutations of RAS in 12% to 20% of cSCCs.[122,123] The use of targeted BRAF inhibition in melanoma has led to additional insights into the role of RAS in cSCC. About 25% of patients receiving vemurafenib develop squamoproliferative lesions, including well-differentiated cSCC, which have an increased frequency of gain of function RAS mutations (35%–60%) compared with sporadic cSCC.[28]

KNSTRN

UV radiation signature mutations in KNSTRN, a kinetochore protein have been detected in 19% of cSCC in 1 study. Point mutations of KNSTRN disrupt sister chromatid cohesion and chromosome segregation, leading to aneuploidy. KNSTRN mutations are also identified in the normal epidermis in addition to AK and cSCC, suggesting that KNSTRN dysregulation can be an early event in squamous carcinogenesis.[124]

p300

Higher expression of the transcriptional coactivator p300 has been found in cSCC compared with the adjacent histologically normal skin. Moreover, high p300 expression has been correlated positively with lymph node metastasis, advanced clinical stage, and poor patient outcomes in terms of recurrence-free survival and overall survival, leading to a suggestion that p300 expression can be a biomarker for predicting clinical outcomes in cSCC patients.[125]

TERT

TERT promoter mutations are frequent in cSCC. Heterogeneity of TERT promoter mutations were found in SCC of different anatomic sites, giving rise to the hypothesis that different tumor development mechanisms are operational in SCC of different sites.[126,127]

CARD11

In 1 study, CARD11 was found to be mutated in more than 38% of 111 cSCCs. CARD11 regulates nuclear factor κB signaling cascade and point mutations of CARD11 can lead to constitutive activation of the nuclear factor κB pathway, which in turn can lead to the transformation of keratinocytes. Consistent with that, CARD11 messenger RNA and protein expression were detectable in normal skin and increased in cSCC. CARD11 mutations are also identified in the peritumoral and sun-exposed skin, suggesting that these mutations may also be early events in tumor development as with TP53, NOTCH1, and KNSTRN.[128]

MicroRNA Alterations

MicroRNAs (miRNA) are small noncoding RNAs that negatively regulate protein expression. Several studies have found that altered expression of miRNAs contribute to the initiation and progression of cSCC. In cSCC, miRNAs that are downregulated include miR1, miR-34a, MiR-124a, miR-125b, miR-155, miR-193b/365a, MiR-199a, MiR-361-5p, and miR-483-3p. The miRNAs that are specifically upregulated in cSCC include miR-21, miR-31, miR-135b, miR205, miR-223, miR-365, miR-424, and miR-766.[129,130] One study has found significant upregulation of miR-4286, miR-200a-3p, and miR-148-3p, and down-regulation of miR-1915-3p, miR-205-5p, miR-4516, and miR-150-5p in metastatic cSCC as compared with nonmetastatic primary cSCC.[131]

SUMMARY

Cutaneous SCC is one of the most common malignancies worldwide, with a trend toward an increasing incidence. It is important to distinguish well-differentiated cSCC from several other benign and reactive squamoproliferative lesions, identify the common histologic variants to avoid diagnostic pitfalls, as well as to detect and report the well-known high-risk histologic features predictive of an aggressive tumor behavior. A better understanding of the molecular pathways that drive the development and progression of cSCC would provide us with new markers for the diagnostic and prognostic assessment, and molecular targets for newer therapeutic modalities.

REFERENCES

1. Elder DE. Lever's histopathology of the skin. 10th edition. Philadelphia: Wolters Kluwer/Lippincott Williams & Williams; 2008.
2. Miller DL, Weinstock MA. Nonmelanoma skin cancer in the United States: incidence. J Am Acad Dermatol 1994;30(5 Pt 1):774–8.
3. Rogers HW, Weinstock MA, Feldman SR, et al. Incidence estimate of nonmelanoma skin cancer (keratinocyte carcinomas) in the U.S. Population, 2012. JAMA Dermatol 2015;151(10):1081–6.
4. Staples M, Marks R, Giles G. Trends in the incidence of non-melanocytic skin cancer (NMSC) treated in Australia 1985-1995: are primary prevention programs starting to have an effect? Int J Cancer 1998;78(2):144–8.

5. Casey AS, Kennedy CE, Goldman GD. Mohs micrographic surgery: how ACMS fellowship directors practice. Dermatol Surg 2009;35(5):747–56.
6. Nestor MS, Zarraga MB. The incidence of nonmelanoma skin cancers and actinic keratoses in South Florida. J Clin Aesthet Dermatol 2012;5(4):20–4.
7. Karagas MR, Greenberg ER, Spencer SK, et al. Increase in incidence rates of basal cell and squamous cell skin cancer in New Hampshire, USA. New Hampshire Skin Cancer Study Group. Int J Cancer 1999;81(4):555–9.
8. Gray DT, Suman VJ, Su WP, et al. Trends in the population-based incidence of squamous cell carcinoma of the skin first diagnosed between 1984 and 1992. Arch Dermatol 1997;133(6):735–40.
9. Karia PS, Han J, Schmults CD. Cutaneous squamous cell carcinoma: estimated incidence of disease, nodal metastasis, and deaths from disease in the United States, 2012. J Am Acad Dermatol 2013;68(6):957–66.
10. Berg D, Otley CC. Skin cancer in organ transplant recipients: epidemiology, pathogenesis, and management. J Am Acad Dermatol 2002;47(1):1–17 [quiz: 18–20].
11. Jensen P, Hansen S, Møller B, et al. Skin cancer in kidney and heart transplant recipients and different long-term immunosuppressive therapy regimens. J Am Acad Dermatol 1999;40(2 Pt 1):177–86.
12. Ramsay HM, Reece SM, Fryer AA, et al. Seven-year prospective study of nonmelanoma skin cancer incidence in U.K. renal transplant recipients. Transplantation 2007;84(3):437–9.
13. Silverberg MJ, Leyden W, Warton EM, et al. HIV infection status, immunodeficiency, and the incidence of non-melanoma skin cancer. J Natl Cancer Inst 2013;105(5):350–60.
14. Akguner M, Barutçu A, Yilmaz M, et al. Marjolin's ulcer and chronic burn scarring. J Wound Care 1998;7(3):121–2.
15. Carli P, Cattaneo A, De Magnis A, et al. Squamous cell carcinoma arising in vulval lichen sclerosus: a longitudinal cohort study. Eur J Cancer Prev 1995; 4(6):491–5.
16. Jellouli-Elloumi A, Kochbati L, Dhraief S, et al. Cancers arising from burn scars: 62 cases. Ann Dermatol Venereol 2003;130(4):413–6 [in French].
17. Knackstedt TJ, Collins LK, Li Z, et al. Squamous cell carcinoma arising in hypertrophic lichen planus: a review and analysis of 38 cases. Dermatol Surg 2015; 41(12):1411–8.
18. Lavogiez C, Delaporte E, Darras-Vercambre S, et al. Clinicopathological study of 13 cases of squamous cell carcinoma complicating hidradenitis suppurativa. Dermatology 2010;220(2):147–53.
19. Sulica VI, Kao GF. Squamous-cell carcinoma of the scalp arising in lesions of discoid lupus erythematosus. Am J Dermatopathol 1988;10(2):137–41.
20. Trent JT, Kirsner RS. Wounds and malignancy. Adv Skin Wound Care 2003; 16(1):31–4.
21. Kraemer KH, Lee MM, Scotto J. Xeroderma pigmentosum. Cutaneous, ocular, and neurologic abnormalities in 830 published cases. Arch Dermatol 1987; 123(2):241–50.
22. Kromberg JG, Castle D, Zwane EM, et al. Albinism and skin cancer in Southern Africa. Clin Genet 1989;36(1):43–52.
23. Majewski S, Jablonska S. Skin autografts in epidermodysplasia verruciformis: human papillomavirus-associated cutaneous changes need over 20 years for malignant conversion. Cancer Res 1997;57(19):4214–6.

24. Gallagher RP, Bajdik CD, Fincham S, et al. Chemical exposures, medical history, and risk of squamous and basal cell carcinoma of the skin. Cancer Epidemiol Biomarkers Prev 1996;5(6):419–24.

25. Karagas MR, Stukel TA, Morris JS, et al. Skin cancer risk in relation to toenail arsenic concentrations in a US population-based case-control study. Am J Epidemiol 2001;153(6):559–65.

26. Quint KD, Genders RE, de Koning MN, et al. Human beta-papillomavirus infection and keratinocyte carcinomas. J Pathol 2015;235(2):342–54.

27. Wang J, Aldabagh B, Yu J, et al. Role of human papillomavirus in cutaneous squamous cell carcinoma: a meta-analysis. J Am Acad Dermatol 2014;70(4): 621–9.

28. Su F, Viros A, Milagre C, et al. RAS mutations in cutaneous squamous-cell carcinomas in patients treated with BRAF inhibitors. N Engl J Med 2012;366(3): 207–15.

29. Adams CC, Thomas B, Bingham JL. Cutaneous squamous cell carcinoma with perineural invasion: a case report and review of the literature. Cutis 2014;93(3): 141–4.

30. Hussein MR. Skin cancer in Egypt: a word in your ear. Cancer Biol Ther 2005; 4(5):593–5.

31. Mora RG, Perniciaro C. Cancer of the skin in blacks. I. A review of 163 black patients with cutaneous squamous cell carcinoma. J Am Acad Dermatol 1981;5(5): 535–43.

32. Marks R. The role of treatment of actinic keratoses in the prevention of morbidity and mortality due to squamous cell carcinoma. Arch Dermatol 1991;127(7): 1031–3.

33. Marks R, Rennie G, Selwood TS. Malignant transformation of solar keratoses to squamous cell carcinoma. Lancet 1988;1(8589):795–7.

34. Cockerell CJ. Histopathology of incipient intraepidermal squamous cell carcinoma ("actinic keratosis"). J Am Acad Dermatol 2000;42(1 Pt 2):11–7.

35. Stockfleth E. Actinic keratoses. Cancer Treat Res 2009;146:227–39.

36. Goldberg LH, Joseph AK, Tschen JA. Proliferative actinic keratosis. Int J Dermatol 1994;33(5):341–5.

37. Švajdler M Jr, Mezencev R, Kašpírková J, et al. Human papillomavirus infection and p16 expression in extragenital/extraungual Bowen disease in immunocompromised patients. Am J Dermatopathol 2016;38(10):751–7.

38. Al-Arashi MY, Byers HR. Cutaneous clear cell squamous cell carcinoma in situ: clinical, histological and immunohistochemical characterization. J Cutan Pathol 2007;34(3):226–33.

39. Memezawa A, Okuyama R, Tagami H, et al. p63 constitutes a useful histochemical marker for differentiation of pagetoid Bowen's disease from extramammary Paget's disease. Acta Derm Venereol 2008;88(6):619–20.

40. Cassarino DS, Derienzo DP, Barr RJ. Cutaneous squamous cell carcinoma: a comprehensive clinicopathologic classification–part two. J Cutan Pathol 2006; 33(4):261–79.

41. Quaedvlieg PJ, Creytens DH, Epping GG, et al. Histopathological characteristics of metastasizing squamous cell carcinoma of the skin and lips. Histopathology 2006;49(3):256–64.

42. Cassarino DS, Derienzo DP, Barr RJ. Cutaneous squamous cell carcinoma: a comprehensive clinicopathologic classification. Part one. J Cutan Pathol 2006; 33(3):191–206.

43. Driemel O, Müller-Richter UD, Hakim SG, et al. Oral acantholytic squamous cell carcinoma shares clinical and histological features with angiosarcoma. Head Face Med 2008;4:17.
44. Johnson WC, Helwig EB. Adenoid squamous cell carcinoma (adenoacanthoma). A clinicopathologic study of 155 patients. Cancer 1966;19(11):1639–50.
45. Lever WF. Adenocanthoma of sweat glands; carcinoma of sweat glands with glandular and epidermal elements: report of four cases. Arch Derm Syphilol 1947;56(2):157–71.
46. Muller SA, Wilhelmj CM Jr, Harrison EG Jr, et al. Adenoid squamous cell carcinoma (adenoacanthoma of lever). Report of seven cases and review. Arch Dermatol 1964;89:589–97.
47. Ogawa T, Kiuru M, Konia TH, et al. Acantholytic squamous cell carcinoma is usually associated with hair follicles, not acantholytic actinic keratosis, and is not "high risk": diagnosis, management, and clinical outcomes in a series of 115 cases. J Am Acad Dermatol 2017;76(2):327–33.
48. Banks ER, Cooper PH. Adenosquamous carcinoma of the skin: a report of 10 cases. J Cutan Pathol 1991;18(4):227–34.
49. Cubilla AL, Ayala MT, Barreto JE, et al. Surface adenosquamous carcinoma of the penis. A report of three cases. Am J Surg Pathol 1996;20(2):156–60.
50. Weidner N, Foucar E. Adenosquamous carcinoma of the skin. An aggressive mucin- and gland-forming squamous carcinoma. Arch Dermatol 1985;121(6):775–9.
51. Gartrell R, Pauli J, Zonta M. Primary cutaneous mucoepidermoid carcinoma: a case study with a review of the literature. Int J Surg Pathol 2015;23(2):161–4.
52. Evans HL, Smith JL. Spindle cell squamous carcinomas and sarcoma-like tumors of the skin: a comparative study of 38 cases. Cancer 1980;45(10):2687–97.
53. Silvis NG, Swanson PE, Manivel JC, et al. Spindle-cell and pleomorphic neoplasms of the skin. A clinicopathologic and immunohistochemical study of 30 cases, with emphasis on "atypical fibroxanthomas". Am J Dermatopathol 1988;10(1):9–19.
54. Martin HE, Stewart FW. Spindle cell epidermoid carcinoma. Am J Cancer Res 1935;24(2):273–98.
55. Petter G, Haustein UF. Histologic subtyping and malignancy assessment of cutaneous squamous cell carcinoma. Dermatol Surg 2000;26(6):521–30.
56. Ha Lan TT, Chen SJ, Arps DP, et al. Expression of the p40 isoform of p63 has high specificity for cutaneous sarcomatoid squamous cell carcinoma. J Cutan Pathol 2014;41(11):831–8.
57. Sigel JE, Skacel M, Bergfeld WF, et al. The utility of cytokeratin 5/6 in the recognition of cutaneous spindle cell squamous cell carcinoma. J Cutan Pathol 2001;28(10):520–4.
58. Breuninger H, Holzschuh J, Schaumburg Lever G, et al. Desmoplastic squamous epithelial carcinoma of the skin and lower lip. A morphologic entity with great risk of metastasis and recurrence. Hautarzt 1998;49(2):104–8 [in German].
59. Breuninger H, Schaumburg-Lever G, Holzschuh J, et al. Desmoplastic squamous cell carcinoma of skin and vermilion surface: a highly malignant subtype of skin cancer. Cancer 1997;79(5):915–9.
60. Kuo T. Clear cell carcinoma of the skin. A variant of the squamous cell carcinoma that simulates sebaceous carcinoma. Am J Surg Pathol 1980;4(6):573–83.
61. Swanson PE, Marrogi AJ, Williams DJ, et al. Tricholemmal carcinoma: clinicopathologic study of 10 cases. J Cutan Pathol 1992;19(2):100–9.

62. Cramer SF, Heggeness LM. Signet-ring squamous cell carcinoma. Am J Clin Pathol 1989;91(4):488–91.
63. McKinley E, Valles R, Bang R, et al. Signet-ring squamous cell carcinoma: a case report. J Cutan Pathol 1998;25(3):176–81.
64. Bastian BC, Kutzner H, Ts Yen, et al. Signet-ring cell formation in cutaneous neoplasms. J Am Acad Dermatol 1999;41(4):606–13.
65. Malviya N, Wickless H. CD30+ primary cutaneous post-transplant lymphoproliferative disorder with signet-ring cell features. Hematol Rep 2016;8(2):6433.
66. Jurado I, Saez A, Luelmo J, et al. Pigmented squamous cell carcinoma of the skin: report of two cases and review of the literature. Am J Dermatopathol 1998;20(6):578–81.
67. Morgan MB, Lima-Maribona J, Miller RA, et al. Pigmented squamous cell carcinoma of the skin: morphologic and immunohistochemical study of five cases. J Cutan Pathol 2000;27(8):381–6.
68. Chapman MS, Quitadamo MJ, Perry AE. Pigmented squamous cell carcinoma. J Cutan Pathol 2000;27(2):93–5.
69. Pool SE, Manieei F, Clark WH Jr, et al. Dermal squamo-melanocytic tumor: a unique biphenotypic neoplasm of uncertain biological potential. Hum Pathol 1999;30(5):525–9.
70. Aird I, Johnson HD, Lennox B, et al. Epithelioma cuniculatum: a variety of squamous carcinoma peculiar to the foot. Br J Surg 1954;42(173):245–50.
71. Schwartz RA. Verrucous carcinoma of the skin and mucosa. J Am Acad Dermatol 1995;32(1):1–21 [quiz: 22–4].
72. Hodak E, Jones RE, Ackerman AB. Solitary keratoacanthoma is a squamous-cell carcinoma: three examples with metastases. Am J Dermatopathol 1993; 15(4):332–42 [discussion: 343–52].
73. Schwartz RA. Keratoacanthoma. J Am Acad Dermatol 1994;30(1):1–19 [quiz: 20–2].
74. Skalova A, Michal M. Patterns of cell proliferation in actinic keratoacanthomas and squamous cell carcinomas of the skin. Immunohistochemical study using the MIB 1 antibody in formalin-fixed paraffin sections. Am J Dermatopathol 1995;17(4):332–4.
75. Shah K, Kazlouskaya V, Lal K, et al. Perforating elastic fibers ('elastic fiber trapping') in the differentiation of keratoacanthoma, conventional squamous cell carcinoma and pseudocarcinomatous epithelial hyperplasia. J Cutan Pathol 2014;41(2):108–12.
76. Ahmed MM, Moore BA, Schmalbach CE. Utility of head and neck cutaneous squamous cell carcinoma sentinel node biopsy: a systematic review. Otolaryngol Head Neck Surg 2014;150(2):180–7.
77. Farasat S, Yu SS, Neel VA, et al. A new American Joint Committee on Cancer staging system for cutaneous squamous cell carcinoma: creation and rationale for inclusion of tumor (T) characteristics. J Am Acad Dermatol 2011;64(6): 1051–9.
78. Szewczyk M, Pazdrowski J, Golusiński P, et al. Analysis of selected risk factors for nodal metastases in head and neck cutaneous squamous cell carcinoma. Eur Arch Otorhinolaryngol 2015;272(10):3007–12.
79. Brantsch KD, Meisner C, Schönfisch B, et al. Analysis of risk factors determining prognosis of cutaneous squamous-cell carcinoma: a prospective study. Lancet Oncol 2008;9(8):713–20.

80. Brougham ND, Dennett ER, Cameron R, et al. The incidence of metastasis from cutaneous squamous cell carcinoma and the impact of its risk factors. J Surg Oncol 2012;106(7):811–5.
81. Greene FL, Page DL, Fleming ID, et al, editors. AJCC cancer staging manual. 6th edition. New York: Springer; 2002.
82. Sobin L, Gospodarowicz M, Wittekind C, editors. UICC International Union Against Cancer TNM classification of malignant tumors. 7th edition. West Sussex (United Kingdom): Wiley-Blackwell; 2009.
83. Karia PS, Jambusaria-Pahlajani A, Harrington DP, et al. Evaluation of American Joint Committee on Cancer, International Union Against Cancer, and Brigham and Women's Hospital tumor staging for cutaneous squamous cell carcinoma. J Clin Oncol 2014;32(4):327–34.
84. Bichakjian CK, Farma JM, Schmults CD, et al. NCCN Clinical Practice Guidelines in Oncology (NCCN Guidelines) squamous cell skin cancer. Fort Washington (PA): National Comprehensive Cancer Network, Inc; 2016.
85. Stratigos A, Garbe C, Lebbe C, et al. Diagnosis and treatment of invasive squamous cell carcinoma of the skin: European consensus-based interdisciplinary guideline. Eur J Cancer 2015;51(14):1989–2007.
86. Cherpelis BS, Marcusen C, Lang PG. Prognostic factors for metastasis in squamous cell carcinoma of the skin. Dermatol Surg 2002;28(3):268–73.
87. Rowe DE, Carroll RJ, Day CL Jr. Prognostic factors for local recurrence, metastasis, and survival rates in squamous cell carcinoma of the skin, ear, and lip. Implications for treatment modality selection. J Am Acad Dermatol 1992;26(6): 976–90.
88. Thompson AK, Kelley BF, Prokop LJ, et al. Risk factors for cutaneous squamous cell carcinoma recurrence, metastasis, and disease-specific death: a systematic review and meta-analysis. JAMA Dermatol 2016;152(4):419–28.
89. Edwards MJ, Hirsch RM, Broadwater JR, et al. Squamous cell carcinoma arising in previously burned or irradiated skin. Arch Surg 1989;124(1):115–7.
90. Mullen JT, Feng L, Xing Y, et al. Invasive squamous cell carcinoma of the skin: defining a high-risk group. Ann Surg Oncol 2006;13(7):902–9.
91. Ross AS, Schmults CD. Sentinel lymph node biopsy in cutaneous squamous cell carcinoma: a systematic review of the English literature. Dermatol Surg 2006; 32(11):1309–21.
92. Clayman GL, Lee JJ, Holsinger FC, et al. Mortality risk from squamous cell skin cancer. J Clin Oncol 2005;23(4):759–65.
93. Krediet JT, Beyer M, Lenz K, et al. Sentinel lymph node biopsy and risk factors for predicting metastasis in cutaneous squamous cell carcinoma. Br J Dermatol 2015;172(4):1029–36.
94. Levine DE, Karia PS, Schmults CD. Outcomes of patients with multiple cutaneous squamous cell carcinomas: a 10-year single-institution cohort study. JAMA Dermatol 2015;151(11):1220–5.
95. Hartevelt MM, Bavinck JN, Kootte AM, et al. Incidence of skin cancer after renal transplantation in The Netherlands. Transplantation 1990;49(3):506–9.
96. Euvrard S, Kanitakis J, Claudy A. Skin cancers after organ transplantation. N Engl J Med 2003;348(17):1681–91.
97. Smith KJ, Hamza S, Skelton H. Histologic features in primary cutaneous squamous cell carcinomas in immunocompromised patients focusing on organ transplant patients. Dermatol Surg 2004;30(4 Pt 2):634–41.

98. Zwald FO, Brown M. Skin cancer in solid organ transplant recipients: advances in therapy and management: part II. Management of skin cancer in solid organ transplant recipients. J Am Acad Dermatol 2011;65(2):263–79 [quiz: 280].

99. Bovill ES, Banwell PE. Re-excision of incompletely excised cutaneous squamous cell carcinoma: histological findings influence prognosis. J Plast Reconstr Aesthet Surg 2012;65(10):1390–5.

100. Garcia C, Crowson AN. Acantholytic squamous cell carcinoma: is it really a more-aggressive tumor? Dermatol Surg 2011;37(3):353–6.

101. Salmon PJ, Hussain W, Geisse JK, et al. Sclerosing squamous cell carcinoma of the skin, an underemphasized locally aggressive variant: a 20-year experience. Dermatol Surg 2011;37(5):664–70.

102. Savage JA, Maize JC Sr. Keratoacanthoma clinical behavior: a systematic review. Am J Dermatopathol 2014;36(5):422–9.

103. Carter JB, Johnson MM, Chua TL, et al. Outcomes of primary cutaneous squamous cell carcinoma with perineural invasion: an 11-year cohort study. JAMA Dermatol 2013;149(1):35–41.

104. Ross AS, Whalen FM, Elenitsas R, et al. Diameter of involved nerves predicts outcomes in cutaneous squamous cell carcinoma with perineural invasion: an investigator-blinded retrospective cohort study. Dermatol Surg 2009;35(12):1859–66.

105. Goepfert H, Dichtel WJ, Medina JE, et al. Perineural invasion in squamous cell skin carcinoma of the head and neck. Am J Surg 1984;148(4):542–7.

106. Moore BA, Weber RS, Prieto V, et al. Lymph node metastases from cutaneous squamous cell carcinoma of the head and neck. Laryngoscope 2005;115(9):1561–7.

107. Peat B, Insull P, Ayers R. Risk stratification for metastasis from cutaneous squamous cell carcinoma of the head and neck. ANZ J Surg 2012;82(4):230–3.

108. Asgari MM, Wang W, Ioannidis NM, et al. Identification of susceptibility loci for cutaneous squamous cell carcinoma. J Invest Dermatol 2016;136(5):930–7.

109. Purdie KJ, Harwood CA, Gulati A, et al. Single nucleotide polymorphism array analysis defines a specific genetic fingerprint for well-differentiated cutaneous SCCs. J Invest Dermatol 2009;129(6):1562–8.

110. Leufke C, Leykauf J, Krunic D, et al. The telomere profile distinguishes two classes of genetically distinct cutaneous squamous cell carcinomas. Oncogene 2014;33(27):3506–18.

111. Bolshakov S, Walker CM, Strom SS, et al. p53 mutations in human aggressive and nonaggressive basal and squamous cell carcinomas. Clin Cancer Res 2003;9(1):228–34.

112. Kress S, Sutter C, Strickland PT, et al. Carcinogen-specific mutational pattern in the p53 gene in ultraviolet B radiation-induced squamous cell carcinomas of mouse skin. Cancer Res 1992;52(22):6400–3.

113. Giglia-Mari G, Sarasin A. TP53 mutations in human skin cancers. Hum Mutat 2003;21(3):217–28.

114. Bukhari MH, Niazi S, Chaudhry NA. Relationship of immunohistochemistry scores of altered p53 protein expression in relation to patient's habits and histological grades and stages of squamous cell carcinoma. J Cutan Pathol 2009;36(3):342–9.

115. Brown VL, Harwood CA, Crook T, et al. p16INK4a and p14ARF tumor suppressor genes are commonly inactivated in cutaneous squamous cell carcinoma. J Invest Dermatol 2004;122(5):1284–92.

116. Gray SE, Kay E, Leader M, et al. Analysis of p16 expression and allelic imbalance/loss of heterozygosity of 9p21 in cutaneous squamous cell carcinomas. J Cell Mol Med 2006;10(3):778–88.
117. Okuyama R, Tagami H, Aiba S. Notch signaling: its role in epidermal homeostasis and in the pathogenesis of skin diseases. J Dermatol Sci 2008;49(3):187–94.
118. Chin SS, Romano RA, Nagarajan P, et al. Aberrant epidermal differentiation and disrupted DeltaNp63/Notch regulatory axis in Ets1 transgenic mice. Biol Open 2013;2(12):1336–45.
119. Ota T, Takekoshi S, Takagi T, et al. Notch signaling may be involved in the abnormal differentiation of epidermal keratinocytes in psoriasis. Acta Histochem Cytochem 2014;47(4):175–83.
120. Wang NJ, Sanborn Z, Arnett KL, et al. Loss-of-function mutations in Notch receptors in cutaneous and lung squamous cell carcinoma. Proc Natl Acad Sci U S A 2011;108(43):17761–6.
121. South AP, Purdie KJ, Watt SA, et al. NOTCH1 mutations occur early during cutaneous squamous cell carcinogenesis. J Invest Dermatol 2014;134(10):2630–8.
122. Balmain A, Ramsden M, Bowden GT, et al. Activation of the mouse cellular Harvey-ras gene in chemically induced benign skin papillomas. Nature 1984; 307(5952):658–60.
123. Durinck S, Ho C, Wang NJ, et al. Temporal dissection of tumorigenesis in primary cancers. Cancer Discov 2011;1(2):137–43.
124. Lee CS, Bhaduri A, Mah A, et al. Recurrent point mutations in the kinetochore gene KNSTRN in cutaneous squamous cell carcinoma. Nat Genet 2014; 46(10):1060–2.
125. Chen MK, Cai MY, Luo RZ, et al. Overexpression of p300 correlates with poor prognosis in patients with cutaneous squamous cell carcinoma. Br J Dermatol 2015;172(1):111–9.
126. Cheng KA, Kurtis B, Babayeva S, et al. Heterogeneity of TERT promoter mutations status in squamous cell carcinomas of different anatomical sites. Ann Diagn Pathol 2015;19(3):146–8.
127. Griewank KG, Murali R, Schilling B, et al. TERT promoter mutations are frequent in cutaneous basal cell carcinoma and squamous cell carcinoma. PLoS One 2013;8(11):e80354.
128. Watt SA, Purdie KJ, den Breems NY, et al. Novel CARD11 mutations in human cutaneous squamous cell carcinoma lead to aberrant NF-kappaB regulation. Am J Pathol 2015;185(9):2354–63.
129. Bruegger C, Kempf W, Spoerri I, et al. MicroRNA expression differs in cutaneous squamous cell carcinomas and healthy skin of immunocompetent individuals. Exp Dermatol 2013;22(6):426–8.
130. Sand M, Skrygan M, Georgas D, et al. Microarray analysis of microRNA expression in cutaneous squamous cell carcinoma. J Dermatol Sci 2012;68(3):119–26.
131. Gillespie J, Skeeles LE, Allain DC, et al. MicroRNA expression profiling in metastatic cutaneous squamous cell carcinoma. J Eur Acad Dermatol Venereol 2016;30(6):1043–5.

Cutaneous T-cell Lymphoma

Melissa Pulitzer, MD

KEYWORDS

- Cutaneous lymphoma • Mycosis fungoides • Sézary syndrome
- Anaplastic large cell lymphoma • Lymphomatoid papulosis
- Reflective confocal microscopy • Flow cytometry

KEY POINTS

- Primary cutaneous T-cell lymphoma (CTCL) comprises a group of diseases characterized by different recognizable clinicopathologic patterns.
- The vast majority of clinically recognizable cutaneous lymphoma can be diagnostically supported by routine morphologic analysis with a few ancillary studies.
- Dermoscopic, confocal, and flow cytometric analysis (FCA) may add useful information in the evaluation of CTCL in the correct context.

INTRODUCTION

CTCLs consist of a heterogeneous group of clinicopathologically definable monoclonal T-cell proliferations involving the skin. Although a majority of CTCLs are nonaggressive diseases that can be adequately clinically managed with minimal toxicity to patients, knowledge of the basic classification of these disorders by key clinical and pathologic distinguishing features is important and achievable. The occasionally encountered rapidly progressive and aggressive CTCL subtypes are also identifiable with the use of ancillary studies, allowing appropriate and timely therapeutic intervention.

The 2005 World Health Organization–European Organisation for Research and Treatment of Cancer classification for cutaneous lymphomas,[1] along with the 2008 World Health Organization blue book revised in 2016,[2,3] is the basis for the current standardized classification of CTCL, offering both accepted and provisional categories (**Table 1**), and the understanding that the appropriate stratification of these diseases is an ongoing process as new technologies help diagnose and treat CTCL more effectively.

Sources of Support: This research was funded in part through the NIH/NCI Cancer Center support grant P30 CA008748.
Department of Pathology, Memorial Sloan Kettering Cancer Center, 1275 York Avenue, New York, NY 10065, USA
E-mail address: pulitzem@mskcc.org

Clin Lab Med 37 (2017) 527–546
http://dx.doi.org/10.1016/j.cll.2017.06.006
0272-2712/17/© 2017 Elsevier Inc. All rights reserved.

labmed.theclinics.com

Table 1
Cutaneous T-cell lymphomas according to the 2016 update of the World Health Organization classification

	Variant/Subtype
Distinct entity	
MF	Pilotropic MF
	Granulomatous slack skin
	Localized pagetoid reticulosis
SS	
Primary cutaneous CD30$^+$ T-cell LPDs	LyP
	pcALCL
Primary cutaneous GDTCL	
Provisional entity	
Primary cutaneous CD8$^+$ aggressive epidermotropic cytotoxic T-cell lymphoma	
Primary cutaneous acral CD8$^+$ T-cell lymphoma	
Primary cutaneous CD4$^+$ SMTCL	
EBV+ mucocutaneous ulcer	

Data from Swerdlow SH, Campo E, Pileri SA, et al. The 2016 revision of the World Health Organization classification of lymphoid neoplasms. Blood 2016:127(20):2375–90.

The most common CTCLs (mycosis fungoides [MF]/Sézary syndrome [SS] and the CD30$^+$ lymphoproliferative disorders [LPDs] [primary cutaneous anaplastic large cell lymphoma (pcALCL) and lymphomatoid papulosis (LyP)]) are addressed with consideration to diagnostic modalities, including dermoscopy, reflectance confocal microscopy (RCM), and flow cytometry.

Gamma-delta T-cell lymphoma (GDTCL), subcutaneous panniculitis-like T-cell lymphoma (SPTCL), and provisional entities primary cutaneous CD4$^+$ small/medium T-cell LPD (SMTCL),[4] primary cutaneous acral CD8$^+$ T-cell lymphoma (PCAL), and primary cutaneous CD8$^+$ aggressive epidermotropic cytotoxic T-cell lymphoma (AECTCL) are also addressed briefly to enhance recognition of these less common LPDs.

ETIOLOGY/PATHOGENESIS

The vast number of T cells residing in skin (estimated to be 20 billion per normal adult)[5] underlies a significant potential for neoplasia. Genetic factors, such as an individual's HLA type, may predispose some people to develop CTCL[6] by abetting the inappropriate activation and accumulation of T cells via antigen presentation. Environmental mechanisms that may deregulate tumor suppressor or pro-oncogenic pathways include viral or other microbial pathogens (human T-cell lymphotropic virus type 1, Epstein-Barr virus [EBV], herpes simplex virus, *Staphylococcus aureus*, dermatophytes, *Mycobacterium leprae*, and *Chlamydia pneumoniae*).[7,8] Regional variations in incidence of disease, geographic or familial (eg, married couples) clustering, drug triggers (antihistamines, antiepileptics, antihypertensives, and selective serotonin reuptake inhibitors),[9] and occupational/nutritional associations, including exposure to aromatic hydrocarbons or vitamin D deficiency, support an environmental role in the evolution of CTCL.[10–16] In some patients, a shift of helper T Helper 1 (TH1) and T Helper 2 (TH2) cytokines may drive progression of CTCL in a positive feedback loop, for example, by providing a favorable milieu for *Staphylococcus aureus* with additional subsequent activation of oncogenic Jak/Stat[17] and T-cell receptor (TCR) signaling.

CLINICAL PRESENTATION
Mycosis Fungoides/Sézary Syndrome

MF is the most common CTCL, can usually be distinguished from SS with complete clinicopathologic evaluation, and is not a difficult diagnostic challenge when clinical and ancillary information are properly integrated. MF is most often an indolent, progressive monoclonal proliferation of skin-homing memory T cells that occurs predominantly in patients over the age of 60 years. MF is most typically characterized by a slow evolution from scattered epidermotropic lymphocytic infiltrates manifesting as a few patches or plaques of scaly erythema to more widespread epidermal involvement, resulting in patches, plaques, or erythroderma. In some patients, lymphoid tumors grow to become pandermal and subcutaneous nodules and tumors, rarely spreading to regional or distant lymph nodes, bone marrow, and other organs. Peripheral blood involvement by disease can occur in different degrees and has a bearing on prognosis and treatment, as reflected in staging algorithms (**Tables 2** and **3**).

Table 2			
Mycosis fungoides/Sézary syndrome staging adapted per International Society for Cutaneous Lymphomas/European Organisation for Research and Treatment of Cancer revision			
Skin	T1		Limited patches, papules, plaques <10% body surface area[a]
	T2		Patches, papules, plaques >10%[b]
	T3		One or more tumors >1 cm diameter
	T4		Confluent erythema >80% body surface area
Node	N0		No clinically abnormal peripheral lymph nodes; no biopsy required
	N1	N1a	Clinically abnormal peripheral lymph nodes biopsied: Dutch grade 1[c]/NCI LN0-2; clone negative
		N1b	Clinically abnormal peripheral lymph nodes biopsied: Dutch grade 1/NCI LN0-2; clone positive
	N2	N2a	Clinically abnormal peripheral lymph nodes biopsied: Dutch grade 2[d]/NCI LN3; clone negative
		N2b	Clinically abnormal peripheral lymph nodes biopsied: Dutch grade 2/NCI LN3; clone positive
	N3		Clinically abnormal peripheral lymph nodes biopsied: Dutch grade $^3/_4$[e]/NCI LN4; clone positive or negative
	Nx		Clinically abnormal peripheral lymph nodes, not biopsied
Visceral	M0		No visceral organ involvement
	M1		Visceral organ involvement (pathologically confirmed)[f]
Blood	B0	B0a	Absent peripheral blood involvement (<5% Sézary cells); clone negative
		B0b	Absent peripheral blood involvement (<5% Sézary cells); clone positive
	B1	B1a	Low blood tumor burden >5% Sézary cells, but not B2; clone negative
		B1b	Low blood tumor burden >5% Sézary cells, but not B2; clone positive
	B2		High blood tumor burden, >1000 Sézary cells/ul[g]; clone positive

Abbreviations: LN, lymph node; NCI, National Cancer Institute; uL, microliter.
[a] May be divided into T1a patch or T1b patch/plaque.
[b] May be divided into T2a patch or T2b patch/plaque.
[c] Dutch grade 1 includes dermatopathic lymphadenopathy.
[d] Dutch grade 2 includes early presence of cerebriform nuclei in aggregates.
[e] Dutch grades 3 and 4 are partial and complete effacement of lymph node architectures.
[f] Spleen/liver may be considered involved by imaging.
[g] If Sezary cells cannot be measured, then expanded CD3+/CD4+ cells with CD4:CD8 greater than 10:1 or loss of CD7 or CD26 in the presence of T-cell clonality can be used for B2.
From Olsen E, Vonderheid E, Pimpinelli N, et al. Revisions to the staging and classification of mycosis fungoides and Sezary syndrome: a proposal of the International Society for Cutaneous Lymphomas (ISCL) and the cutaneous lymphoma task force of the European Organization of Research and Treatment of Cancer (EORTC). Blood 2007:110(6):1715; with permission.

Table 3
TNM staging according to International Society for Cutaneous Lymphomas/European Organisation for Research and Treatment of Cancer revision for mycosis fungoides/Sézary syndrome

Clinical Stage	T	N	M	B
IA	1	0	0	0, 1
IB	2	0	0	0, 1
IIA	1–2	1,2	0	0, 1
IIB	3	0–2	0	0, 1
IIIA	4	0–2	0	0
IIIB	4	0–2	0	1
IVA1	1–4	0–2	0	2
IVA2	1–4	3	0	0–2
IVB	1–4	0–3	1	0–2

From Olsen E, Vonderheid E, Pimpinelli N, et al. Revisions to the staging and classification of mycosis fungoides and Sezary syndrome: a proposal of the International Society for Cutaneous Lymphomas (ISCL) and the cutaneous lymphoma task force of the European Organization of Research and Treatment of Cancer (EORTC). Blood 2007;110(6):1719; with permission.

Late progression of disease is often characterized by an accompanying decrease in the functional immunity of the patient, with susceptibility to widespread infection and tumoral mass and cytokine-related clinical distress.

Characteristic skin lesions in MF patients show a cigarette paper–like wrinkly scale, are flat to slightly indurated, and may be round to oval or serpiginous in appearance. Later, tumor lesions may exhibit less scale and more shiny induration as the infiltrates expand the underlying dermis and cease to extend into the epidermal compartment. Tumors may ulcerate when they are very large. Superinfection is common. Erythroderma encompassing greater than 80% of body surface area may mimic severe atopic dermatitis, drug eruption, or psoriasis. Clinical variants, including follicle-based pilotropic,[18] unilesional,[19,20] hyperpigmented or hypopigmented,[21] erythrodermic, or poikilodermatous MF, are not uncommon. Less common clinical manifestations include alopecia, leonine facies, nail involvement, and acral hyperkeratosis.

SS is a leukemic variant of CTCL characterized by atypical malignant Sézary cells with a central memory T-cell phenotype, different from MF, in blood, lymph nodes, and skin. Patients are typically 55 to 60 years old and present with erythroderma (>80% body surface area), itching, and lymph node enlargement. Median overall survival is 63 months, and 5-year survival may be as low as 28%.[22]

CD30+ Lymphoproliferative Disorders

The primary cutaneous CD30+ LPDs include LyP and CD30+ pcALCL. Although patients can present with lesions of LyP and pcALCL at the same time, the different disorders individually exhibit distinct clinical behaviors and warrant distinct therapeutic interventions. LyP is characterized by a clear pattern of recurrent, regressing crops of macules, and papules with superficial ulceration and a variable distribution. LyP may leave scars but usually goes away without intervention. Conversely, pcALCL most often presents as a solitary nodule or a few nodules, tumors, or plaques in the skin (in particular extremities), which may or may not resolve on their own after a period of time. pcALCL may also ulcerate and can appear shiny and violaceous as expansion of the skin by the underlying aggregates of lymphocytes occurs. ALCL can occasionally progress to involve the regional lymph nodes and may recur over time in the skin. It uncommonly progresses to a more aggressive disease process. LyP has been described in the lymph nodes on a rare occasion.[23] Some patients present with lesions with intermediate behavior to these 2 entities or with lesions of both entities and sometimes with another lymphoma, such as MF, which may share clonal T-cell gene rearrangements suggesting a common origin of the diseases.[24–26] These patients and their skin lesions need to be approached at a granular level with attention to what is happening with their disease process at the time.

Non–Mycosis Fungoides/Sézary Syndrome/CD30+ Lymphoma/Lymphoproliferative Disorders

Aggressive primary cutaneous lymphomas, aside from the occasional indolent variant that evolves to a more high-grade disease, include the GDTCLs[27] and the CD8+ aggressive epidermotropic cytotoxic T-cell lymphomas. These lymphomas clinically present with rapidly progressive clinical lesions of variable morphology (patch/plaque/tumor), with widespread distribution and ulceration of individual lesions. Because of the concomitant vasodestruction that often occurs with these infiltrates, lesions may appear dusky, hemorrhagic, red, or violaceous. Either entity may exhibit scale and surface alteration due to extensive epidermal involvement. Although a long-standing history of patch-stage disease is more indicative of progressing MF, there are some cases of cytotoxic CTCL that evolve in the setting of a previously indolent presentation.[28] Primary cutaneous gamma-delta (GD) lymphomas may be associated with autoimmune syndromes and systemic symptoms, including hemophagocytic syndrome.

  Primary cutaneous CD8+ acral lymphoma and CD4+ SMTCLs have been proposed as immunophenotypic counterparts of the same clinical processes. Both entities may present as a solitary papule, nodule, or tumor, often on an acral site (including ears, face, extremities, and limbs), which has some bearing on the theory that these processes may represent lymphoid reactions to antigen exposure typical for this type of physical milieu (ear piercing, Borrelia infection, or arthropod bite, for example). CD4+ SMTCL is particularly more likely to present as several nodules, perhaps in a less distal distribution (face, neck, or upper trunk) in the sixth decade. Although both entities are characteristically dermal processes, effacing the overlying epidermis, the CD4+ lesions more frequently involve follicular epithelium and extend into overlying epidermis. Of the 30 or so cases reported of primary cutaneous CD8+ acral lymphoma, presentation on ear, nose, face, feet, and hands have been well described. There is a 2:1 male:female predominance and a wide age distribution among adults (29–87 years). Clinically a discrete papule or nodule is noted to grow slowly, which may be bilateral and symmetric. Patches or plaques characteristic of MF are not seen in either of these entities, both of which are indolent in course. **Table 4** lists classic clinical features helpful for the clinicopathologic correlation of the CTCLs.

Dermoscopy

When compared with chronic inflammatory dermatitis, dermoscopic examination of early-stage MF has been reported to display a dotted pattern,[29] with fine short linear vessels, orange-yellow patchy areas, and vascular structures resembling spermatozoa.[30] A description of poikilodermatous MF included polygonal lobules with white storiform streaks studded with fine dots or hairpin vessels, septal pigmented dots,

Table 4
Classic clinical presentation of cutaneous T-cell lymphoma

Mycosis fungoides	Patches, plaques, tumors
Anaplastic large cell lymphoma	Tumors
LyP	Recurrent papules, crusted, crops
CD4$^+$ SMTCL	Solitary or few nodules or tumors
CD8$^+$ acral T-cell lymphoma	Solitary nodule or papule
SPTCL	Subcutaneous nodules — single or multiple
GDTCL	Subcutaneous nodules — multiple, ulcerated
CD8$^+$ AECTCL	Patches, plaques, tumors, ulcerated

and red and yellow smudges.[31] Dermoscopic examination of alopecia associated with CTCL showed follicular or diffuse scaling and reduced numbers of follicular openings with broken hairs, short hairs, or keratotic filiform spicules.[32]

One study evaluated the varying stages of LyP using dermoscopy[33] and found tortuous irregular vessels radiating from the center to the periphery with a surrounding white structure-less area in the initial inflammatory lesion. Persistence of the white structure-less area but without the vascular central component was seen in more mature hyperkeratotic papules, with a brown-gray structure-less area corresponding to a fibrin-imbued ulcer bed with peripheral vessels in the ulcerated stage, which persisted into the last cicatricial phase.

Reflectance Confocal Microscopy

It has been suggested that noninvasive imaging, such as RCM, could be used to aid in selection of biopsy sites for MF, to decrease false-negative pathology test results.[34] Primary diagnosis may be limited at this time using this technique, because most prominent confocal features were in well-developed plaque lesions but not patch lesions of MF and correlation with histology has been moderate in the larger studies.[34,35] RCM correlation was found with histologically atypical lymphocytes in the epidermis (weakly refractile oval to round structures in the spinous layer), dermoepidermal junction and dermis, and Pautrier microabscesses (vesicle-like dark spaces with monomorphous weakly refractile oval to round cells). Junctional bright roundish and large pleomorphic cells, epidermal disarray, and spongiosis were most significantly histologically correlated using RCM, with an 84% to 90% specificity for MF versus parapsoriasis or normal skin but not versus other CTCLs, such as SS or LyP. Other findings include the loss of edged papillae (basal cells around dermal papillae look hyporefractile) in erythematous patch-stage MF, hyperreflective dermal papillae in hyperpigmented MF, and disrupted dermal papillae rings in tumor-stage MF.[34–36] Limitations at this time include that thick plaques and tumors cannot be analyzed using usual histologic correlates due to the thickened epidermal architecture preventing RCM access to the dermoepidermal junction. Furthermore, there is disagreement among researchers as to the sensitivity and specificity of epidermal alteration, such as epidermal disarray.

In vivo RCM has been described in LyP with a high grade of correspondence to histopathology. Inflammatory cells in the upper epidermis, nonrimmed papillary rings, and enlarged bright cells correspond with atypical lymphocytes in the dermis, supporting consideration of the use of RCM in LyP as an aid in biopsy site selection[37] when clinical assessment is insufficient.

Microscopic Features

Histologically, MF varies with clinical stage. Patch/plaque lesions comprise epidermotropic infiltrates of medium-size lymphocytes with mildly atypical to hyperconvoluted cerebriform nuclei (**Fig. 1A, B**). These cells tend to increase in size and become less epitheliotropic as lesions progress to plaque and tumor stage (see **Fig. 1C**). Although intraepidermal Pautrier microabscesses can be seen in any stage, they are most common earlier on and are not sensitive for the diagnosis. Spongiosis, interface dermatitis, and intervening histiocytes may be seen. Dermal fibrosis is typical.

The most common variant of MF is pilotropic (follicular) MF (FMF), which most often shows a folliculocentric atypical lymphocytic infiltrate with sparing of the interfollicular epidermis and a mixed inflammatory infiltrate. Syringotropism, follicular mucinosis, suppurative folliculitis, cyst formation, and granulomatous change may be seen.[38]

SS shows similar cytologic features to MF — although sometimes the cerebriform atypia is more striking and epidermotropism less marked. Overlying acanthosis and dermal fibrosis are typical.

Distinct from MF, lesions of ALCL almost always look like tumors, presenting with cohesive sheets of greater than 75% CD30$^+$ cells in the dermis, often involving intratumoral vessels or peritumoral intravascular structures. Histologic evidence of ulceration with abundant apoptotic debris is common when the infiltrates are close to

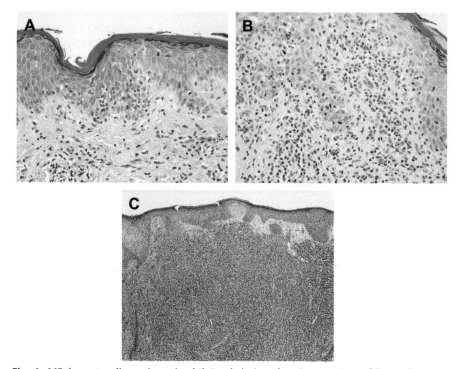

Fig. 1. MF, hematoxylin-eosin stain. (*A*) Patch lesion showing tagging of hyperchromatic lymphocytes out of proportion to spongiosis in a hyperkeratotic epidermis (original magnification ×200). (*B*) Plaque lesion; hyperchromatic lymphocytes with cerebriform atypia are present in the epidermis as well as in the superficial dermis (original magnification ×200). (*C*) Tumor lesion; lymphocytes mostly spare the epidermis and are present in sheets extending throughout the dermis, obscuring adnexal [hair] structures (original magnification ×40).

the epidermis. Most lesions are comprised by medium to large-size lymphocytes, with intranuclear protrusions, horseshoe-shaped or kidney bean–shaped nuclei, and multi-nucleation. A small cell variant of ALCL has been described. Eosinophils and/or neu-trophils may be prominent.

LyP can be challenging to commit to diagnostically. At least 5 histologic subtypes of LyP have been described to date, all of which may occur synchronously or metachro-nously in the same individual. Type A LyP is a wedge-shaped mixed cell infiltrate with the broad base of the wedge oriented along the epidermis. These lesions may be associated with epidermal hyperplasia, ulceration, and epidermotropism. In type A le-sions, lymphocytes are small–intermediate and large-sized cells in a polymorphous background of neutrophils and eosinophils. The large cells label with CD30 and gener-ally make up less than 50% of the infiltrate. Type B LyP is a lichenoid and epidermo-tropic infiltrate of cerebriform Lutzner cells, lymphocytes that may or may not be CD30+. Type C LYP is made up of sheets of large anaplastic CD30+lymphocytes, which are histologically indistinguishable from lesions of anaplastic large cell lym-phoma. Type D LyP is the lichenoid and epidermotropic form of LyP characterized by CD8+, TCR-beta–positive, cytotoxic marker–positive T cells, sometimes histolog-ically indistinguishable from a CD8+ AECTCL or CD8+ MF. LyP type E (angioinvasive LyP) is an oligolesional, characteristically ulcerated, large necrotic eschar-like and self-healing lesion with prominent angioinvasion and angiodestruction by small to medium-size atypical CD8+, CD30+ T cells.

Of the more aggressive lymphomas, CD8+ AECTCL can be histologically striking. With these lesions, MF might initially be thought of but exaggerated features (cell size and epidermotropism) are noted. Typically larger (medium to large-size) lympho-cytes invade the epidermis in a dense front with high level pagetosis and may extend into the dermis and/or subcutis with destruction of adnexa, angiocentricity, and angio-destruction. Lymphocytes cluster around dyskeratotic, necrotic basilar epidermis.

GD-TCL can show either a similarly dramatic or a confounding nonspecific appear-ance, particularly when the malignant infiltrates are deeper than the reactive compo-nent that is often captured by a superficial biopsy. The lymphocytes are most commonly small to medium in size but may be medium to large. Interface alteration or other features of cytotoxicity, including hemorrhage, necrosis, and vasculitis, may occur. GD-TCL should be considered when there is strong suspicion of CTCL clinically, but the histologic features do not add up convincingly to MF.

SPTCL in the most diagnostic cases comprises diffuse sheets of atypical lympho-cytes, which eradicate the fat lobules as in a lobular panniculitis pattern, with some septal involvement. The dermis and epidermis are not involved by lymphoma, although reactive periadnexal lymphocytes are often seen. Classic but not sensitive of specific histologic features include rimming of adipocytes by tumor cells in which lymphoma cells protrude into adipocyte cytoplasm. Cytology of the lymphocytes varies from small to large/pleomorphic and ranges from bland to bizarre with cytotoxic damage, including karyorrhexis and cytophagia (causing bean bag cells or emperipol-esis), and granulomatous infiltrates. Angiocentricity is often common. Lymphoid folli-cles with germinal centers and plasma cells are usually absent and, if found, suggest collagen vascular disease.

The acral clustering CD4+ SMTCL and CD8+ PCAL suggest reactive infiltrates at first glance. Perivascular dermal diffuse or nodular infiltrates of small to medium-size lymphocytes predominate in both. The CD4+ lesions are more polymorphous in cell composition and pleomorphic in cell shape, harboring many histiocytes and B cells as well as large cells making up as much as 30% of infiltrates. Adnexal structures may be affected and epidermotropism and Pautrier-like microabscesses can be seen. CD8$^+$ acral lesions are monomorphous in size and composition, lacking histiocytes and B cells and sparing epithelial structures. Large cells are uncommon.

Immunohistochemistry

MF is a CD4$^+$ memory T-helper cell process. Pan–T-cell antigens CD2, CD3, and CD5 are retained in early lesions and lost later, although CD7 is lost early (**Fig. 2, Table 5**). CD8 is the predominant phenotype in some lesions of MF, often in younger patients, and in poikilodermatous, hyperpigmented, and hypopigmented lesion. TCR-beta is typically expressed on the atypical lymphocytes of MF, reflecting a monoclonal rearrangement of the TCR-alpha and TCR-beta chains. Variants with both TCR-beta and TCR-gamma or TCR-gamma alone have been described (**Fig. 3**A–C).[39] TCR-delta can be seen on gamma-expressing MF (see **Fig. 3**D). Ki-67 proliferation indices are not typically high until disease is advanced at which point Ki-67 may correlate with prognosis (**Fig. 4**A–C).[40] CD25 (the interleukin-2 receptor) can be seen in later-stage MF but tends to be mild in intensity, with a vague cytoplasmic staining pattern in contrast to the crisp cytoplasmic and membranous pattern seen in adult T-cell leukemia/lymphoma. The majority of MF is CD30$^-$ by routine immunohistochemistry (IHC) (see **Fig. 4**D). MF with CD30 positivity has been described in a low number of cases of non-transformed MF[40] and in 40% of transformed MF[41] with multiple patterns of labeling

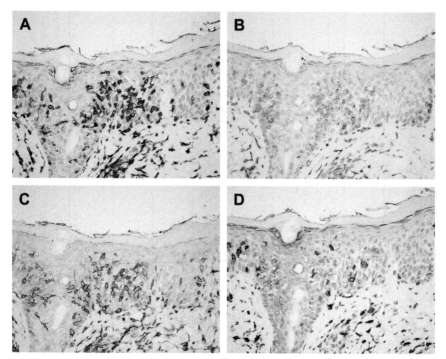

Fig. 2. MF, classic, IHC. (*A*) CD3 labels numerous lymphocytes extending into the mid and upper levels of the epidermis and tagging the dermoepidermal junction (original magnification ×400). (*B*) CD7 shows complete negativity in the CD3$^+$ cells (original magnification ×400). (*C*) CD4 highlights the same population labeled by CD3 (original magnification ×400). (*D*) CD8 shows a rare scattered lymphocyte in the epidermis but more notably highlights scattered reactive dermal cells (original magnification ×400).

Table 5
Helpful immunohistochemistry and flags in evaluating cutaneous T-cell lymphoma

	CD4/CD8	CD20	Pan-T-cell Issues	CD68/163	CD30	T-cell Receptor	Flags
MF	CD4	Clusters in advanced MF or TFH IHC	Loss CD7	If GSS or GMF, after TX	+/–	AB, rare GD	Null-type; Loss CD3, retain CD7, strong CD25, strong CD30; TFH markers, positive EBER
SS	CD4	Scattered	Loss CD7		+/–	AB, rare GD	See MF
ALCL	CD8	No	Loss CD3, Loss TCR-beta, Loss CD45RA	Yes	+	AB, rare GD	Strong CD25; Strong FOXp3, positive EBER; TCR-delta
LYP	CD4/8	No		Yes	+	AB, rare GD	TCR-delta
CD8 AECTCL	CD8	No	Retain CD7	No	Rare, limited	AB	TCR-delta; Positive EBER; CD30
GDTCL	None	No		Yes	Rare, limited	GD	CD8; CD30; TCRB Positive EBRR
SPTCL	CD8	No		Yes	Rare, limited	AB	GD; Positive EBER; CD30
CD4 SMTCL	CD4	Clusters		Yes		AB	CD30; Positive EBER; GD
CD8CAL	CD8	No	Retain CD2/5/7	No	No	AB	CD30; Positive EBER; GD

Abbreviations: AB, alpha-beta; AECTCL, primary cutaneous CD8+ aggressive epidermotropic cytotoxic T-cell lymphoma; ALCL, anaplastic large cell lymphoma; CAL, cutaneous acral lymphoma; EBER, EBV-encoded ribonucleic acid; GD, gamma delta; GDTCL, gamma-delta T-cell lymphoma; GMF, granulomatous mycosis fungoides; GSS, granulomatous slack skin; LyP, lymphomatoid papulosis; SMTCL, small/medium T-cell lymphoma; SPTCL, subcutaneous panniculitis like T-cell lymphoma; SS, Sezary syndrome; TCR, T-cell receptor; TFH, T-follicular helper; TX, therapy.

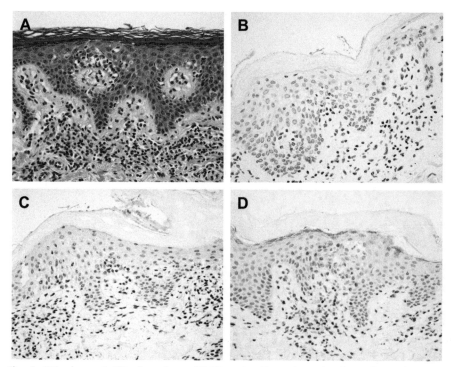

Fig. 3. MF, aberrant GD phenotype. (*A*) Hematoxylin-eosin stain shows hyperchromatic atypical lymphocytes tagging the dermoepidermal junction, in midlayers of the epidermis and within papillary dermis. (*B*) TCR-beta is negative in the junctional lymphocytes but positive in some small reactive papillary dermal lymphocytes. (*C*) TCR-gamma labels junctional lymphocytes, as does (*D*) TCR-delta [*A–D*, original magnification ×400].

and localization noted (scattered, clusters, epidermis, and dermis). Higher proportions of dermal CD30 have been found associated with higher stage at diagnosis and associated with an adverse prognosis although other studies have shown the converse.[42,43]

PD-1 is the best studied T-follicle helper (TFH) phenotype marker in MF and seems to be the most sensitive, followed by ICOS, CXCL-13, Bcl-6, and CD10.[44,45] A TFH phenotype is not uncommon in MF or SS, seems to remain concordant among MF biopsies from the same patient, and is not dependent on disease stage with a cutoff of at least 10% of neoplastic cells expressing at least 3 antigens.[46]

Distinct from MF, the loss of pan–T-cell antigens, such as CD3, CD5, and CD7, is common in ALCL, which may also be CD45RA⁻.[47] CD2 and CD45RO are often positive. TCR-beta is the usual TCR heterodimer expressed in ALCL, although TCR-gamma and/or TCR-delta may be occasionally seen in these cases, which can be particularly difficult to interpret when cases also show a CD4/CD8 null immunophenotype.[48] CD30 labels at least 75% of ALCL cells (**Fig. 5**) and ALK-1 is typically negative, although positivity in children or with aberrant (cytoplasmic) expression has been noted.[49] Cytotoxic markers, TIA-1, perforin, and granzyme B, are abundant.

Lesions of LYP typically express CD30, regardless of the subtype (A–E). Types A, B, C, and E all show a CD4⁺ predominant but mixed T-cell population whereas type D is

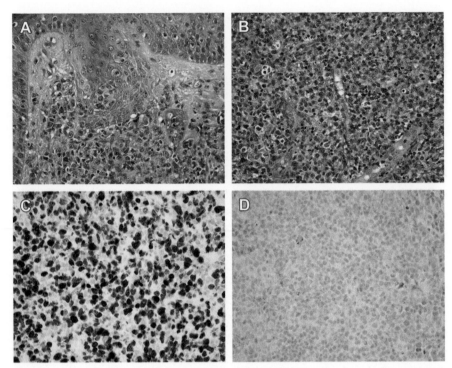

Fig. 4. Tumor-stage MF, showing large cell transformation. (*A, B*) Hematoxylin-eosin stain shows large Pautrier microabscesses comprising cells that are 3× to 4× larger than intervening small reactive lymphocytes. Similar cells efface the dermis in sheets and large clusters. (*C*) Ki-67 proliferation index is high in these lesion, probably 85% in this case. (*D*) Only a rare CD30⁺ lymphocyte is noted, underscoring the oft absence of CD30 in cases of transformed MF [*A–D*, original magnification ×400].

characteristically CD8⁺. Cytotoxic markers can be positive, including CD56.[50] TCR-beta or TCR-gamma[39] can be found.

CD8⁺ AECTCL is strongly CD3⁺ and CD8⁺; additional findings include preservation of CD7 (**Fig. 6**) and expression of TCR-beta, although it has been suggested that TCR-gamma expression can be seen. As with MF, other pan–T-cell markers are lost.[51] Cytotoxic granules (TIA1⁺, granzyme B, and perforin) are expressed. CD56 is usually negative.

GD-TCL may be difficult to diagnose on routine IHC, particularly if sampling is superficial, as discussed previously. The hallmark finding is the absence of TCR-beta expression in the context of positive TCR-gamma or TCR-delta staining (**Fig. 7**C, D). The author has found that moderate increases of TCR-gamma and TCR-delta expression can be seen at all stages of the disease and should raise suspicion if found in any biopsy specimen. Most GD-TCL shows a null immunophenotype (CD3⁺ but CD4⁻ and CD8⁻) (see **Fig. 7**A, B), although CD8 can be seen in some lesions and may vary with time.

CD4⁺ SMTCL (**Fig. 8**A) may express 1 or more TFH markers, PD-1⁺, ICOS⁺, CXCL13⁺, and bcl-6⁺. Tumors contain numerous CD20⁺ B-cell aggregates and CD163⁺ macrophages. There is loss of pan–T-cell antigens and a Ki-67 proliferation index less than 30%. Monoclonal T-cell gene rearrangements are common.

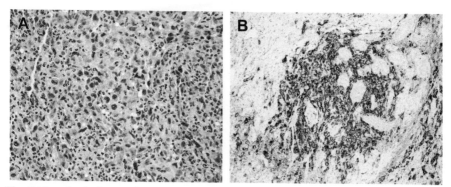

Fig. 5. Anaplastic large cell lymphoma, DUSP22 rearranged. (*A*) Hematoxylin-eosin stain shows a mixed large and small cell population. Large cells are atypical with kidney bean–shaped and donut-shaped nuclei. (*B*) CD30 labels greater than 75% of lesional (large) atypical lymphocytes [*A–B*, original magnification ×400].

The immunophenotype of primary cutaneous acral CD8$^+$ lymphoma (see **Fig. 8**B) is that of a nonactivated cytotoxic T-cell (CD8$^+$, CD3$^+$, or CD45RO/RA$^+$), which is negative for CD30, CD56, and TFH markers. CD2, CD5, or CD7 may be positive or negative. MIB-1/Ki-67 labeling is often less than 10%. Rare CD20$^+$ B cells may be seen.

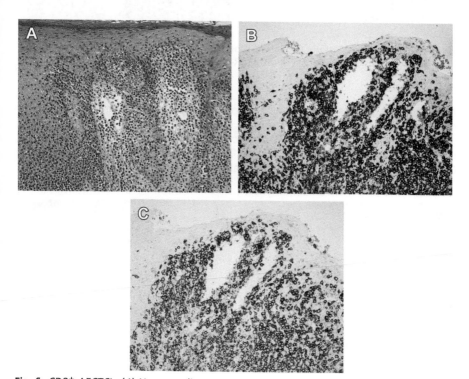

Fig. 6. CD8$^+$ AECTCL. (*A*) Hematoxylin- eosin stain showing a florid front of monomorphic large atypical lymphocytes effacing the dermoepidermal junction and involving the underlying dermis (original magnification ×200). (*B*) CD7 is retained, strong, and diffuse (original magnification ×400). (*C*) CD8 is typically strong and diffuse (original magnification ×400).

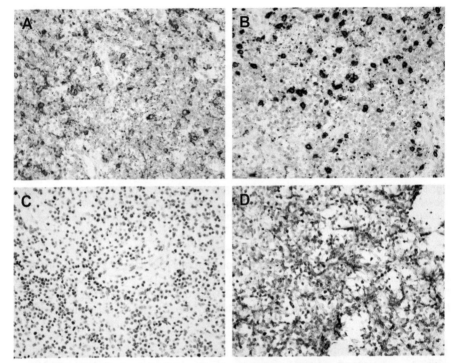

Fig. 7. GDTCL, IHC. (*A–C*, original magnification ×400) CD4, CD8, and TCR-beta are negative in a majority of lesional lymphocytes. (*D*) TCR-delta is strongly and diffusely positive in lesional lymphocytes.

Most but not all cases show monoclonal TCR-gamma and/or TCR-beta gene rearrangements.

Immunophenotypically, SPTCL is characterized by a CD3[+] CD8[+] TCR-beta[+] and often TIA-1[+] phenotype. EBV, CD30, and TCR-gamma and TCR-delta are negative. Clonal TCR gene rearrangement is detectable in most cases.

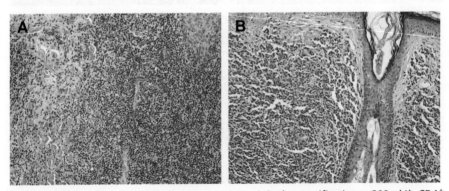

Fig. 8. Indolent LPDs, hematoxylin-eosin stain, original magnification ×200. (*A*) CD4[+] SMTCL shows a mixed cell morphology with histiocytes and variably sized lymphocytes, effacing epithelial structures. (*B*) Primary cutaneous CD8[+] acral lymphoma demonstrates sparing of epithelial structures by a monomorphic small cell population in dermis.

Flow Cytometry

FCA is used to evaluate peripheral blood specimens of patients with MF for staging purposes and in SS for diagnosis. Patients with SS have higher percentages of CD4+/CD7− cells compared with patients with benign dermatoses and significantly higher CD4:CD8 ratios than patients with benign dermatoses or no LPDs. MF patients do not show differences in either ratio or percentage.[52] FCA could detect aberrant CD2, CD3, or CD5 in 66% of SS and 30% of MF patients. As with other mature T-cell lymphomas, loss of expression of a pan–T-cell marker greater than 25% is abnormal, and loss of 2 antigens or a single antigen greater than 50% is worrisome for a T-cell LPD. These abnormalities have been found to have a sensitivity of 78% and specificity of 89% compared with non-MF or indeterminate histologies.[53]

The use of CD26 for diagnosis of MF on FCA is challenging because MF can be CD26+ or CD26− and reactive T cells can show a loss of CD26.[54] The use of V-beta FCA may make this issue moot. Monoclonal TCR gene rearrangements can be assessed for with a set of monoclonal antibodies to 23 V-beta segments covering 70% of the known V-beta repertoire. A clonal T-cell population shows either restriction of one of these V-beta chains or is negative for all tested chains. V-beta FCA may be more sensitive than molecular clonality analysis in the assessment of a monoclonal T-cell population and can be used when CD4:CD8 ratio is greater than 10 or with CD4+/CD26− or CD7− cells to upstage blood staging to B2.[55,56]

Skin biopsy specimens (eg, digested with collagenase) from patients with diagnostic International Society for Cutaneous Lymphomas (ISCL) scores for MF seem to have correlative diagnostic findings by FCA, whereas subdiagnostic ISCL scores or histology were normal by FCA and polyclonal on TCR PCR.[57] FCA has identified both small and large cell shared monoclonal populations in MF not seen by IHC, with CD3+/CD26− T cells accounting for 70% of MF cases and absent CD7 in only 57% of cases.[58] The large cell size and complexity identified by increased forward and side-scatter properties, or high-scatter T-cells, are have been said to be specific for the FC diagnosis of MF.[59]

GDTCL can be identified by FCA, with the findings of CD2+, surface (epsilon) CD3+, TCR-GD, and CD4 and CD8 negativity, as seen in IHC. CD5 and CD7 are variable. NK markers CD16, CD56, CD57, and Killer cell Ig-like receptors (KIRs) are said to be acquired by some GDTCL.

Molecular

Karyotypic, cytogenetic, and array comparative genomic hybridization studies of SS have revealed a complex karyotype with structural and numerical abnormalities thought to reflect gross chromosomal instability, involving chromosomes 10 and 6 as well as chromosomes 3, 7, 9, 17, 1, 12, 8, 11, and 13. In transformed or tumor MF, the most common (but not specific) finding may be loss of 9p21, with gains in 1p, 1q, 7q, and 8/8q. Loss of 9p21/CDKn2A or 19q26 and gains in 8q have been suggested to correlated with worsened outcome in tumor or transformed MF, but these effects may be attributable in part to selection bias.[60–62] Additional products noted to be gained in CTCL include Nav3 (12q21), JunB (chr19), c-MYC/MAX, p53, PTEN/Fas, p15, p16, NFKB, bcl-2, and Stat2. Overall SS shows numerous nonrecurrent complex unbalanced translocations but no disease-specific balanced translocations. Copy number variations are typically numerous and may be recurrent.[22] Microsatellite instability has been reported to be increased in stage IIB MF and in large cell transformation and has been reported in 24% of CTCL overall. Mutational data continue to be gathered and analyzed on this diverse group of disease showing alterations in multiple pathways, including TCR signaling and chromatin modification (eg, ARID1A, CTCL, and DNMT3a).[63]

The ALK/NPM translocation typically seen in systemic ALCL is only rarely seen in pcALCL. Diagnostically, IRF4 alterations identified in 75% of ALCL[64] are helpful but not entirely specific, because rare MF (Pham-Ledard) showed IRF4 translocation.[65] ALCL/LyP may show DUSP22-IRF4 locus on 6p25.3 rearrangements, with characteristic dimorphic cytology. These are not diagnostic or prognostic but may be helpful in ruling out high-grade ALK-negative extracutaneous disease.[66] Other characteristic genetic anomalies include Nav3 in SPTCL and Stat5B/STAT3 mutations in GDTCL.[67]

Molecular characterization of CTCL is an evolving field and requires close scrutiny in regard to disease course and response to therapy, in relationship to all clinical, laboratory, and other pathologic data as they become incorporated into current diagnostic and therapeutic algorithms.

Prognosis

Numerous prognostic markers have been sought for CTCL, including age greater than 60, clinical stage, lactate dehydrogenase, β2-microglobulin, neutrophil-lymphocyte ratio, *Staphylococcus aureus* infection, cell size (small or large, depending on subtype), IHC or flow cytometric documentation of differentiation marker anomalies, proliferation indices (for example, ki-67), and molecular features (p53 and CDKN2A[61]).[68–70] With most cases, the appropriate diagnostic stratification and clinical staging remain the most reliable discriminators at this point, particularly because many studies are small and/or cannot adequately control for the effect of prior therapies. As molecular (eg, TCR sequence and mutational data) and flow cytometric data are gathered, multivariate analysis of large groups will be needed to better assess prognostic features for CTCL.

Diagnosis

The differential diagnosis of cutaneous lymphomas is broad and has been well reviewed previously for individual entities. Disease mimics range from infection, autoimmune or hypersensitivity reactions, and solid tumors to secondary involvement of the skin by other peripheral T-cell lymphoma, and T-cell–rich B-cell lymphoma. A good rule of thumb is to maintain alertness for features that do not follow the usual clinical and histopathologic patterns described for these entities here (see **Table 4**, **Table 5**). When the diagnostic features are not clear, the most prudent course is to ensure clear communication between clinicians and pathologists and to consider the acquisition of additional biopsy material over time as the disease evolves to a more clearly diagnostic phenotype.

REFERENCES

1. Willemze R, Jaffe ES, Burg G, et al. WHO-EORTC classification for cutaneous lymphomas. Blood 2005;105(10):3768–85.

2. Swerdlow SH, Campo E, Harris NL, et al. WHO classification of tumours of haematopoietic and lymphoid tissues. 4th edition. Lyon (France): IARC Press; 2008.

3. Swerdlow SH, Campo E, Pileri SA, et al. The 2016 revision of the World Health Organization classification of lymphoid neoplasms. Blood 2016;127(20):2375–90.

4. Beltraminelli H, Leinweber B, Kerl H, et al. Primary cutaneous CD4+ small-/medium-sized pleomorphic T-cell lymphoma: a cutaneous nodular proliferation of

pleomorphic T lymphocytes of undetermined significance? A study of 136 cases. Am J Dermatopathol 2009;31(4):317–22.

5. Clark RA. Skin-resident T cells: the ups and downs of on site immunity. J Invest Dermatol 2010;130(2):362–70.

6. Jackow CM, Cather JC, Hearne V, et al. Association of erythrodermic cutaneous T-cell lymphoma, superantigen-positive Staphylococcus aureus, and oligoclonal T-cell receptor V beta gene expansion. Blood 1997;89(1):32–40.

7. Mirvish JJ, Pomerantz RG, Falo LD Jr, et al. Role of infectious agents in cutaneous T-cell lymphoma: facts and controversies. Clin Dermatol 2013;31(4):423–31.

8. Abrams JT, Balin BJ, Vonderheid EC. Association between Sezary T cell-activating factor, Chlamydia pneumoniae, and cutaneous T cell lymphoma. Ann N Y Acad Sci 2001;941:69–85.

9. Litvinov IV, Shtreis A, Kobayashi K, et al. Investigating potential exogenous tumor initiating and promoting factors for Cutaneous T-Cell Lymphomas (CTCL), a rare skin malignancy. Oncoimmunol 2016;5(7):e1175799.

10. Korgavkar K, Xiong M, Weinstock M. Changing incidence trends of cutaneous T-cell lymphoma. JAMA Dermatol 2013;149(11):1295–9.

11. Scarisbrick JJ, Prince HM, Vermeer MH, et al. Cutaneous lymphoma international Consortium study of outcome in advanced stages of mycosis fungoides and sezary syndrome: effect of specific prognostic markers on survival and Development of a prognostic Model. J Clin Oncol 2015;33(32):3766–73.

12. Litvinov IV, Tetzlaff MT, Rahme E, et al. Demographic patterns of cutaneous T-cell lymphoma incidence in Texas based on two different cancer registries. Cancer Med 2015;4(9):1440–7.

13. Litvinov IV, Tetzlaff MT, Rahme E, et al. Identification of geographic clustering and regions spared by cutaneous T-cell lymphoma in Texas using 2 distinct cancer registries. Cancer 2015;121(12):1993–2003.

14. Ghazawi FM, Netchiporouk E, Rahme E, et al. Comprehensive analysis of cutaneous T-cell lymphoma (CTCL) incidence and mortality in Canada reveals changing trends and geographic clustering for this malignancy. Cancer 2017. [Epub ahead of print].

15. Slodownik D, Moshe S, Sprecher E, et al. Occupational mycosis fungoides - a case series. Int J Dermatol 2017;56(7):733–7.

16. Talpur R, Cox KM, Hu M, et al. Vitamin D deficiency in mycosis fungoides and Sezary syndrome patients is similar to other cancer patients. Clin Lymphoma Myeloma Leuk 2014;14(6):518–24.

17. Litvinov IV, Hegazy RA, Gawdat HI, et al. Analysis of STAT4 expression in cutaneous T-cell lymphoma (CTCL) patients and patient-derived cell lines. Cell Cycle 2014;13(18):2975–82.

18. Demirkesen C, Esirgen G, Engin B, et al. The clinical features and histopathologic patterns of folliculotropic mycosis fungoides in a series of 38 cases. J Cutan Pathol 2015;42(1):22–31.

19. Kempf W, et al. Unilesional follicular mycosis fungoides: report of two cases with progression to tumor stage and review of the literature. J Cutan Pathol 2012; 39(9):853–60.

20. Amitay-Laish I, Tavallaee M, Kim J, et al. Unilesional folliculotropic mycosis fungoides: a unique variant of cutaneous lymphoma. J Eur Acad Dermatol Venereol 2016;30(1):25–9.

21. Castano E, Glick S, Wolgast L, et al. Hypopigmented mycosis fungoides in childhood and adolescence: a long-term retrospective study. J Cutan Pathol 2013; 40(11):924–34.

22. Izykowska K, Przybylski GK, Gand C, et al. Genetic rearrangements result in altered gene expression and novel fusion transcripts in Sezary syndrome. Oncotarget 2017. [Epub ahead of print].

23. Eberle FC, Song JY, Xi L, et al. Nodal involvement by cutaneous CD30-positive T-cell lymphoma mimicking classical Hodgkin lymphoma. Am J Surg Pathol 2012;36(5):716–25.

24. Basarab T, Fraser-Andrews EA, Orchard G, et al. Lymphomatoid papulosis in association with mycosis fungoides: a study of 15 cases. Br J Dermatol 1998; 139(4):630–8.

25. de la Garza Bravo MM, Patel KP, Loghavi S, et al. Shared clonality in distinctive lesions of lymphomatoid papulosis and mycosis fungoides occurring in the same patients suggests a common origin. Hum Pathol 2015;46(4):558–69.

26. Zackheim HS, Jones C, Leboit PE, et al. Lymphomatoid papulosis associated with mycosis fungoides: a study of 21 patients including analyses for clonality. J Am Acad Dermatol 2003;49(4):620–3.

27. Ralfkiaer E, Wollf-Sneedorff A, Thomsen K, et al. T-cell receptor gamma delta-positive peripheral T-cell lymphomas presenting in the skin: a clinical, histological and immunophenotypic study. Exp Dermatol 1992;1(1):31–6.

28. Berti E, Tomasini D, Vermeer MH, et al. Primary cutaneous CD8-positive epidermotropic cytotoxic T cell lymphomas. A distinct clinicopathological entity with an aggressive clinical behavior. Am J Pathol 1999;155(2):483–92.

29. Bosseila M, Sayed Sayed K, El-Din Sayed SS, et al. Evaluation of angiogenesis in early mycosis fungoides patients: dermoscopic and immunohistochemical study. Dermatology 2015;231(1):82–6.

30. Lallas A, Apalla Z, Lefaki I, et al. Dermoscopy of early stage mycosis fungoides. J Eur Acad Dermatol Venereol 2013;27(5):617–21.

31. Xu P, Tan C. Dermoscopy of poikilodermatous mycosis fungoides (MF). J Am Acad Dermatol 2016;74(3):e45–7.

32. Miteva M, El Shabrawi-Caelen L, Fink-Puches R, et al. Alopecia universalis associated with cutaneous T cell lymphoma. Dermatology 2014;229(2):65–9.

33. Moura FN, Thomas L, Balme B, et al. Dermoscopy of lymphomatoid papulosis. Arch Dermatol 2009;145(8):966–7.

34. Agero AL, Gill M, Ardigo M, et al. In vivo reflectance confocal microscopy of mycosis fungoides: a preliminary study. J Am Acad Dermatol 2007;57(3):435–41.

35. Mancebo SE, Cordova M, Myskowski PL, et al. Reflectance confocal microscopy features of mycosis fungoides and Sezary syndrome: correlation with histopathologic and T-cell receptor rearrangement studies. J Cutan Pathol 2016;43(6): 505–15.

36. Lange-Asschenfeldt S, Babilli J, Beyer M, et al. Consistency and distribution of reflectance confocal microscopy features for diagnosis of cutaneous T cell lymphoma. J Biomed Opt 2012;17(1):016001.

37. Ardigo M, Donadio C, Vega H, et al. Concordance between in vivo reflectance confocal microscopy and optical histology of lymphomatoid papulosis. Skin Res Technol 2013;19(3):308–13.

38. Gerami P, Guitart J. The spectrum of histopathologic and immunohistochemical findings in folliculotropic mycosis fungoides. Am J Surg Pathol 2007;31(9): 1430–8.

39. Rodriguez-Pinilla SM, Ortiz-Romero PL, Monsalvez V, et al. TCR-gamma expression in primary cutaneous T-cell lymphomas. Am J Surg Pathol 2013;37(3): 375–84.

40. Edinger JT, Clark BZ, Pucevich BE, et al. CD30 expression and proliferative fraction in nontransformed mycosis fungoides. Am J Surg Pathol 2009;33(12): 1860–8.
41. Arulogun SO, Prince HM, Ng J, et al. Long-term outcomes of patients with advanced-stage cutaneous T-cell lymphoma and large cell transformation. Blood 2008;112(8):3082–7.
42. Barberio E, Barbosa HS, Vieira MD, et al. Transformed mycosis fungoides: clinicopathological features and outcome. Br J Dermatol 2007;157(2):284–9.
43. Pulitzer M, Myskowski PL, Horwitz SM, et al. Mycosis fungoides with large cell transformation: clinicopathological features and prognostic factors. Pathology 2014;46(7):610–6.
44. Meyerson HJ, Awadallah A, Pavlidakey P, et al. Follicular center helper T-cell (TFH) marker positive mycosis fungoides/Sezary syndrome. Mod Pathol 2013; 26(1):32–43.
45. Guitart J, Gammon B. The difficulties in defining follicular T helper phenotype in cutaneous lymphomas. Am J Dermatopathol 2013;35(6):691.
46. Bosisio FM, Cerroni L. Expression of T-follicular helper markers in sequential biopsies of progressive mycosis fungoides and other primary cutaneous T-cell lymphomas. Am J Dermatopathol 2015;37(2):115–21.
47. Fierro MT, Novelli M, Savoia P, et al. CD45RA+ immunophenotype in mycosis fungoides: clinical, histological and immunophenotypical features in 22 patients. J Cutan Pathol 2001;28(7):356–62.
48. Hodak E, David M, Maron L, et al. CD4/CD8 double-negative epidermotropic cutaneous T-cell lymphoma: an immunohistochemical variant of mycosis fungoides. J Am Acad Dermatol 2006;55(2):276–84.
49. Pulitzer M, Ogunrinade O, Lin O, et al. ALK-positive (2p23 rearranged) anaplastic large cell lymphoma with localization to the skin in a pediatric patient. J Cutan Pathol 2015;42(3):182–7.
50. Poppe H, Kerstan A, Bockers M, et al. Childhood mycosis fungoides with a CD8+ CD56+ cytotoxic immunophenotype. J Cutan Pathol 2015;42(4):258–64.
51. Lee AD, Cohen PR. What is Woringer-Kolopp disease? Skinmed 2013;11(1): 17–20.
52. Harmon CB, Witzig TE, Katzmann JA, et al. Detection of circulating T cells with CD4+CD7- immunophenotype in patients with benign and malignant lymphoproliferative dermatoses. J Am Acad Dermatol 1996;35(3 Pt 1):404–10.
53. Jokinen CH, Fromm JR, Argenyi ZB, et al. Flow cytometric evaluation of skin biopsies for mycosis fungoides. Am J Dermatopathol 2011;33(5):483–91.
54. Pierson DM, Jones D, Muzzafar T, et al. Utility of CD26 in flow cytometric immunophenotyping of T-cell lymphomas in tissue and body fluid specimens. Cytometry B Clin Cytom 2008;74(6):341–8.
55. Olsen E, Vonderheid E, Pimpinelli N, et al. Revisions to the staging and classification of mycosis fungoides and sezary syndrome: a proposal of the International Society for Cutaneous Lymphomas (ISCL) and the cutaneous lymphoma task force of the European Organization of Research and Treatment of Cancer (EORTC). Blood 2007;110(6):1713–22.
56. Feng B, Jorgensen JL, Jones D, et al. Flow cytometric detection of peripheral blood involvement by mycosis fungoides and Sezary syndrome using T-cell receptor Vbeta chain antibodies and its application in blood staging. Mod Pathol 2010;23(2):284–95.
57. Oshtory S, Apisarnthanarax N, Gilliam AC, et al. Usefulness of flow cytometry in the diagnosis of mycosis fungoides. J Am Acad Dermatol 2007;57(3):454–62.

58. Novelli M, Fierro MT, Quaglino P, et al. Flow cytometry immunophenotyping in mycosis fungoides. J Am Acad Dermatol 2008;59(3):533–4.
59. Clark RA, Chong BF, Mirchandani N, et al. High-scatter T cells: a reliable biomarker for malignant T cells in cutaneous T-cell lymphoma. Blood 2011; 117(6):1966–76.
60. Laharanne E, Oumouhou N, Bonnet F, et al. Genome-wide analysis of cutaneous T-cell lymphomas identifies three clinically relevant classes. J Invest Dermatol 2010;130(6):1707–18.
61. Laharanne E, Chevret E, Idrissi Y, et al. CDKN2A-CDKN2B deletion defines an aggressive subset of cutaneous T-cell lymphoma. Mod Pathol 2010;23(4): 547–58.
62. Salgado R, Servitje O, Gallardo F, et al. Oligonucleotide array-CGH identifies genomic subgroups and prognostic markers for tumor stage mycosis fungoides. J Invest Dermatol 2010;130(4):1126–35.
63. Choi J, Goh G, Walradt T, et al. Genomic landscape of cutaneous T cell lymphoma. Nat Genet 2015;47(9):1011–9.
64. Kiran T, Demirkesen C, Eker C, et al. The significance of MUM1/IRF4 protein expression and IRF4 translocation of CD30(+) cutaneous T-cell lymphoproliferative disorders: a study of 53 cases. Leuk Res 2013;37(4):396–400.
65. Pham-Ledard A, Prochazkova-Carlotti M, Laharanne E, et al. IRF4 gene rearrangements define a subgroup of CD30-positive cutaneous T-cell lymphoma: a study of 54 cases. J Invest Dermatol 2010;130(3):816–25.
66. Karai LJ, Kadin ME, Hsi ED, et al. Chromosomal rearrangements of 6p25.3 define a new subtype of lymphomatoid papulosis. Am J Surg Pathol 2013;37(8): 1173–81.
67. Kucuk C, Jiang B, Hu XZ, et al. Activating mutations of STAT5B and STAT3 in lymphomas derived from gammadelta-T or NK cells. Nat Commun 2015;6:6025.
68. Eren R, Nizam N, Doğu MH, et al. Evaluation of neutrophil-lymphocyte ratio in patients with early-stage mycosis fungoides. Ann Hematol 2016;95(11):1853–7.
69. Takahashi Y, Takata K, Kato S, et al. Clinicopathological analysis of 17 primary cutaneous T-cell lymphoma of the gammadelta phenotype from Japan. Cancer Sci 2014;105(7):912–23.
70. Cengiz FP, Emiroglu N, Ozkaya DB, et al. Prognostic evaluation of neutrophil/ lymphocyte ratio in patients with mycosis fungoides. Ann Clin Lab Sci 2017; 47(1):25–8.

Primary Cutaneous B-cell Lymphomas

Charity B. Hope, MD[a], Laura B. Pincus, MD[a,b],*

KEYWORDS

- Primary cutaneous B-cell lymphoma • Primary cutaneous marginal zone lymphoma
- Primary cutaneous follicle center lymphoma
- Primary cutaneous diffuse large B-cell lymphoma • Leg type
- Intravascular diffuse large B-cell lymphoma

KEY POINTS

- Among cutaneous lymphomas, B-cell lymphomas are not uncommon, representing approximately 20% to 25% of primary cutaneous lymphomas.
- Primary cutaneous marginal zone lymphoma is an indolent lymphoma characterized by a nodular or diffuse pleomorphic infiltrate of small to medium centrocyte-like cells with admixed plasmacytoid cells, larger centroblasts/immunoblasts, and reactive cells. Reactive follicles are often present. Plasma cells with light chain restriction at the periphery of nodules are characteristic.
- Primary cutaneous follicle center lymphoma (pcFCL) is a low-grade lymphoma characterized by a proliferation of medium to large neoplastic centrocytes arranged in either a follicular, diffuse, or mixed configuration. Neoplastic cells are typically positive for B-cell markers and Bcl-6 and negative for MUM-1.
- Primary cutaneous diffuse large B-cell lymphoma, leg type carries an intermediate prognosis and is composed of diffuse sheets of large atypical centroblasts and/or immunoblasts. The immunophenotype is typically positive for B-cell markers, Bcl-2, and MUM-1.
- Intravascular large B-cell lymphoma is a rare, aggressive B-cell malignancy characterized by neoplastic B-lymphocytes confined to the lumina of blood vessels.

Disclosure Statement: The authors have no commercial or financial conflicts of interest to disclose.
[a] Department of Pathology, UCSF Dermatopathology Section, University of California, San Francisco, 1701 Divisidero Street, Room 280, San Francisco, CA 94115, USA; [b] Department of Dermatology, UCSF Dermatopathology Section, University of California, San Francisco, 1701 Divisidero Street, Room 280, San Francisco, CA 94115, USA
* Corresponding author. UCSF Dermatopathology Section, 1701 Divisidero Street, Room 280, San Francisco, CA 94115.
E-mail address: laura.pincus@ucsf.edu

Clin Lab Med 37 (2017) 547–574
http://dx.doi.org/10.1016/j.cll.2017.05.009
labmed.theclinics.com

INTRODUCTION

Widely disparate classification schemas were used in the diagnosis of cutaneous lymphomas until relatively recently.[1,2] A major breakthrough in the development of a more standardized classification system occurred in 2005 when the 2 major international groups involved in this effort, the European Organization of Research and Treatment of Cancer (EORTC) and the World Health Organization (WHO), developed a consensus statement.[3] Three main categories of B-cell lymphoma that commonly arise as primary cutaneous lesions are included in this classification: primary cutaneous marginal zone lymphoma, primary cutaneous follicle center lymphoma (pcFCL), and primary cutaneous diffuse large B-cell lymphoma, leg type. Together, these represent the vast majority of B-cell lymphomas in the skin, which in turn account for approximately 20%-25% of primary cutaneous lymphomas.[1-4] This classification formed the basis of the 2008 WHO publication[5] with the exception that primary cutaneous marginal zone lymphoma did not receive its own diagnostic category and was instead lumped together with extranodal marginal zone lymphoma of the mucosa-associated lymphoid tissue (MALT), which to many authorities was somewhat problematic (see marginal zone lymphoma section for further details). The 2016 revision of the WHO is largely unchanged.[6] A variety of other B-cell lymphomas, although rarer, may also present primarily in the skin, such as intravascular lymphoma and plasmablastic lymphoma.

The current classification system relies primarily on architectural, cellular morphologic, and immunophenotypic features to distinguish between various neoplastic and reactive B-cell infiltrates in the skin. Clinicopathologic correlation is essential. Importantly, no morphologic, immunologic, or molecular features can reliably differentiate any primary cutaneous lymphoma from secondary cutaneous involvement by nodal or extranodal-noncutaneous disease. Negative staging is thus a prerequisite to the diagnosis of a primary cutaneous lymphoma (**Box 1**).

Unlike other areas in hematopathology in which molecular and cytogenetic studies may offer essential diagnostic and prognostic information, molecular assays in the realm of cutaneous lymphoma outside of a research setting have more limited practical utility and are less frequently performed. Clonality studies are an exception and are commonly used to support a diagnosis of lymphoma, although even these may not be definitive. Selected information on molecular features of cutaneous lymphoma, particularly those of diagnostic utility and those which may distinguish cutaneous lymphomas from nodal counterparts, is presented here. For a more detailed review of developments in this arena, the reader is referred to several recent reviews, which address this topic in more depth.[7,8]

PRIMARY CUTANEOUS MARGINAL ZONE LYMPHOMA

Primary cutaneous marginal zone lymphoma accounts for approximately 30% of cutaneous B-cell lymphomas in most large studies (range 24%–57%)[9-13] and encompasses entities previously known as cutaneous plasmacytoma, immunocytoma, and

---

Box 1
Potential pitfall: primary versus secondary cutaneous lymphoma

No morphologic, immunologic, or molecular features can reliably differentiate any primary cutaneous lymphoma from secondary cutaneous involvement by nodal or extranodal noncutaneous disease. Negative staging is a prerequisite to the diagnosis of a primary cutaneous B-cell lymphoma.

cutaneous follicular lymphoid hyperplasia with monotypic plasma cells.[14–17] Primary cutaneous marginal zone lymphoma is not recognized as a separate, distinct entity in the WHO. Rather, marginal zone lymphoma of the skin is classified within the category "extranodal marginal zone lymphoma of mucosal-associated lymphoid tissue (MALT)."[5,6] Although the name is somewhat imprecise (the skin is not a mucosal site), there are some commonalties between entities in the extranodal MALT category that seem to support this grouping. In particular, these are a group of low-grade lymphomas with an excellent prognosis, with characteristic histopathologic and immunologic features and with a hypothesized etiologic role for chronic immune stimulation leading to neoplastic transformation.[18] At least in some cases, an association between cutaneous marginal zone lymphoma and infection has been found, as with some cases of MALT lymphomas of the gastrointestinal tract and the eye.[19–22] However, there are differences between marginal zone lymphomas of the skin and MALT lymphomas in other organs, including the following: the prognosis of cutaneous marginal zone lymphomas is significantly better than MALT lymphomas at other sites[23]; there appear to be site-related differences in molecular features and immunoglobulin expression[24,25]; and it now appears that a small number of cutaneous cases only in Europe are due to infection. Given these differences, many cutaneous lymphoma authorities have criticized grouping primary cutaneous marginal zone lymphoma with extranodal MALT. The authors think that this grouping is problematic for the above reasons as well.

CLINICAL FEATURES

Patients are most commonly young to middle-aged adults (median age 39–55 years),[3,9–13] although reports of occurrence during childhood have been documented.[26–29] Some studies have documented that is more prevalent in men.[9,10,13,30] Patients typically present with solitary or grouped red-brown papules and plaques with a predilection for the trunk and upper extremities[17,30–32] (**Fig. 1**). As mentioned above, an association with *Borrelia burgdorferi* infection has been documented in some cases, but mostly in studies originating out of endemically infected areas in Europe. Others have failed to identify this link, including studies originating in North America and Asia. Differences in *Borrelia* strains may account for this disparity.[15,33–37]

Treatment is most often local skin-directed therapy, including surgical excision, radiation therapy, and intralesional steroids. As the disease is indolent, watchful waiting can also be an option in some cases. Reports have also been published of treatment of this condition with immunomodulators, such as intralesional interferon alpha and systemic or intralesional rituximab, when lesions are multiple and widespread.[30,38,39] In cases with a documented association with *Borrelia* infection, some clinicians have used systemic antibiotics alone with success.[20,30] In general, recurrences are common (44%–71% of patients) and may present at distant sites from the initial presentation.[9–12,40] The prognosis is excellent, with disease-specific survival of 98% to 100% across studies.[3,10–12]

As with all lymphomas that present in the skin, staging is required to exclude secondary cutaneous involvement by a primary MALT lymphoma of another extranodal site, or cutaneous involvement by multiple myeloma or lymphoplasmacytic lymphoma, all of which may rarely occur.[41–43] According to consensus recommendations for management of cutaneous B-cell lymphomas developed by the International Society for Cutaneous Lymphomas (ISCL) and the EORTC, staging should include a complete history and physical examination, computed tomographic imaging, and, in some cases, select laboratory studies including serum electrophoresis, flow cytometry, and

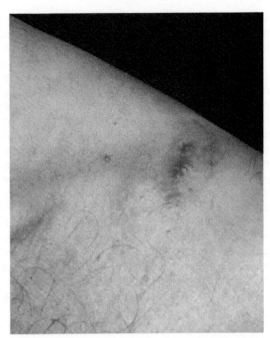

Fig. 1. Primary cutaneous marginal zone shows clustered erythematous papules without overlying epidermal change on the shoulder of a young adult, a typical clinical presentation.

lactate dehydrogenase.[39] Bone marrow biopsy, however, has been shown to have limited value because bone marrow involvement is very rarely detected in cutaneous marginal zone lymphoma.[44]

HISTOPATHOLOGY

Microscopically, this condition often presents at low power as a nodular and/or diffuse dermal infiltrate, in some cases extending into the subcutis. A perivascular or periadnexal pattern of infiltration is sometimes present (**Fig. 2**A). The infiltrate is often polymorphous, composed of small to medium-sized neoplastic "marginal zone cells" (centrocyte-like cells), with indented nuclei and abundant clear cytoplasm, together with a few larger neoplastic cells (centroblast-like or plasmablasts) and various numbers of admixed plasmacytoid lymphocytes and plasma cells, often distributed at the periphery of the infiltrate (**Fig. 2**B). Plasma cells may also commonly be observed in the superficial dermis lining up along a grenz zone (**Fig. 2**C). Admixed reactive T-lymphocytes are usually present and sometimes numerous. Other inflammatory cells, including histiocytes and eosinophils, may be present as well. The epidermis is typically spared. Cases of cutaneous marginal zone lymphoma showing epidermotropism have been reported but are exceedingly rare,[30,45,46] such that concurrent mycoses fungoides is thought to be a more likely explanation for epidermotropism if it is encountered.[20,30,40]

Reactive lymphoid follicles are often apparent at low power, surrounded by pale-appearing zones of expanded "marginal zone cells" (**Fig. 3**). At times, colonization of reactive lymphoid follicles by neoplastic plasma cells may be seen.[20,30,47]

In other cases, the infiltrate may be more monomorphous and diffuse rather than polymorphous and nodular. In some cases, the infiltrate is composed almost

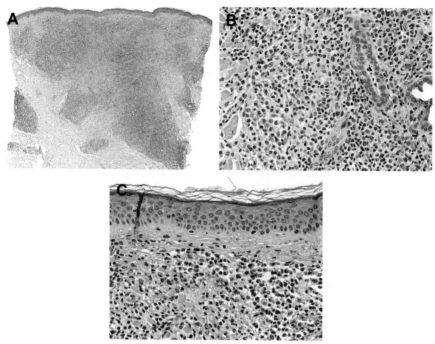

Fig. 2. Marginal zone lymphoma shows nodular diffuse infiltrates within the dermis, with accentuation around follicular structures (*A*, H&E, original magnification ×40); plasma cells are characteristically present at the periphery of nodules (*B*, H&E, original magnification ×100); and additionally are often seen lining up along a grenz zone in the superficial dermis (*C*, H&E, original magnification ×100).

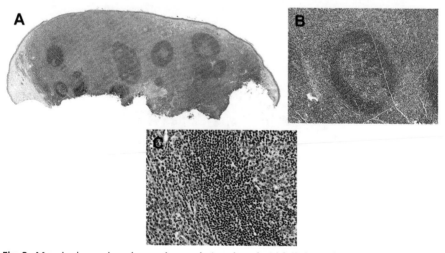

Fig. 3. Marginal zone lymphoma shows obvious lymphoid follicles at low power surrounded by an expanded pale-staining zone of "centrocyte-like cells" (*A*, H&E, original magnification ×20). Follicles have characteristic features of reactive follicles with well-developed mantle zone (*B*, H&E, original magnification ×200) as well as tingible body macrophages and mitotic figures (*C*, H&E, original magnification ×200).

exclusively of plasma cells (**Fig. 4**A, B), and such cases have been referred to as the plasmacytic variant of primary cutaneous marginal zone lymphoma by authorities. Plasma cells with intranuclear periodic acid-Schiff (PAS) + inclusions (Dutcher bodies) are occasionally present (see **Fig. 4**B, C). Many examples of the plasmacytic variant in the past were classified as plasmacytomas. In other cases, a diffuse infiltrate is composed of a combination of lymphocytes, lymphoplasmacytoid cells, and plasma cells. Some authorities have referred to such cases as the lymphoplasmacytic variant and have suggested that this variant may more commonly be associated with somewhat distinct clinical features compared with cutaneous marginal zone lymphomas as a whole, such as a higher age at onset, more common presentation on the lower extremity, and a stronger association with *Borrelia* infection. Less commonly, a blastic variant can be seen in which most neoplastic cells are large and resemble plasmablasts, although admixed neoplastic plasma cells and reactive cells are usually present as well.[30,48]

Overall, most histopathologic variants present and behave similarly, although cases of the blastic variant that represent large-cell transformation from a previously diagnosed marginal zone lymphoma have been shown to have an aggressive course, including in some cases death from disseminated disease. Of note, this contrasts

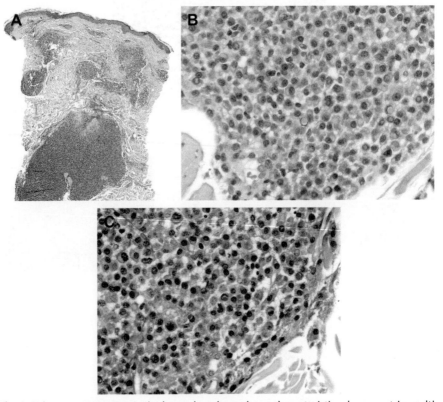

Fig. 4. Primary cutaneous marginal zone lymphoma has a characteristic adnexocentric, multinodular configuration at low power (*A*, H&E, original magnification ×20) and is composed of sheets of neoplastic plasma cells with numerous intranuclear inclusions (Dutcher bodies) (*B*, H&E, original magnification ×400), which are positive for PAS-D (*C*, H&E, original magnification ×400).

with de novo blastic variant marginal zone lymphoma because such cases generally have a prognosis similar to conventional marginal zone lymphoma.[48]

IMMUNOPHENOTYPE

To summarize immunophenotype, primary cutaneous marginal zone lymphoma is positive for B-cell and/or plasma cell markers, positive for Bcl-2, and negative for Bcl-6, CD10, and CD5. Monoclonal light chains are detected in nearly every case. More detailed information for these and other markers is as follows[30,47,49]:

- B-cell and plasma cell markers: The immunophenotype reflects the polymorphous nature of the infiltrate. Neoplastic lymphocytes and plasmacytoid lymphocytes are positive for B-cell markers, including CD20 and CD79a (**Fig. 5**A). Neoplastic plasma cells, in contrast, may be negative for these markers but will be positive for plasma cells markers such as CD138 (**Fig. 5**B). Numerous admixed CD3-positive T-lymphocytes are sometimes present, and there may be more of them than the neoplastic lymphocytes (**Fig. 5**C). This can cause diagnostic uncertainty at times because a primary T-cell process might be misdiagnosed. It is important to note that CD20 expression may be lost following rituximab treatment.[50]
- Monoclonal light chains are almost invariably detected in neoplastic plasma cells, a key diagnostic feature, and characteristically highlight monotypic cells

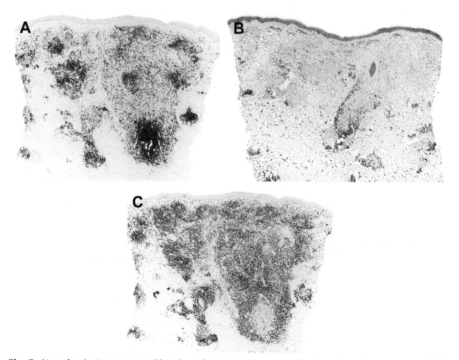

Fig. 5. Neoplastic "centrocyte-like" lymphocytes are positive for B-cell markers such as CD20 (A, CD20 immunoperoxidase stain, ×20), whereas neoplastic plasma cells are typically present at the periphery of aggregates and are positive for plasma cell markers such as CD138 (B, CD128 immunoperoxidase stain, ×20). There are often numerous CD3-positive reactive T cells, as in this case (C, CD3 immunoperoxidase stain, ×20).

at the periphery of nodules (**Fig. 6**A–F). In this regard, a ratio of 10:1 kappa to lambda (or lambda to kappa) is generally used as a threshold for monoclonality.[30]

- Germinal center markers: Bcl-6 and CD10 stains are negative in the neoplastic cells but positive in reactive lymphoid follicles if present.
- CD5 and Bcl-1 stains are negative, which are helpful in excluding mantle cell lymphoma.
- Bcl-2 stains are generally positive.

MOLECULAR FEATURES

Monoclonal rearrangement of immunoglobulin heavy chains is detected in 50% to 60% of cases.[30] Regarding other genetic aberrations, there is evidence of significant site-related differences between the MALT lymphomas, including cutaneous marginal zone lymphoma. Cutaneous marginal zone lymphoma has only rarely been found to harbor the t(11;18) more commonly isolated from MALT lymphomas of lung and gastrointestinal tract. However, a subset of cases has been shown to harbor translocations involving IGH (immunoglobulin heavy chain) and various partners, including a t(14;18) translocation between *IGH* and *MALT1* (which is also seen in ocular, hepatic, and salivary gland MALT lymphomas), the t(14;18) translocation with *BCL2* more commonly seen in nodal follicular lymphoma and diffuse large B-cell lymphoma, and a t(3;14) translocation involving *IGH* and *FOXP1*.[24,51,52]

In contrast to noncutaneous extranodal marginal zone lymphomas, which generally express immunoglobulin M (IgM), most cutaneous marginal zone lymphoma displays class-switched immunoglobulins, including IgG (including IgG4 in some cases), IgA,

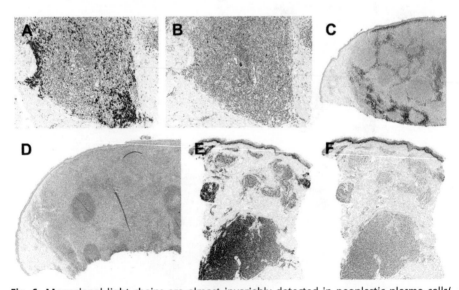

Fig. 6. Monoclonal light chains are almost invariably detected in neoplastic plasma cells/plasmacytoid lymphocytes in primary cutaneous marginal zone lymphoma, with a 10:1 ratio considered significant. The case depicted in **Fig. 2** shows a predominance of lambda (*A*, Lambda in situ hybridization, ×200) over kappa (*B*, Kappa in situ hybridization, ×200). The case depicted in **Fig. 3** shows monoclonality for kappa (*C*, Kappa in situ hybridization, ×100) with negligible staining for lambda (*D*, Lambda in situ hybridization, ×100). The plasmacytic variant shown in **Fig. 4** shows strong and diffuse staining for kappa (*E*, Kappa in situ hybridization, ×20) and is negative for lambda (*F*, Lambda in situ hybridization, ×20).

and IgE. IgM expression has been found to occur in a minority of cases of marginal zone lymphoma, and when present, has been found to be associated with extracutaneous spread.[25,53]

DIFFERENTIAL DIAGNOSIS

The differential diagnosis posed by primary cutaneous marginal zone lymphoma depends on the pattern of the infiltrate. In cases in which obvious lymphoid follicles are present, the differential diagnosis includes cutaneous lymphoid hyperplasia and follicular center lymphoma. In cases in which the infiltrate is nodular or diffuse but without obvious lymphoid follicles, the differential diagnosis includes primary cutaneous CD4$^+$ small/medium T-cell lymphoproliferative disorder and T-cell pseudolymphoma. Guidelines to distinguish these entities are presented in **Table 1**.

PRIMARY CUTANEOUS FOLLICLE CENTER LYMPHOMA
Clinical Features

pcFCL accounts for approximately 50% to 60% of primary cutaneous B-cell lymphomas[3,9,10] and typically occurs in middle aged to older people,[9–11,13] with a slight male predominance reported in some studies.[10] Although pcFCL can be seen occasionally in young adults,[54] the disease is extremely rare in children.[27–29] Clinically, patients with this condition typically present with erythematous papules, plaques, or

---

Table 1
Primary cutaneous marginal zone lymphoma, characteristic features contrasting with conditions on the differential diagnosis

Morphology: Lymphoid follicles

Marginal zone lymphoma	Cutaneous lymphoid hyperplasia	Primary cutaneous follicle center lymphoma
Monoclonal plasma cells at periphery	Lacks monoclonal plasma cells	Monoclonal plasma cells
Shows reactive follicle morphology:	Shows reactive follicle morphology:	Shows abnormal/neoplastic follicle morphology:
• Well-formed, well-spaced follicles	• Well-formed, well-spaced follicles	• Irregular, overlapping follicles
• Well-formed mantle zones	• Well-formed mantle zones	• Attenuated mantle zones
• Tingible body macrophages	• Tingible body macrophages	• Few/absent tangible body macrophages
• Normal polarity (light and dark zones)	• Normal polarity (light and dark zones)	• Absent polarity
• High proliferation rate	• High proliferation rate	• Low proliferation rate
• Bcl-6 within CD21$^+$ follicular networks only	• Bcl-6 within CD21$^+$ follicular networks only	• Bcl-6 within and beyond CD21$^+$ follicular networks

Morphology: Nodular or diffuse without obvious lymphoid follicles

Marginal zone lymphoma	T-cell pseudolymphoma	Primary cutaneous CD4$^+$ small/medium T-cell lymphoproliferative disorder
Monoclonal plasma cells at periphery	Lacks monoclonal plasma cells	Lacks monoclonal plasma cells

Potential pitfall: Reactive T cells may predominate in primary cutaneous marginal zone lymphoma.

tumors on the head, neck, or trunk (**Fig. 7**). However, any site can be involved, including the leg. The clinical lesions can be either solitary or multiple. If there are multiple lesions, they are often grouped, although they can be widely distributed as well.[13,55] pcFCL is associated with an excellent prognosis, with studies documenting an overall 5-year survival at 86.7% to 96.1%, and disease-specific survival at approximately 95%.[3,9,10] If left untreated, the condition usually slowly progresses, although there are rare reports of spontaneous regression.[38,55,56]

With regard to treatment, for a solitary lesion, skin-directed therapies are typically used, in particular, focused radiotherapy or surgical excision. Intralesional steroid injection and targeted cryotherapy at sensitive sites have been reported as well.[38,55] If there are multiple lesions that are relatively few in total number, then treatment is usually radiation. By contrast, if there is widespread disease, then systemic medications, such as rituximab and chemotherapeutic agents, are sometimes used with varying success.[57] Cutaneous recurrences have been reported in half of patients,[9] which are often re-treated with localized therapies.[38,55] Spread to extracutaneous sites has been reported in approximately 10% of patients after initial diagnosis of primary disease.[9,10] Of note, the prognosis of primary cutaneous follicular center lymphoma arising on the legs is worse at other sites, with a prognosis similar to that seen in diffuse large B-cell lymphoma, leg type.[10,58,59] Therefore, for treatment and prognostic purposes, patients with disease on the legs should probably be considered similar to those with diffuse large B-cell lymphoma, leg type.

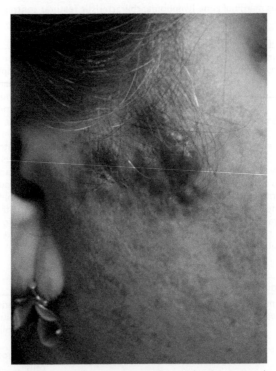

Fig. 7. pcFCL shows multiple erythematous papules coalescing into a large plaque in the preauricular region of the face without overlying epidermal change. This is a typical clinical presentation of pcFCL.

Staging recommendations are similar to those of marginal zone lymphoma in most respects, although the role of bone marrow biopsy is more controversial. In 2008, a study showed that of a cohort of 193 patients with follicle center lymphoma first identified in the skin, 5% of patients had bone marrow involvement as the only identified extracutaneous site involved at staging, and thus without a bone marrow biopsy would have been diagnosed incorrectly with skin-limited indolent disease. These patients had a significantly worse 5-year disease-specific survival at 63% versus 95% in patients with pcFCL.[44] In response to this finding, ISCL/EORTC acknowledge there is no consensus recommendation, but suggest that bone marrow biopsy should be considered for all cases of follicle center lymphoma first presenting in the skin. In their words, "the clinician is advised to follow the standard of care of his or her regional practice" with regard to whether to perform a bone marrow biopsy.[39]

Histopathology

Primary cutaneous follicular center lymphoma shows variation in cytomorphologic features as well as architecture. The architecture may be follicular/nodular, diffuse, or mixed. The follicular pattern of growth shows a neoplastic infiltrate of centrocytes with some admixed reactive small lymphocytes involving the dermis and often the subcutis but sparing the epidermis (**Fig. 8**). Neoplastic infiltrates are arranged in irregular, enlarged, poorly formed and overlapping follicles or nodules (**Fig. 9**). Abnormal follicles lack light and dark zones (follicle polarity), well-formed mantle zones, and easily identified body macrophages, which are characteristic of reactive follicles (**Fig. 10**). Neoplastic centrocytes are frequently present within interfollicular zones as well, another distinguishing feature from reactive follicles.[55,60,61]

The diffuse pattern of growth lacks follicular or nodular morphology and thus may be more difficult to immediately recognize as follicular lymphoma, yet is reported to be the most common pattern seen in the skin,[10] in contrast with nodal disease, in which a purely diffuse microscopic pattern is thought to be rare and attributed to sampling error.[5] The diffuse pattern is not associated with a worse prognosis[10] when located on all body sites other than the leg. In this pattern, there are sheets of large centrocytes with fewer numbers of admixed centroblasts or immunoblasts,

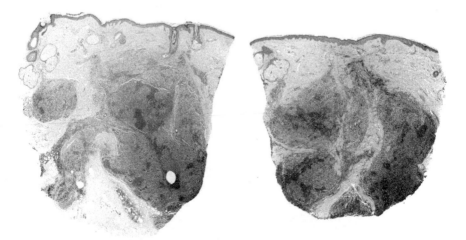

Fig. 8. At low power, this case of pcFCL, follicular pattern, shows dermal involvement by multiple, irregular, coalescing nodules. There is no involvement of the epidermis (H&E, original magnification ×20).

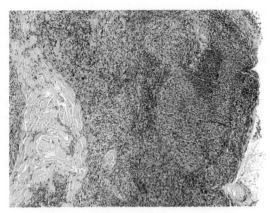

Fig. 9. The neoplastic follicles in this case of pcFCL show large, irregular, and overlapping follicles without well-developed mantle zones (H&E, original magnification ×200).

extending throughout the full thickness of the dermis, often into the subcutis (**Fig. 11**). A grenz zone is usually present. Some small reactive lymphocytes may be present, and occasionally reactive follicles may be present at the periphery of the proliferation.[3,5,55]

Regardless of architectural pattern, the predominant neoplastic cells are medium to large centrocytes (cleaved cells) with angulated, irregular, and sometimes multilobulated nuclei (see **Fig. 10**; **Fig. 12**). Variable numbers of (sometimes many) admixed centroblasts (round cells) with round vesicular nuclei and multiple peripheral nucleoli may also be seen, as may a few immunoblasts with large, central nucleoli. Sheets of centroblasts or immunoblasts should not be present; if seen, such cases are better classified as primary cutaneous diffuse large B-cell lymphoma, leg type.[3,5] It is important to note that unlike nodal follicle center lymphoma, increasing numbers of centroblasts do not portend a worse prognosis, and thus pcFCL are not graded.[5]

Other growth patterns and morphologic variants that have been reported are a mixed pattern of growth, with both follicular and diffuse areas,[55] and a spindle

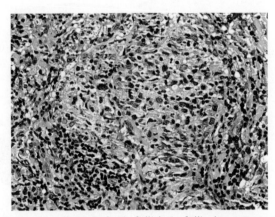

Fig. 10. A high-power view of a neoplastic follicle in follicular pattern pcFCL shows large centrocytes with few centroblasts, and a lack of tangible body macrophages (H&E, original magnification ×400).

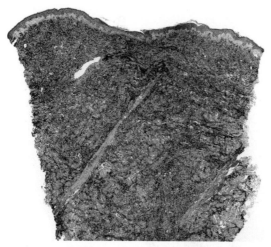

Fig. 11. At low power, this case of diffuse pattern of pcFCL shows a diffuse infiltrate extending throughout the entire dermis. Follicles are not apparent (H&E, original magnification ×20).

cell variant composed of diffuse sheets of large, spindled cells. The latter was formerly thought to be a form of diffuse large B-cell lymphoma but is now recognized as a rare morphologic variant of pcFCL, which despite its alarming appearance behaves similarly to conventional variants.[62,63]

Immunophenotype

To summarize immunophenotype (**Figs. 13** and **14**), all histopathologic variants of pcFCL are characteristically positive for standard B-cell markers and Bcl-6 with variable positivity for CD10. Unlike nodal follicle center lymphoma, most cases are Bcl-2 negative. Staining for MUM-1 is usually negative, in contrast with diffuse large B-cell lymphoma, leg type. More detailed information for these and other markers is listed below:

- B-cell markers: Positive for pan B-cell markers including CD20, CD79a, and PAX-5.

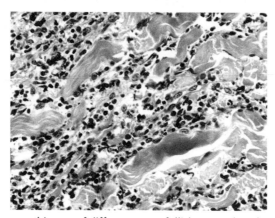

Fig. 12. At high power, this case of diffuse pattern follicle center lymphoma shows medium to large angulated centrocytes with fewer admixed centroblasts and scattered small reactive lymphocytes (H&E, original magnification ×400).

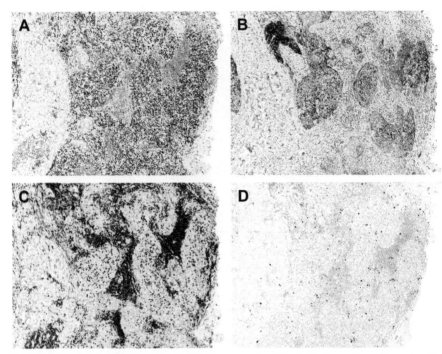

Fig. 13. Immunohistochemical results for the case of pcFCL, follicular pattern (hematoxylin-eosin, original magnification in **Figs. 8–10**). Bcl-6 is positive in neoplastic cells within follicles and small clusters within interfollicular zones (*A*, Bcl6 immunoperoxidase stain, original magnification ×100), highlighted by extension beyond CD21-positive dendritic cell networks (*B*, CD21 immunoperoxidase stain, original magnification ×100); Bcl-2 is negative in neoplastic cells (note: staining in mantle zones and by admixed reactive T cells should not be overcalled) (*C*, Bcl2 immunoperoxidase stain, original magnification ×100); MUM-1 is negative (*D*, MUM-1 immunoperoxidase stain, original magnification ×100).

- Germinal center markers: Bcl-6 is positive in the large majority of cases,[10,58,64] in contrast with marginal zone lymphoma, in which the neoplastic cells are usually negative. CD10 may be positive as well, although many cases are negative, particularly diffuse pattern cases.[10] BCL6/CD10 positivity within follicles does not distinguish between reactive and neoplastic processes, because reactive follicles are also positive. However, positive staining in clusters between follicular zones (highlighted by staining outside CD21-positive dendritic cell networks) strongly supports pcFCL.[62]
- CD21 highlights the dendritic cell network of neoplastic follicles, in cases with follicular pattern pcFCL. Some diffuse pattern cases may also have reactive or neoplastic follicles not evident on hematoxylin and eosin–stained sections but highlighted with CD21, particularly in peripheral zones.[55] Importantly, reactive follicles, such as those commonly seen in primary cutaneous marginal zone lymphoma, are positive for CD21 as well. Alternative markers can also be used to highlight follicular dendritic cells, such as CD23.
- Ki-67 often reveals a lower proliferation rate within neoplastic follicles (<50%) compared with reactive follicles (often >90%).[62]
- Stains for Bcl-2 are usually negative or stain only weakly in a minority of cells, in contrast with node-based follicle center lymphoma, which is characteristically

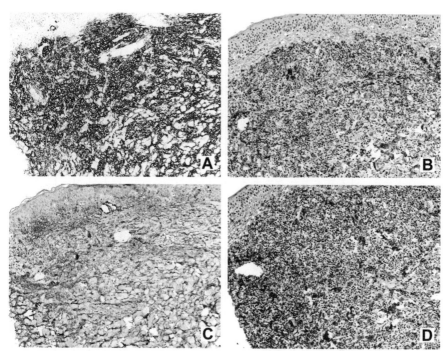

Fig. 14. Immunohistochemical results for the case of pcFCL, diffuse pattern (hematoxylin-eosin, original magnification in **Figs. 11** and **12**). CD20 shows strong, diffuse positivity (*A*, CD20 immunoperoxidase stain, original magnification ×100). Bcl-6 is positive as well (*B*, Bcl-6 immunoperoxidase stain, original magnification ×100), and IgM and MUM-1 are negative (*C* [IgM immunoperoxidase stain, original magnification ×100], *D* [MUM-1 immunoperoxidase stain, original magnification ×100]).

positive. However, positive staining has been documented as high as 11% to 23% in pcFCL.[10,58,64] Thus, positive staining does not necessarily imply that the patient has nodal disease. Positive staining within follicles strongly argues for lymphoma, because reactive follicles do not show this pattern, but there is a possible interpretive pitfall in misinterpreting positive staining of lymphocytes in the follicular mantle (a normal finding). Of note, although some researchers in the past suggested that Bcl-2 positivity implies a worse prognosis,[65,66] studies using current classification criteria have not found that this feature retains independent prognostic significance.[10,58,67]

- MUM-1, FOX-P1, IgM, P63: Most researchers consider greater than 30% of cells staining the threshold for positivity. Using 30% as a benchmark, these markers are usually negative in pcFCL, in contrast with primary cutaneous diffuse large B-cell lymphoma, leg type. Any one marker, however, may be rarely positive; the frequency of positive staining in pcFCL versus primary cutaneous diffuse large B-cell lymphoma is outlined in **Table 2**.[10,55,64,68,69]

- Kappa and lambda light chains: Usually clonality is not present (in contrast with marginal zone lymphoma), but rarely, a small monoclonal population of plasma cells may be identified.[55] This potential pitfall with marginal zone lymphoma is generally easily avoided based on other immunologic and phenotypic characteristics (see **Table 2**).

Table 2
Primary cutaneous follicle center lymphoma, characteristic features contrasting with conditions on the differential diagnosis

Morphology: Lymphoid follicles or irregular nodules		
Primary cutaneous follicle center lymphoma (follicular)	Cutaneous lymphoid hyperplasia	Marginal zone lymphoma
Abnormal/neoplastic follicle morphology: • Irregular, overlapping follicles • Attenuated mantle zones • Few/absent tangible body macrophages • Absent polarity • Low proliferation rate • Bcl-6 within and beyond CD21+ follicular networks Polytypic plasma cells	Reactive follicle morphology: • Well-formed, well-spaced follicles • Well-formed mantle zones • Tingible body macrophages • Normal polarity (light and dark zones) • High proliferation rate • Bcl-6 within CD21+ follicular networks only Polytypic plasma cells	Reactive follicle morphology: • Well-formed, well-spaced follicles • Well-formed mantle zones • Tingible body macrophages • Normal polarity (light and dark zones) • High proliferation rate • Bcl-6 within CD21+ follicular networks only Monoclonal plasma cells at periphery

Morphology: Diffuse, with medium to large B-lymphocytes	
Primary cutaneous follicle center lymphoma (diffuse)	Primary cutaneous diffuse large B-cell lymphoma, leg type
Irregular, angulated, or multilobulated centrocytes with lesser numbers of admixed centroblasts or immunoblasts Immunohistochemistry (IHC): Usually negative for bcl-2, MUM-1, Fox-P1, IgM, and p63	Centroblasts or immunoblasts predominate; may form monotonous sheets IHC: Usually positive for bcl-2, MUM-1, Fox-P1, IgM, and p63

Potential pitfall: Overlap in positive staining for any given marker				
	MUM-1	IgM	Fox-P1	P63
Primary cutaneous follicle center lymphoma, %	2–10	9	4–10	12
Diffuse large B-cell lymphoma, leg type, %	90	100	70–80	70

Molecular Features

Monoclonal rearrangement of immunoglobulin genes may be detected in a subset of cases and may be helpful in supporting a diagnosis of lymphoma, although quoted sensitivity for clonality testing varies considerably (30%–91%) between studies and detection methods.[62,70,71]

The characteristic t(14;18) translocation present in nodal follicle center lymphoma is much less common in pcFCL. Two recent series, for example, identified the translocation in only 8.5% to 10% of cases of pcFCL,[72,73] although estimates have in the past varied considerably and some have been much higher.[74] Other reported cytogenetic abnormalities include translocations between *IGH* and *BCL6* and single cases with novel translocations at t(12;21)(q13;q22) and t(2;14;9;3)(p11.2;q32;p13;q27).[74–76] Testing for translocations is not routinely performed in clinical practice.

Differential Diagnosis

The differential diagnosis for pcFCL includes reactive cutaneous lymphoid hyperplasia, marginal zone lymphoma, and primary cutaneous diffuse large B-cell lymphoma, leg type. Detailed guidelines for distinguishing these entities are presented in **Table 2**.

PRIMARY CUTANEOUS DIFFUSE LARGE B-CELL LYMPHOMA, LEG TYPE
Clinical Features

Primary cutaneous diffuse large B-cell lymphoma, leg type represents approximately 10% to 20% of primary cutaneous lymphomas.[3,9–11] The elderly are most often affected, with a median age at presentation of 70 to 82.[9–13,58,77] Some studies suggest it is more common in women; other studies have not duplicated this finding.[9–19,77] It does not occur in children. The clinical presentation is a rapidly growing nodule or plaque, which may be solitary or multiple and may have surface ulceration (**Fig. 15**). Usually these lesions present on the leg (or rarely, bilateral legs), but a significant minority of cases (approximately 12%) occur at sites other than the legs.[9,10,58,78] Although some studies have found that clinical site and distribution make a difference in patient outcome, with patients with multiple lesions or lesions on the leg having a worse prognosis,[67] others have not duplicated these findings.[9,10] The prognosis is significantly worse primary cutaneous marginal zone or follicle center lymphoma, with a 5-year disease-specific survival between 40% and 60%.[3,10–12,58,77] Most patients (55%–70%) will have recurrence,[9,10,12,77] and in as many as 40% of cases extracutaneous progression may occur, including to the central nervous system.[10,77]

Full staging at diagnosis is required and includes selected laboratory tests, full body imaging, and a bone marrow biopsy. Treatment is also more aggressive from the onset, and a regimen of combination chemotherapy with rituximab (R-CHOP [cyclophosphamide, doxorubicin, vincristine, and prednisone]) is often used, sometimes in combination with local radiation.[39]

Histopathology

Histopathologically, primary cutaneous diffuse large B-cell lymphoma, leg type typically shows overtly malignant histopathologic features, with diffuse involvement of the full dermis and often subcutis with sheets of immunoblasts and/or centroblasts (round cells) and easily identified mitotic figures (**Figs. 16** and **17**). The epidermis may be spared or surface ulceration may be present. Epidermotropism (in a pattern mimicking mycosis fungoides) has been reported but is rare.[78,79] Diffuse large B-cell lymphoma, leg type is more monomorphous than the diffuse pattern of diffuse pattern of follicle center lymphoma and typically lacks the admixed reactive small lymphocytes

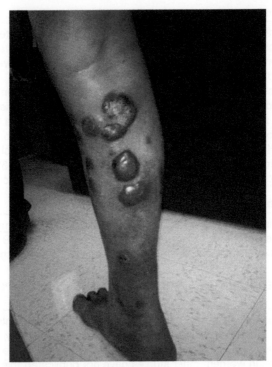

Fig. 15. Primary cutaneous diffuse large B-cell lymphoma, leg type presented in a classic pattern of red-blue nodules and plaques on the leg.

that are seen in the latter. Other distinctive histopathologic features that have been reported include anaplastic or spindled cytomorphology (although most such cases have been found to be follicle center lymphoma), a "starry sky" pattern that mimics Burkitt lymphoma at low power, or growth patterns that show extensive sclerosis, areas of geographic necrosis, or angiotropism/angioinvasion.[5,63,78,79]

More subtle histopathologic presentations have been reported that may be quite challenging to differentiate from inflammatory dermatoses in some cases. Large cells may be present only in a sparse perivascular distribution in early lesions.[78] In one series, the combination of an unusual clinical presentation of annular patches and thin plaques with microscopy showing a superficial and deep perivascular mixed infiltrate of small lymphocytes and variable numbers of large B cells created a significant diagnostic challenge. An abnormal phenotype in the neoplastic large B cells with expression of Bcl-2 and MUM-1 helped to solidify the diagnosis.[80]

Immunophenotype

To summarize immunophenotype (**Fig. 18**), primary cutaneous diffuse large B-cell lymphoma is typically positive for pan-B-cell markers. Other common positive markers include Bcl-2, in contrast with pcFCL, which is most often Bcl-2 negative. MUM-1 is typically positive, as is IgM. Additional immunophenotypic features are outlined below:

- B-cell markers: Standard B-cell markers such as CD20, Pax-5, and CD79a are usually positive, although expression of one or more of these may occasionally be lost.[78]

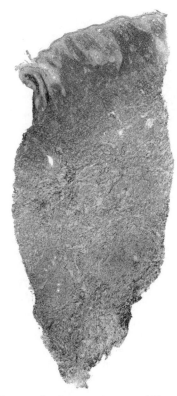

Fig. 16. At low power, this case of primary cutaneous diffuse large B-cell lymphoma, leg type shows sheets of cells throughout the full thickness of the dermis (H&E, original magnification ×20).

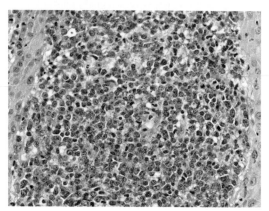

Fig. 17. At high power, sheets of centroblasts and immunoblasts are present in this case of primary cutaneous diffuse large B-cell lymphoma, leg type. There are numerous mitoses (H&E, original magnification ×400).

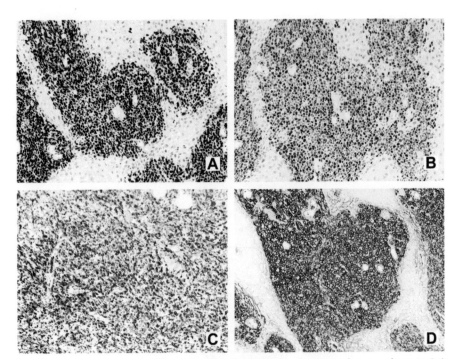

Fig. 18. Primary cutaneous diffuse large B-cell lymphoma, leg type shows a characteristic immunohistochemical profile with positivity for Pax-5 (*A*, original magnification ×100), MUM-1 (*B*, original magnification ×100), Bcl-2 (*C*, original magnification ×100), and IgM (*D*, IgM immunoperoxidase stain, original magnification ×100).

- Germinal center markers: Although CD10 is usually negative, Bcl-6 is frequently positive (45%–75% of cases reported).[10,58,64]
- Bcl-2: Positive staining for Bcl-2 is typical (85%–90% of cases).[10,67] Some researchers, in fact, require Bcl-2 positivity for the diagnosis of primary cutaneous diffuse large B-cell lymphoma, leg type assigning all Bcl-2-negative cases to the category "primary cutaneous diffuse large B-cell lymphoma, other."[12,58,79] Other researchers do not invoke the category "other" in this context.[9,10,67] As there do not appear to be significant differences in outcome between Bcl-2-positive and Bcl-2-negative cases,[10,58] in the authors' practice, they follow the latter. Regardless of preferred diagnostic terminology, the most important concern in this setting is not to render an erroneous diagnosis of diffuse pattern of pcFCL, because the treatment implications would be significant.
- MUM-1, FOX-P1, IgM, P63: Most cases of primary cutaneous diffuse large B-cell lymphoma, leg type are positive for these markers, in contrast with primary cutaneous follicle center lymphoma, in which positive staining is uncommon.[58,64,68,69] Frequency of positive staining in pcFCL versus primary cutaneous diffuse large B-cell lymphoma is outlined in **Table 2**.

Molecular Features

Monoclonal rearrangement of immunoglobulin genes is detected in most cases,[78] with variable detection depending on method of detection as previously discussed.

Currently, most other molecular assays remain in the research realm, but some recurrent molecular alterations with apparent prognostic utility have been identified, which may in the future become more relevant in clinical practice. Some of these include somatic mutations in *MYD88* (present in 40%–75% of cases and associated with decreased survival),[81,82] and inactivation of 9p21.3 (associated with *CDKN2A* gene), which also seems to be associated with a worse prognosis.[83]

Differential Diagnosis

The differential diagnosis for primary cutaneous diffuse large B-cell lymphoma, leg type includes the diffuse pattern of pcFCL and other large B-cell lymphomas, which may uncommonly present in the skin. Detailed guidelines for distinguishing these entities are presented in **Table 3**.

Intravascular Large B-cell Lymphoma

Intravascular large B-cell lymphoma is characterized by malignant B-lymphocytes within vascular lumina.[5] Intravascular large B-cell lymphoma is rare, present in less than 1 per million older adults, with a median age of presentation of 67 years. A variety of organs can be involved, most commonly the central nervous system and skin, and most patients have systemic disease at diagnosis.[84,85] However, cutaneous manifestations may be the first harbinger of the disease, and a significant minority of cases (25%) may be confined to the skin.[85,86] Clinically, skin lesions may be solitary or multiple patches, plaques, or telangiectasias.[87] Intravascular large B-cell lymphoma carries a poor prognosis with a 3-year survival of 22% if the disease is systemic; if the disease is limited to the skin, the prognosis, although still poor, is improved at 56% 3-year survival.[86] Patients are treated with systemic chemotherapy and rituximab.

Microscopically, sections show blood vessel lumina containing large, atypical B-lymphocytes, often with numerous mitotic figures. The immunophenotype shows positivity for pan-B-cell antigens including CD20 and CD79a. Most cases are positive for MUM1 and BCL2 (95% and 91%, respectively). Other markers that may be positive are CD5 in 38%, CD10 in 13%, and Bcl-6 in 26% of cases[88] (**Fig. 19**).

Table 3
Diffuse large B-cell lymphoma, leg type characteristic features contrasting with conditions on the differential diagnosis

Morphology: Diffuse, with large B-lymphocytes		
Primary cutaneous diffuse large B-cell lymphoma, leg type • Centroblasts or immunoblasts predominate; may form monotonous, tumorous sheets • IHC: Usually positive for bcl-2, MUM-1, Fox-P1, IgM, and p63. Negative for EBV	Primary cutaneous follicle center lymphoma (diffuse) • Irregular, angulated, or multilobulated centrocytes with lesser numbers of admixed centroblasts or immunoblasts • IHC: Usually negative for bcl-2, MUM-1, Fox-P1, IgM, and p63	Rare large B-cell lymphomas in the skin • EBV+ diffuse large B-cell lymphoma: EBV+ • Lymphomatoid granulomatosis: EBV+ • Plasmablastic lymphoma: EBV+, may lack B-cell markers • Intravascular diffuse large B-cell lymphoma: intravascular rather than diffuse • B-cell acute lymphoblastic leukemia: TdT+, CD34+/−

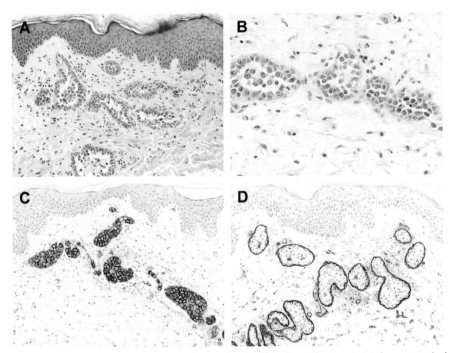

Fig. 19. Intravascular large B-cell lymphoma shows dilated vessels containing large, atypical oval cells (*A*, H&E, original magnification ×100). Atypical cells have pale, vacuolated cytoplasm and large nuclei, some with prominent nucleoli. Several mitotic figures are present (*B*, H&E, original magnification ×400). Atypical cells are positive for CD20 (*C*, CD20 immunoperoxidase stain, original magnification ×100). A CD31 stain highlights the intravascular location of the lymphoma cells (*D*, CD21 immunoperoxidase stain, original magnification ×100).

To date, it is not clear why lymphoma cells are confined within vessels. Researchers have proposed a variety of explanations, including tumor expression of angiogenic factors, lack of adhesion molecules or matrix metalloproteinases required for transendothelial migration or tissue invasion, or aberrant chemokine receptor expression leading to enhanced endothelial cell binding.[89–92]

REFERENCES

1. Willemze R, Kerl H, Sterry W, et al. EORTC classification for primary cutaneous lymphomas: a proposal from the Cutaneous Lymphoma Study Group of the European Organization for Research and Treatment of Cancer. Blood 1997;90(1): 354–71.

2. Fink-Puches R, Zenahlik P, Bäck B, et al. Primary cutaneous lymphomas: applicability of current classification schemes (European Organization for Research and Treatment of Cancer, World Health Organization) based on clinicopathologic features observed in a large group of patients. Blood 2002;99(3):800–5.

3. Willemze R, Jaffe ES, Burg G, et al. WHO-EORTC classification for cutaneous lymphomas. Blood 2005;105(10):3768–85.

4. Bradford PT, Devesa SS, Anderson WF, et al. Cutaneous lymphoma incidence patterns in the United States: a population-based study of 3884 cases. Blood 2009;113(21):5064–73.

5. Swerdlow SH, Campo E, Harris NL, et al. IARC WHO classification of tumours, No 2. Fourth edition. WHO Classification of Tumours of Haematopoietic and Lymphoid Tissues, Vol. 2. WHO Classification of Tumours. Lyon (France): IARC Press; 2008.

6. Swerdlow SH, Campo E, Pileri SA, et al. The 2016 revision of the World Health Organization classification of lymphoid neoplasms. Blood 2016;127(20):2375–90.

7. Hope CB, Pincus LB. Primary cutaneous B-cell lymphomas with large cell predominance-primary cutaneous follicle center lymphoma, diffuse large B-cell lymphoma, leg type and intravascular large B-cell lymphoma. Semin Diagn Pathol 2016;34(1):85–98.

8. Swerdlow SH. Cutaneous marginal zone lymphomas. Semin Diagn Pathol 2016; 34(1):76–84.

9. Zinzani PL, Quaglino P, Pimpinelli N, et al. Prognostic factors in primary cutaneous B-cell lymphoma: the Italian Study Group for cutaneous lymphomas. J Clin Oncol 2006;24(9):1376–82.

10. Senff NJ, Hoefnagel JJ, Jansen PM, et al. Reclassification of 300 primary cutaneous B-cell lymphomas according to the new WHO-EORTC classification for cutaneous lymphomas: comparison with previous classifications and identification of prognostic markers. J Clin Oncol 2007;25(12):1581–7.

11. Golling P, Cozzio A, Dummer R, et al. Primary cutaneous B-cell lymphomas - clinicopathological, prognostic and therapeutic characterisation of 54 cases according to the WHO-EORTC classification and the ISCL/EORTC TNM classification system for primary cutaneous lymphomas other than mycosis fungoides and Sezary syndrome. Leuk Lymphoma 2008;49(6):1094–103.

12. Bessell EM, Humber CE, O'Connor S, et al. Primary cutaneous B-cell lymphoma in Nottinghamshire U.K.: prognosis of subtypes defined in the WHO-EORTC classification. Br J Dermatol 2012;167(5):1118–23.

13. Haverkos B, Tyler K, Gru AA, et al. Primary cutaneous B-cell lymphoma: management and patterns of recurrence at the multimodality cutaneous lymphoma clinic of the Ohio state university. Oncologist 2015;20(10):1161–6.

14. Rijlaarsdam JU, van der Putte SC, Berti E, et al. Cutaneous immunocytomas: a clinicopathologic study of 26 cases. Histopathology 1993;23(2):117–25.

15. LeBoit PE, McNutt NS, Reed JA, et al. Primary cutaneous immunocytoma. A B-cell lymphoma that can easily be mistaken for cutaneous lymphoid hyperplasia. Am J Surg Pathol 1994;18(10):969–78.

16. Schmid U, Eckert F, Griesser H, et al. Cutaneous follicular lymphoid hyperplasia with monotypic plasma cells. a clinicopathologic study of 18 patients. Am J Surg Pathol 1995;19(1):12–20.

17. Duncan LM, LeBoit PE. Are primary cutaneous immunocytoma and marginal zone lymphoma the same disease? Am J Surg Pathol 1997;21(11):1368–72.

18. Suarez F, Lortholary O, Hermine O, et al. Infection-associated lymphomas derived from marginal zone B cells: a model of antigen-driven lymphoproliferation. Blood 2006;107(8):3034–44.

19. Foster LH, Portell CA. The role of infectious agents, antibiotics, and antiviral therapy in the treatment of extranodal marginal zone lymphoma and other low-grade lymphomas. Curr Treat Options Oncol 2015;16(6):28.

20. Cerroni L, Zöchling N, Pütz B, et al. Infection by Borrelia burgdorferi and cutaneous B-cell lymphoma. J Cutan Pathol 1997;24(8):457–61.

21. de la Fouchardiere A, Vandenesch F, Berger F. Borrelia-associated primary cutaneous MALT lymphoma in a nonendemic region. Am J Surg Pathol 2003;27(5): 702–3.

22. Goodlad JR, Davidson MM, Hollowood K, et al. Primary cutaneous B-cell lymphoma and Borrelia burgdorferi infection in patients from the highlands of Scotland. Am J Surg Pathol 2000;24(9):1279–85.
23. Olszewski AJ, Castillo JJ. Survival of patients with marginal zone lymphoma: analysis of the surveillance, epidemiology, and end results database. Cancer 2013; 119(3):629–38.
24. Streubel B, Simonitsch-Klupp I, Müllauer L, et al. Variable frequencies of MALT lymphoma-associated genetic aberrations in MALT lymphomas of different sites. Leukemia 2004;18(10):1722–6.
25. van Maldegem F, van Dijk R, Wormhoudt TA, et al. The majority of cutaneous marginal zone B-cell lymphomas expresses class-switched immunoglobulins and develops in a T-helper type 2 inflammatory environment. Blood 2008;112(8): 3355–61.
26. Taddesse-Heath L, Pittaluga S, Sorbara L, et al. Marginal zone B-cell lymphoma in children and young adults. Am J Surg Pathol 2003;27(4):522–31.
27. Amitay-Laish I, Tavallaee M, Kim J, et al. Paediatric primary cutaneous marginal zone B-cell lymphoma: does it differ from the adult counterpart? Br J Dermal 2016;176(4):1010–20.
28. Kempf W, Kazakov DV, Belousova IE, et al. Paediatric cutaneous lymphomas: a review and comparison with adult counterparts. J Eur Acad Dermatol Venereol 2015;29(9):1696–709.
29. Fink-Puches R, Chott A, Ardigó M, et al. The spectrum of cutaneous lymphomas in patients less than 20 years of age. Pediatr Dermatol 2004;21(5):525–33.
30. Cerroni L. Cutaneous marginal zone lymphoma (cutaneous MALT lymphoma) and variants. In: Skin lymphoma. 4th edition. Chichester (United Kingdom): John Wiley & Sons; 2014. p. 201–19.
31. Cerroni L, Signoretti S, Höfler G, et al. Primary cutaneous marginal zone B-cell lymphoma: a recently described entity of low-grade malignant cutaneous B-cell lymphoma. Am J Surg Pathol 1997;21(11):1307–15.
32. Hoefnagel JJ, Vermeer MH, Jansen PM, et al. Primary cutaneous marginal zone B-cell lymphoma: clinical and therapeutic features in 50 cases. Arch Dermatol 2005;141(9):1139–45.
33. Goteri G, Ranaldi R, Simonetti O, et al. Clinicopathological features of primary cutaneous B-cell lymphomas from an academic regional hospital in central Italy: no evidence of Borrelia burgdorferi association. Leuk Lymphoma 2007;48(11): 2184–8.
34. Ponzoni M, Ferreri AJ, Mappa S, et al. Prevalence of Borrelia burgdorferi infection in a series of 98 primary cutaneous lymphomas. Oncologist 2011;16(11):1582–8.
35. Wood GS, Kamath NV, Guitart J, et al. Absence of Borrelia burgdorferi DNA in cutaneous B-cell lymphomas from the United States. J Cutan Pathol 2001; 28(10):502–7.
36. Takino H, Li C, Hu S, et al. Primary cutaneous marginal zone B-cell lymphoma: a molecular and linicopathological study of cases from Asia, Germany, and the United States. Mod Pathol 2008;21(12):1517–26.
37. Li C, Inagaki H, Kuo TT, et al. Primary cutaneous marginal zone B-cell lymphoma: a molecular and clinicopathologic study of 24 asian cases. Am J Surg Patrol 2003;27(8):1061–9.
38. Suárez AL, Querfeld C, Horwitz S, et al. Primary cutaneous B-cell lymphomas: part II. Therapy and future directions. J Am Acad Dermatol 2013;69(3):343.e1–11.
39. Senff NJ, Noordijk EM, Kim YH, et al. European Organization for Research and Treatment of Cancer and International Society for Cutaneous Lymphoma

consensus recommendations for the management of cutaneous B-cell lymphomas. Blood 2008;112(5):1600–9.

40. Servitje O, Muniesa C, Benavente Y, et al. Primary cutaneous marginal zone B-cell lymphoma: response to treatment and disease-free survival in a series of 137 patients. J Am Acad Dermatol 2013;69(3):357–65.

41. Bailey EM, Ferry JA, Harris NL, et al. Marginal zone lymphoma (low-grade B-cell lymphoma of mucosa-associated lymphoid tissue type) of skin and subcutaneous tissue: a study of 15 patients. Am J Surg Pathol 1996;20(8):1011–23.

42. Requena L, Kutzner H, Palmedo G, et al. Cutaneous involvement in multiple myeloma: a clinicopathologic, immunohistochemical, and cytogenetic study of 8 cases. Arch Dermatol 2003;139(4):475–86.

43. Gerami P, Wickless SC, Querfeld C, et al. Cutaneous involvement with marginal zone lymphoma. J Am Acad Dermatol 2010;63(1):142–5.

44. Senff NJ, Kluin-Nelemans HC, Willemze R. Results of bone marrow examination in 275 patients with histological features that suggest an indolent type of cutaneous B-cell lymphoma. Br J Haematol 2008;142(1):52–6.

45. Magro CM, Momtahen S, Lee BA, et al. Epidermotropic B-cell lymphoma: a unique subset of CXCR3-positive marginal zone lymphoma. Am J Dermatopathol 2016;38(2):105–12.

46. Lee BA, Jacobson M, Seidel G. Epidermotropic marginal zone lymphoma simulating mycosis fungoides. J Cutan Pathol 2013;40(6):569–72.

47. Servitje O, Gallardo F, Estrach T, et al. Primary cutaneous marginal zone B-cell lymphoma: a clinical, histopathological, immunophenotypic and molecular genetic study of 22 cases. Br J Dermatol 2002;147(6):1147–58.

48. Magro CM, Yang A, Fraga G. Blastic marginal zone lymphoma: a clinical and pathological study of 8 cases and review of the literature. Am J Dermatopathol 2013;35(3):319–26.

49. de Leval L, Harris NL, Longtine J, et al. Cutaneous B-cell lymphomas of follicular and marginal zone types: use of Bcl-6, CD10, Bcl-2, and CD21 in differential diagnosis and classification. Am J Surg Pathol 2001;25(6):732–41.

50. Lozzi GP, Coletti G, Peris K. Persistent CD20-negative primary cutaneous marginal zone lymphoma after treatment with intralesional rituximab therapy. J Am Acad Dermatol 2008;59(5 Suppl):S110–2.

51. Palmedo G, Hantschke M, Rütten A, et al. Primary cutaneous marginal zone B-cell lymphoma may exhibit both the t(14;18)(q32;q21) IGH/BCL2 and the t(14;18)(q32;q21) IGH/MALT1 translocation: an indicator for clonal transformation towards higher-grade B-cell lymphoma? Am J Dermatopathol 2007;29(3):231–6.

52. Streubel B, Vinatzer U, Lamprecht A, et al. T(3;14)(p14.1;q32) involving IGH and FOXP1 is a novel recurrent chromosomal aberration in MALT lymphoma. Leukemia 2005;19(4):652–8.

53. Edinger JT, Kant JA, Swerdlow SH. Cutaneous marginal zone lymphomas have distinctive features and include 2 subsets. Am J Surg Pathol 2010;34(12):1830–41.

54. Soon CW, Pincus LB, Ai WZ, et al. Acneiform presentation of primary cutaneous follicle center lymphoma. J Am Acad Dermatol 2011;65(4):887–9.

55. Cerroni L. Cutaneous follicular center lymphoma. In: Cerroni L, editor. Skin lymphoma. 4th edition. Chichester (United Kingdom): John Wiley & Sons; 2014. p. 185–200.

56. Gulia A, Saggini A, Wiesner T, et al. Clinicopathologic features of early lesions of primary cutaneous follicle center lymphoma, diffuse type: implications for early diagnosis and treatment. J Am Acad Dermatol 2011;65(5):991–1000.

57. Morales AV, Advani R, Horwitz SM, et al. Indolent primary cutaneous B-cell lymphoma: experience using systemic rituximab. J Am Acad Dermatol 2008;59(6): 953–7.
58. Kodama K, Massone C, Chott A, et al. Primary cutaneous large B-cell lymphomas: clinicopathologic features, classification, and prognostic factors in a large series of patients. Blood 2005;106(7):2491–7.
59. Grange F, Bekkenk MW, Wechsler J, et al. Prognostic factors in primary cutaneous large B-cell lymphomas: a European multicenter study. J Clin Oncol 2001;19(16):3602–10.
60. Cerroni L, Arzberger E, Pütz B, et al. Primary cutaneous follicle center cell lymphoma with follicular growth pattern. Blood 2000;95(12):3922–8.
61. Leinweber B, Colli C, Chott A, et al. Differential diagnosis of cutaneous infiltrates of B lymphocytes with follicular growth pattern. Am J Dermatopathol 2004;26(1): 4–13.
62. Cerroni L, El-Shabrawi-Caelen L, Fink-Puches R, et al. Cutaneous spindle-cell B-cell lymphoma: a morphologic variant of cutaneous large B-cell lymphoma. Am J Dermatopathol 2000;22(4):299–304.
63. Charli-Joseph Y, Cerroni L, LeBoit PE. Cutaneous spindle-cell B-cell lymphomas:- most are neoplasms of follicular center cell origin. Am J Surg Pathol 2015;39(6): 737–43.
64. Koens L, Vermeer MH, Willemze R, et al. IgM expression on paraffin sections distinguishes primary cutaneous large B-cell lymphoma, leg type from primary cutaneous follicle center lymphoma. Am J Surg Pathol 2010;34(7):1043–8.
65. Hallermann C, Niermann C, Fischer RJ, et al. New prognostic relevant factors in primary cutaneous diffuse large B-cell lymphomas. J Am Acad Dermatol 2007; 56(4):588–97.
66. Grange F, Petrella T, Beylot-Barry M, et al. Bcl-2 protein expression is the strongest independent prognostic factor of survival in primary cutaneous large B-cell lymphomas. Blood 2004;103(10):3662–8.
67. Grange F, Beylot-Barry M, Courville P, et al. Primary cutaneous diffuse large B-cell lymphoma, leg type: clinicopathologic features and prognostic analysis in 60 cases. Arch Dermatol 2007;143(9):1144–50.
68. Demirkesen C, Tüzüner N, Esen T, et al. The expression of IgM is helpful in the differentiation of primary cutaneous diffuse large B cell lymphoma and follicle center lymphoma. Leuk Res 2011;35(9):1269–72.
69. Robson A, Shukur Z, Ally M, et al. Immunocytochemical p63 expression discriminates between primary cutaneous follicle centre cell and diffuse large B cell lymphoma-leg type, and is of theTAp63 isoform. Histopathology 2016;69(1):11–9.
70. Morales AV, Arber DA, Seo K, et al. Evaluation of B-cell clonality using the BIOMED-2 PCR method effectively distinguishes cutaneous B-cell lymphoma from benign lymphoid infiltrates. Am J Dermatopathol 2008;30(5):425–30.
71. Schafernak KT, Variakojis D, Goolsby CL, et al. Clonality assessment of cutaneous B-cell lymphoid proliferations: a comparison of flow cytometry immunophenotyping, molecular studies, and immunohistochemistry/in situ hybridization and review of the literature. Am J Dermatopathol 2014;36(10):781–95.
72. Pham-Ledard A, Cowppli-Bony A, Doussau A, et al. Diagnostic and prognostic value of BCL2 rearrangement in 53 patients with follicular lymphoma presenting as primary skin lesions. Am J Clin Pathol 2015;143(3):362–73.
73. Abdul-Wahab A, Tang SY, Robson A, et al. Chromosomal anomalies in primary cutaneous follicle center cell lymphoma do not portend a poor prognosis. J Am Acad Dermatol 2014;70(6):1010–20.

74. Streubel B, Scheucher B, Valencak J, et al. Molecular cytogenetic evidence of t(14;18)(IGH;BCL2) in a substantial proportion of primary cutaneous follicle center lymphomas. Am J Surg Pathol 2006;30(4):529–36.

75. Jelic TM, Berry PK, Jubelirer SJ, et al. Primary cutaneous follicle center lymphoma of the arm with a novel chromosomal translocation t(12;21)(q13;q22): a case report. Am J Hematol 2006;81(6):448–53.

76. Subramaniyam S, Magro CM, Gogineni S, et al. Primary cutaneous follicle center lymphoma associated with an extracutaneous dissemination: a cytogenetic finding of potential prognostic value. Am J Clin Pathol 2015;144(5):805–10.

77. Grange F, Joly P, Barbe C, et al. Improvement of survival in patients with primary cutaneous diffuse large B-cell lymphoma, leg type, in France. JAMA Dermatol 2014;150(5):535–41.

78. Cerroni L. Cutaneous diffuse large B-cell lymphoma, leg type. In: Cerroni L, editor. Skin lymphoma. 4th edition. Chichester (United Kingdom): John Wiley & Sons; 2014. p. 220–31.

79. Plaza JA, Kacerovska D, Stockman DL, et al. The histomorphologic spectrum of primary cutaneous diffuse large B-cell lymphoma: a study of 79 cases. Am J Dermatopathol 2011;33(7):649–55.

80. Massone C, Fink-Puches R, Wolf I, et al. Atypical clinicopathologic presentation of primary cutaneous diffuse large B-cell lymphoma, leg type. J Am Acad Dermatol 2015;72(6):1016–20.

81. Menguy S, Gros A, Pham-Ledard A, et al. MYD88 somatic mutation is a diagnostic criterion in primary cutaneous large B-cell lymphoma. J Invest Dermatol 2016;136(8):1741–4.

82. Pham-Ledard A, Beylot-Barry M, Barbe C, et al. High frequency and clinical prognostic value of MYD88 L265P mutation in primary cutaneous diffuse large B-cell lymphoma, leg-type. JAMA Dermatol 2014;150(11):1173–9.

83. Senff NJ, Zoutman WH, Vermeer MH, et al. Fine-mapping chromosomal loss at 9p21: correlation with prognosis in primary cutaneous diffuse large B-cell lymphoma, leg type. J Invest Dermatol 2009;129(5):1149–55.

84. Murase T, Nakamura S, Kawauchi K, et al. An Asian variant of intravascular large B-cell lymphoma: clinical, pathological and cytogenetic approaches to diffuse large B-cell lymphoma associated with haemophagocytic syndrome. Br J Haematol 2000;111(3):826–34.

85. Ferreri AJ, Dognini GP, Campo E, et al. Variations in clinical presentation, frequency of hemophagocytosis and clinical behavior of intravascular lymphoma diagnosed in different geographical regions. Haematologica 2007;92(4):486–92.

86. Ferreri AJ, Campo E, Seymour JF, et al. Intravascular lymphoma: clinical presentation, natural history, management and prognostic factors in a series of 38 cases, with special emphasis on the cutaneous variant. Br J Haematol 2004; 127:173–83.

87. Cerroni L. Intravascular large cell lymphomas. In: Skin lymphoma. 4th edition. Chichester (United Kingdom): John Wiley & Sons; 2014. p. 232–6.

88. Murase T, Yamaguchi M, Suzuki R, et al. Intravascular large B-cell lymphoma (IVLBCL): a clinicopathologic study of 96 cases with special reference to the immunophenotypic heterogeneity of CD5. Blood 2007;109(2):478–85.

89. Saurel CA, Personett DA, Edenfield BH, et al. Molecular analysis of intravascular large B-cell lymphoma with neoangiogenesis. Br J Haematol 2011;152(2):234–6.

90. Ponzoni M, Arrigoni G, Gould VE, et al. Lack of CD29 (beta1 integrin) and CD54 (ICAM-1) adhesion molecules in intravascular lymphomatosis. Hum Pathol 2000; 31:220–6.

91. Kinoshita M, Izumoto S, Hashimoto N, et al. Immunohistochemical analysis of adhesion molecules and matrix metalloproteinases in malignant CNS lymphomas:a study comparing primary CNS malignant and CNS intravascular lymphomas. Brain Tumor Pathol 2008;25(2):73–8.
92. Kato M, Ohshima K, Mizuno M, et al. Analysis of CXCL9 and CXCR3 expression in a case of intravascular large B-cell lymphoma. J Am Acad Dermatol 2009; 61(5):888–91.

Myeloid Neoplasms

Antonio Subtil, MD, MBA[a,b,*]

KEYWORDS

- Myeloid • Neoplasms • Skin • Leukemia • Cutis • Acute • Chronic
- Myelomonocytic

KEY POINTS

- Myeloid neoplasms may involve the skin and may be the presenting sign of underlying bone marrow disease.
- Dermal infiltration by neoplastic myeloid cells may occur in otherwise normal skin or in sites of cutaneous inflammation.
- Leukemia cutis may precede evidence of blood and/or bone marrow involvement (aleukemic leukemia cutis).
- The classification of myeloid neoplasms has undergone major changes and currently relies heavily on genetic abnormalities.

INTRODUCTION

Myeloid neoplasms comprise a complex and heterogeneous group of hematopoietic diseases with variable prognosis.[1] The classification of myeloid leukemias has undergone major changes and currently relies heavily on genetic abnormalities (**Box 1**).[2] Cutaneous manifestations may be the presenting sign of underlying bone marrow disease.[3] A variety of patterns may occur in the skin and include cutaneous involvement by acute myeloid leukemia (AML), inflammatory dermatoses with variable association with myelodysplastic and myeloproliferative disorders, cutaneous involvement by chronic myelomonocytic leukemia, and cutaneous involvement by blastic plasmacytoid dendritic cell neoplasm.

Cutaneous Manifestations of Acute Myeloid Leukemia (AML)

Certain inflammatory dermatoses may be associated with underlying myelodysplastic/myeloproliferative disorders and include Sweet syndrome, pyoderma gangrenosum, neutrophilic eccrine hidradenitis, vasculitis, and erythema nodosum.[4] In addition, the skin may be infiltrated by leukemic cells. Myeloid leukemia cutis occasionally precedes

Disclosure: No conflicts of interest or financial relationships.
[a] Department of Dermatology, Yale Dermatopathology Laboratory, 15 York Street, LMP5031, New Haven, CT 06520, USA; [b] Department of Pathology, Yale Dermatopathology Laboratory, 15 York Street, LMP5031, New Haven, CT 06520, USA
* Department of Dermatology, Yale Dermatopathology Laboratory, 15 York Street, LMP5031, New Haven, CT 06520.
E-mail address: antonio.subtil@yale.edu

Clin Lab Med 37 (2017) 575–585
http://dx.doi.org/10.1016/j.cll.2017.05.005
0272-2712/17/© 2017 Elsevier Inc. All rights reserved.

labmed.theclinics.com

Box 1
Subtypes of acute myeloid leukemia.[a]

Acute myeloid leukemia (AML) with recurrent genetic abnormalities
  AML with t(8;21) (q22;q22.1);RUNX1-RUNX1T1
  AML with inv(16) (p13.1q22) or t(16;16) (p13.1;q22);CBFB-MYH11
  Acute promyelocytic leukemia with PML-RARA
  AML with t(9;11) (p21.3;q23.3);MLLT3-KMT2A
  AML with t(6;9) (p23;q34.1);DEK-NUP214
  AML with inv(3) (q21.3q26.2) or t(3;3) (q21.3;q26.2); GATA2, MECOM
  AML (megakaryoblastic) with t(1;22) (p13.3;q13.3);RBM15-MKL1
  Provisional entity: AML with BCR-ABL1
  AML with mutated NPM1(see **Figs. 1** and **2**)
  AML with biallelic mutations of CEBPA
  Provisional entity: AML with mutated RUNX1 (see **Fig. 5**)

AML with myelodysplasia-related changes (see **Fig. 3**)

Therapy-related myeloid neoplasms

AML, NOS (not otherwise specified)
  AML with minimal differentiation
  AML without maturation
  AML with maturation
  Acute myelomonocytic leukemia
  Acute monoblastic/monocytic leukemia
  Pure erythroid leukemia
  Acute megakaryoblastic leukemia
  Acute basophilic leukemia
  Acute panmyelosis with myelofibrosis

Myeloid sarcoma

[a]Three examples are shown in Figs. 1–3, 5
Adapted from Arber DA, Orazi A, Hasserjian R, et al. The 2016 revision to the World Health Organization classification of myeloid neoplasms and acute leukemia. Blood 2016;127(20):2392; with permission.

---

evidence of peripheral blood and/or bone marrow involvement (aleukemic leukemia cutis).[5]

Specific AML subtypes have been refined by focusing on significant cytogenetic and molecular genetic subgroups with variable impact on prognosis and treatment.[1] A large number of recurring, balanced cytogenetic abnormalities are recognized as subtype defining by the World Health Organization (WHO) classification (see **Box 1**).[2] Tissue infiltrates of AML (myeloid sarcoma) may represent a unique clinical presentation of any subtype of AML.[1] Myeloid sarcoma may present de novo, may accompany blood and marrow involvement, may present as relapse of prior AML, or may present as progression of a prior myelodysplastic syndrome, myeloproliferative neoplasm, or myelodysplastic/myeloproliferative neoplasm.[2] In a large series of myeloid leukemia cutis, skin lesions were de novo in 7.5%, concurrent in 26.6%, and subsequent in 60.7%.[6] Although any subtype of AML may involve the skin secondarily, acute myelomonocytic leukemia and acute monocytic leukemia are the most common.[6]

Most patients with myeloid leukemia cutis are adults, but children and neonates may also be affected, particularly in cases of acute leukemia with MLL translocations.[1] Skin lesions may be reddish-brown or violaceous papules, plaques, or tumors. Oral mucosa (especially gingiva) may be involved.[5]

The histopathologic pattern often shows a triple combination of perivascular, interstitial, and periadnexal arrangement of immature mononuclear cells in the reticular dermis with variable pannicular extension (**Fig. 1**). The infiltrate can vary from mild to dense and diffuse, but is generally nonepitheliotropic.[5] Leukemic vasculitis is rare.[7] The atypical mononuclear cells show high nuclear cytoplasmic ratio, delicate chromatin, and prominent nucleoli (**Fig. 2**). Nuclear folds may also be observed.[1] Rarely, the leukemic cells show cytoplasmic granules (**Fig. 3**). An immunohistochemical panel is generally necessary to differentiate among the various diseases with atypical hematolymphoid cells in the skin (**Table 1** and **Fig. 4**). Dermal infiltration by leukemic cells may occur in otherwise normal skin or in sites of cutaneous inflammation (**Fig. 5**).

The immunophenotype is variable depending on the type of AML, but lack of T-cell markers (eg, CD3), B-cell markers (CD20, CD79a), and CD30 associated with CD43 expression is characteristic (see **Fig. 4**). Myeloperoxidase (42%–62.5% of cases), lysozyme, CD13, CD33 (93%), and/or CD68 (94%–100%) expression is common.[6,8,9] There is variable expression of CD117 and HLA-DR.[1] CD34 is often negative, particularly in acute PML-RARA.[1] In 2 series of myeloid leukemia cutis, CD34 and CD117 were insufficiently sensitive (CD34 expression identified in only 6%–17% of cases, and CD117 in 10%–33%).[8,9] CD19, PAX5, and/or cytoplasmic CD79a may be expressed in AML with t(8;21) (q22;q22.1);RUNX1-RUNX1T1.[1] A mixed phenotype (myeloid and lymphoblastic) may be observed in acute leukemias with MLL translocations.[1] CD56 and CD123 are occasionally expressed, and an extended immunohistochemical panel may be needed to differentiate AML from blastic plasmacytoid dendritic cell neoplasm (BPDCN).[10] Myeloid cell nuclear differentiation antigen (MNDA) may be helpful in this differential given its absence in BPDCN.[11] In cases with concurrent or prior systemic AML, there is frequent discrepancy between the immunophenotype (particularly expression of CD34 and CD117) in the skin and in

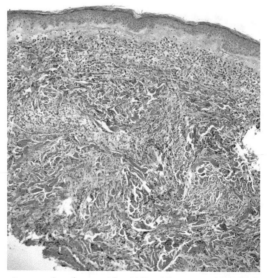

Fig. 1. Secondary cutaneous involvement by AML with mutated NPM1. Perivascular, interstitial, and periadnexal dermal infiltration by leukemic cells. The epidermis is not involved. A grenz zone of uninvolved papillary dermis is present (hematoxylin and eosin, original magnification, ×40).

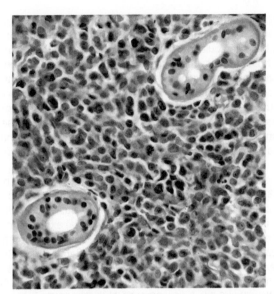

Fig. 2. Secondary cutaneous involvement by AML with mutated NPM1. The infiltrate shows perieccrine infiltration. The atypical mononuclear cells show high nuclear cytoplasmic ratio, delicate chromatin, and prominent nucleolus (hematoxylin and eosin, original magnification ×400).

the bone marrow or peripheral blood.[9] This lack of concordance may result from antigen downregulation by extramedullary or posttreatment blasts as well as from the difference in sensitivity or antibody epitope targets between flow cytometric and immunohistochemical techniques.[6,9,12] Fluorescence in situ hybridization (FISH) for recurrent cytogenetic abnormalities may be performed in skin biopsies (see **Box 1**).[9]

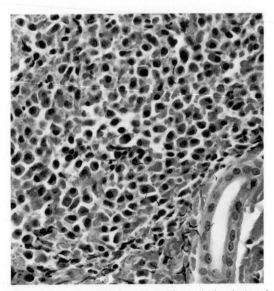

Fig. 3. Secondary cutaneous involvement by AML with myelodysplasia-related changes. The atypical mononuclear cells show cytoplasmic granules (hematoxylin and eosin, original magnification ×400).

Key features: cutaneous involvement by acute myeloid leukemia

- Any subtype of AML may involve the skin secondarily; however, acute myelomonocytic leukemia and acute monocytic leukemia are the most common.

- Myeloid leukemia cutis occasionally precedes evidence of peripheral blood and/or bone marrow involvement (aleukemic leukemia cutis).

- Skin biopsies show a characteristic pattern of dermal infiltration by blasts (triple combination of interstitial, perivascular, and periadnexal patterns).

- The immunophenotype is variable depending on the type of AML, but lack of T-cell markers (CD3), B-cell markers (CD20), and CD30 associated with CD43 expression is characteristic.

- FISH for recurrent cytogenetic abnormalities may be performed in skin biopsies of myeloid leukemia cutis.

Cutaneous Involvement by Chronic Myelomonocytic Leukemia

Chronic myelomonocytic leukemia (CMML) is a clonal hematopoietic neoplasm characterized by both myelodysplastic and myeloproliferative features and generally associated with persistent peripheral blood monocytosis.[1] BCR-ABL1 fusion gene is not present in CMML.[1] ASXL1 mutations are frequent in CMML and are prognostically detrimental.[13]

Table 1
Usual staining pattern of acute myeloid leukemia compared with other atypical cutaneous mononuclear infiltrates

	T-cell Markers (CD3, CD2)	B-cell Markers (CD20, CD79a)	CD30	CD43	TdT	Additional Markers
AML	−	−	−	+	−/+	Variable expression of myeloperoxidase, lysozyme, CD34, CD68, CD13, CD33, CD117, HLA-DR
CTCL	+	−	−/+	+	−	CD4, CD8, TIA1, CD56, CD45RO, CD5, CD7
CBCL	−	+	−	−/+	−	Kappa, lambda, CD21, CD5, CD10, CD23, BCL6, BCL2, MUM1, Cyclin D1, Ki-67
Cutaneous CD30+ lymphoproliferative disorders	+	−	+	+	−	ALK, CD4, CD8, TIA1, CD5, CD7, EMA
T-ALL	+	−	−	NA	+	CD7, CD2, CD5, CD4, CD8, CD34, CD45, CD117
B-ALL	−	+	−	NA	+	CD19, CD10, CD34, CD22, CD38, CD45, HLA-DR

Abbreviations: B-ALL, B acute lymphoblastic leukemia; CBCL, cutaneous B-cell lymphoma; CTCL, cutaneous T-cell lymphoma; NA, not applicable; T-ALL, T acute lymphoblastic leukemia.

Data from Swerdlow SH, Campo E, Harris NL, et al, editors. WHO Classification of tumors of hematopoietic and lymphoid tissues. Lyon (France): IARC; 2008.

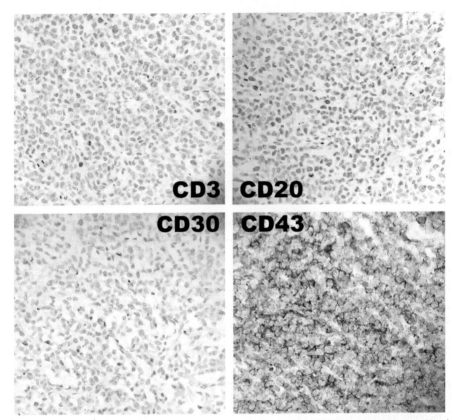

Fig. 4. Usual immunohistochemical staining pattern of AML: CD43 expression associated with negative CD30, B-cell (CD20), and T-cell (CD3) markers (immunoperoxidase, original magnification ×100).

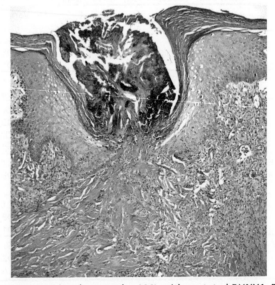

Fig. 5. Secondary cutaneous involvement by AML with mutated RUNX1. Focal dermal infiltration by leukemic cells may occur in sites of cutaneous inflammation. Superficial ulceration with bacterial impetiginization in a patient with AML (hematoxylin and eosin, original magnification ×100).

Secondary cutaneous involvement has been estimated to occur in 10% of patients with CMML and may be associated with disease progression to AML.[14] Pruritus may be a presenting symptom in CMML and may precede the diagnosis by several years.[3] A variety of hematolymphoid neoplasms can present with pruritus as the initial symptom, and resolution of the pruritus after treatment of the underlying disease may occur. This phenomenon has been documented in Hodgkin lymphoma (10%–30% of patients), polycythemia vera (30%–50%), and occasionally in other lymphomas and leukemias.[15]

Secondary cutaneous involvement by CMML usually shows a polymorphous dermal infiltrate including a small subset of immature myeloid cells admixed with histiocytes, lymphocytes, plasma cells, and mature neutrophils. There is often a subset of mature plasmacytoid dendritic cells, which can be highlighted by CD123 stain (**Fig. 6**).[16] A subset of indeterminate dendritic cells (CD1a+, Langerin−) may also be present.[16]

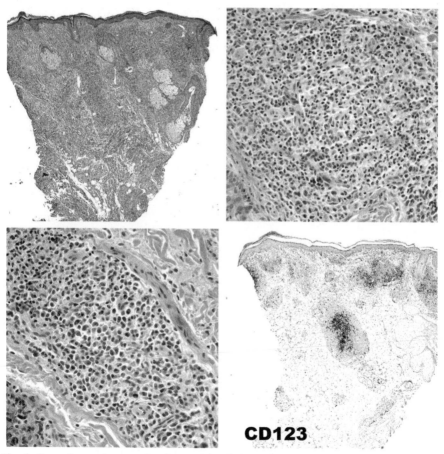

CD123

Fig. 6. Secondary cutaneous involvement by CMML. There is a moderate, polymorphous dermal infiltrate including a small subset of immature myeloid cells admixed with histiocytes, lymphocytes, plasma cells, and neutrophils. CD123 stain highlights a subset of mature plasmacytoid dendritic cells (hematoxylin and eosin and immunoperoxidase, original magnification ×40 and ×100).

Key features: cutaneous involvement by chronic myelomonocytic leukemia

- CMML is a clonal hematopoietic neoplasm characterized by both myelodysplastic and myeloproliferative features and generally associated with persistent peripheral blood monocytosis.

- Secondary cutaneous involvement has been estimated to occur in 10% of patients with CMML and may be associated with disease progression to AML. Pruritus may be a presenting symptom in CMML.

- Skin biopsies show a polymorphous dermal infiltrate including a small subset of immature myeloid cells admixed with histiocytes, lymphocytes, plasma cells, and mature neutrophils. There is often a subset of mature CD123 + plasmacytoid dendritic cells and CD1a+, Langerin-indeterminate dendritic cells.

Blastic Plasmacytoid Dendritic Cell Neoplasm

BPDCN is an aggressive hematopoietic neoplasm derived from precursor plasmacytoid dendritic cells. There is a high frequency of both cutaneous and bone marrow involvement at presentation, and the median survival is 12 to 14 months.[1] Before the cell of origin was elucidated, BPDCN was initially termed blastic NK-cell lymphoma and CD4+/CD56 + hematodermic neoplasm.[17] Since 2008, BPDCN has been classified by the WHO as part of the group of AMLs and related precursor neoplasms.[1]

Patients usually present with multiple nodules and plaques, but presentation with a solitary skin lesion may occur. Bruiselike patches and mucosal involvement have been described.[18] Lymphadenopathy may be seen in 20% of cases.[1] There is a male predominance.[18] Most patients are adults, but children may also be affected.[1]

Microscopically, there is an interstitial, perivascular, periadnexal, and/or diffuse dermal infiltrate of variable density (**Fig. 7**).[19] Pannicular extension may be seen.

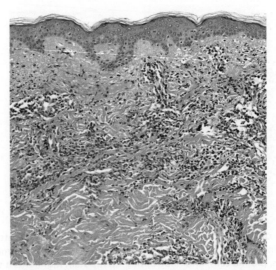

Fig. 7. BPDCN. Perivascular, interstitial, and periadnexal dermal infiltration by leukemic cells. The epidermis is not involved (hematoxylin and eosin, original magnification ×40).

Monomorphous, medium-sized blastoid cells show fine chromatin, 1 to several small nucleoli, and generally scant cytoplasm. A morphologic variant of BPDCN with cleaved nuclei may morphologically resemble cutaneous follicle center lymphoma but is negative with B-cell markers.[19]

An extensive immunohistochemical panel is often necessary to exclude other hematolymphoid neoplasms and to document plasmacytoid dendritic cell origin. The following markers are almost always positive: CD4, CD56, CD43, CD45RA, CD123, and TCL1 (**Fig. 8**), although cases without CD4 or CD56 have been reported.[1] Regularly negative markers include CD3, CD5, CD13, CD16, CD19, CD20, CD79a, CD34, CD117, TIA1, lysozyme, myeloperoxidase, and Epstein-Barr virus (EBV; EBV-encoded small RNA [EBER]). There is variable expression of CD68 (50% of cases; cytoplasmic dot pattern), TdT (33% of cases), CD7, CD2, and CD38. CD33 may be expressed by BPDCN, which may cause diagnostic confusion with myeloperoxidase-negative myeloid leukemia cutis.[10] MNDA may be helpful in the differential with AML given its absence in BPDCN.[11] CD303 expression and high proliferative index (Ki-67) have been reported to be significantly associated with longer survival.[20]

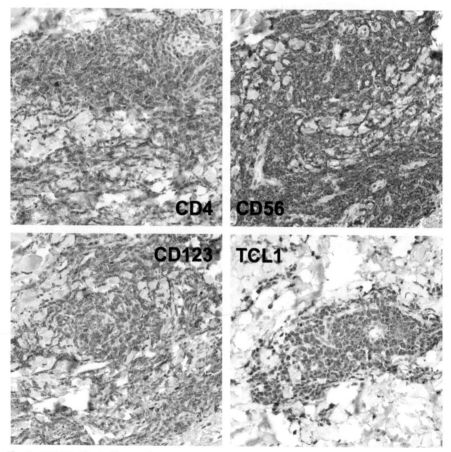

Fig. 8. BPDCN. The infiltrate shows expression of CD4, CD56, CD123, and TCL1 (immunoperoxidase, original magnification ×100).

Key features: blastic plasmacytoid dendritic cell neoplasm

- BPDCN is an aggressive hematopoietic neoplasm derived from precursor plasmacytoid dendritic cells.

- There is a high frequency of both cutaneous and bone marrow involvement.

- Skin biopsies show a variably dense, interstitial, perivascular, periadnexal, and/or diffuse dermal infiltrate of monomorphous, medium-sized blastoid cells.

- An extensive immunohistochemical panel is often necessary to exclude other hematolymphoid neoplasms and to document plasmacytoid dendritic cell origin. However, CD4, CD56, CD43, CD45RA, CD123, and TCL1 are almost always positive.

Pearls and pitfalls: myeloid neoplasms

- The immunophenotype of AML is variable. However, almost all cases show CD43 expression in association with negative CD30, B-cell (CD20), and T-cell (CD3) markers.

- The classification of myeloid neoplasms relies heavily on genetic abnormalities, which may be investigated in a skin biopsy showing a leukemic infiltrate.

- A clue to the diagnosis of BPDCN is an atypical mononuclear dermal infiltrate with multiple negative markers (including CD3, CD20, CD79a, and myeloperoxidase).

- Nonneoplastic (mature) plasmacytoid dendritic cells are negative with CD56 and TdT.

REFERENCES

1. Swerdlow SH, Campo E, Harris NL, et al, editors. WHO classification of tumors of hematopoietic and lymphoid tissues. Lyon (France): IARC; 2008.

2. Arber DA, Orazi A, Hasserjian R, et al. The 2016 revision to the World Health Organization classification of myeloid neoplasms and acute leukemia. Blood 2016; 127(20):2391–405.

3. Peterson AO, Jarratt M. Pruritus and nonspecific nodules preceding myelomonocytic leukemia. J Am Acad Dermatol 1980;2(6):496–8.

4. Winfield HL, Smoller BR. Lymphoproliferative and myeloproliferative diseases. In: Bolognia JL, Jorizzo JL, Schaffer JV, editors. Dermatology. 3rd edition. Philadelphia: Saunders Elsevier; 2012. p. 2037–47.

5. Cerroni L. Skin lymphoma. The illustrated guide. Hoboken (NJ): Wiley-Blackwell; 2014.

6. Benet C, Gomez A, Aguilar C, et al. Histologic and immunohistologic characterization of skin localization of myeloid disorders a study of 173 cases. Am J Clin Pathol 2011;135:278–90.

7. Odell ID, Zeidan AM, Parker TL, et al. Leukaemic vasculitis with myelodysplastic syndrome. Lancet 2015;386(9992):501–2.

8. Cibull TL, Thomas AB, O'Malley DP, et al. Myeloid leukemia cutis: a histologic and immunohistochemical review. J Cutan Pathol 2008;35:180–5.

9. Cronin DM, George TI, Sundram UN. An updated approach to the diagnosis of myeloid leukemia cutis. Am J Clin Pathol 2009;132:101–10.

10. Cronin DM, George TI, Reichard KK, et al. Immunophenotypic analysis of myeloperoxidase-negative leukemia cutis and blastic plasmacytoid dendritic cell neoplasm. Am J Clin Pathol 2012;137(3):367–76.

11. Johnson RC, Kim J, Natkunam Y, et al. Myeloid cell nuclear differentiation antigen (MNDA) expression distinguishes extramedullary presentations of myeloid leukemia from blastic plasmacytoid dendritic cell neoplasm. Am J Surg Pathol 2016; 40(4):502–9.

12. Sachdev R, George TI, Schwartz EJ, et al. Discordant immunophenotypic profiles of adhesion molecules and cytokines in acute myeloid leukemia involving bone marrow and skin. Am J Clin Pathol 2012;138:290–9.

13. Patnaik MM, Itzykson R, Lasho TL, et al. ASXL1 and SETBP1 mutations and their prognostic contribution in chronic myelomonocytic leukemia: a two-center study of 466 patients. Leukemia 2014;28(11):2206–12.

14. Matthew RA, Bennett JM, Liu JJ, et al. Cutaneous manifestations in CMML: indication of disease acceleration or transformation to AML and review of the literature. Leuk Res 2012;36(1):72–80.

15. Weisshaar E, Fleischer AB, Bernhard JD, et al. Pruritus and dysesthesia. In: Bolognia JL, Jorizzo JL, Schaffer JV, editors. Dermatology. 3rd edition. Philadelphia: Saunders Elsevier; 2012. p. 111–25.

16. Vitte F, Fabiani B, Benet C, et al. Specific skin lesions in chronic myelomonocytic leukemia. Am J Surg Pathol 2012;36:1302–16.

17. Petrella T, Comeau MR, Maynadié M, et al. Agranular CD4+ CD56+ hematodermic neoplasm (blastic NK-cell lymphoma) originates from a population of CD56+ precursor cells related to plasmacytoid monocytes. Am J Surg Pathol 2002;26(7): 852–62.

18. Julia F, Petrella T, Beylot-Barry M, et al. Blastic plasmacytoid dendritic cell neoplasm: clinical features in 90 patients. Br J Dermatol 2013;169(3):579–86.

19. Cota C, Vale E, Viana I, et al. Cutaneous manifestations of blastic plasmacytoid dendritic cell neoplasm–morphologic and phenotypic variability in a series of 33 patients. Am J Surg Pathol 2010;34(1):75–87.

20. Julia F, Dalle S, Duru G, et al. Blastic plasmacytoid dendritic cell neoplasms: clinico-immunohistochemical correlations in a series of 91 patients. Am J Surg Pathol 2014;38(5):673–80.

Cutaneous Sweat Gland Carcinomas with Basaloid Differentiation

An Update with Emphasis on Differential Diagnoses

Katharina Flux, MD[a,b], Thomas Brenn, MD, PhD, FRCPath[c,*]

KEYWORDS

- Basaloid • Primary cutaneous • Sweat gland carcinoma • Mucinous carcinoma
- Endocrine • Adenoid-cystic • Apocrine

KEY POINTS

- The clinical behavior of sweat gland carcinomas ranges from indolent to aggressive.
- Sweat gland carcinomas show significant morphologic overlap.
- The histologic features of sweat gland carcinomas do not always correlate well with outcome.
- Separating sweat gland carcinomas from metastases of visceral adenocarcinomas may be impossible on histology alone and careful clinical work-up may be necessary.

INTRODUCTION

Cutaneous sweat gland tumors show a wide range of histologic features and clinical behavior. Most sweat gland tumors are benign and experience with malignant tumors is limited. The clinical behavior of sweat gland carcinomas ranges from indolent with potential for locally destructive growth and recurrence but only rare metastatic disease to those with frankly malignant behavior and associated mortality. Accurate diagnosis and classification is therefore necessary to predict prognosis and guide treatment. A particular diagnostic challenge is the morphologic overlap of some sweat gland carcinomas with benign disorders because of their deceptively bland histologic appearances. Furthermore, the separation of cutaneous metastases from visceral primary adenocarcinomas poses a significant challenge. Although the demonstration of

The authors have nothing to disclose.
[a] Labor für Dermatohistologie und Oralpathologie, Bayersstrasse 69, Munich 80335, Germany;
[b] Department of Dermatology, University of Heidelberg, Neuenheimer Feld 440, Heidelberg 69120, Germany; [c] Department of Pathology, Western General Hospital, The University of Edinburgh, Crewe Road, Edinburgh EH4 2XU, UK
* Corresponding author.
E-mail address: t_brenn@yahoo.com

Clin Lab Med 37 (2017) 587–601
http://dx.doi.org/10.1016/j.cll.2017.05.006
0272-2712/17/© 2017 Elsevier Inc. All rights reserved.

labmed.theclinics.com

a myoepithelial layer is a helpful clue for some primary cutaneous tumors, others can only be separated on clinical grounds with the aid of clinical history and screening.

The following discussion of sweat gland carcinomas with basaloid features highlights these issues. It includes rare and possibly underrecognized neoplasms, such as primary cutaneous cribriform apocrine carcinoma, a tumor of indolent behavior; endocrine mucin-producing sweat gland carcinoma (EMPSGC), a tumor of indolent behavior that may be a precursor to invasive mucinous carcinoma; primary cutaneous adenoid cystic carcinoma, a tumor with high local recurrence rates but infrequent metastasis despite its identical histologic and genetic features to visceral primary neoplasms; spiradenocarcinoma, the behavior of which is predicted by its morphologic appearances, ranging from locally aggressive to outright malignant with associated mortality; and digital papillary adenocarcinoma, characterized by potential for disseminated metastatic disease and mortality despite innocuous and bland histologic features. The salient diagnostic features and pitfalls of these neoplasms with emphasis on differential diagnosis are discussed here.

PRIMARY CUTANEOUS CRIBRIFORM APOCRINE CARCINOMA

Primary cutaneous cribriform apocrine carcinoma is a poorly documented and rare neoplasm. It has been proposed to represent part of a morphologic spectrum with apocrine carcinoma.[1] Its entirely indolent and benign behavior raises the question whether it should truly be regarded as a carcinoma.

Clinical Presentation

The tumors are slowly growing firm nodules, measuring 1 cm to 3 cm in diameter. There is a strong predilection for the proximal extremities of middle-aged adults and females are twice as frequently affected as males.[1–3] The clinical behavior is entirely benign with as yet no documented recurrences or metastases.[1,2]

Histologic Features

This well-circumscribed, nodular but unencapsulated neoplasm is centered in the dermis (**Fig. 1**A). It is composed of interconnecting islands and strands of medium-sized cuboidal tumor cells showing prominent duct formation, giving rise to a cribriform architecture (see **Fig. 1**B). There is little cytologic atypia and nuclear pleomorphism is not a feature (see **Fig. 1**C). The mitotic activity is low. Focal decapitation secretion may be present as evidence of its apocrine differentiation.

Immunohistochemistry

Tumor cells express cytokeratins, AE1/3, MNF116, Cam5.2, and cytokeratin 7 (CK7). Epithelial membrane antigen (EMA) and carcinoembryonic antigen (CEA) staining highlights luminal differentiation. S100 staining shows patchy positivity in tumor cells but smooth muscle actin (SMA) and calponin fail to demonstrate a surrounding myoepithelial cell layer.

Differential Diagnosis

Primary cutaneous cribriform apocrine carcinoma shows a characteristic and reproducible histologic appearance. It is separated from adenoid cystic carcinoma by lack of an infiltrative architecture and absence of the characteristic mucin-filled pseudocysts. Aggressive digital papillary adenocarcinoma is characterized by a solid and cystic growth with macropapillae. Furthermore, it is confined to the distal extremities.

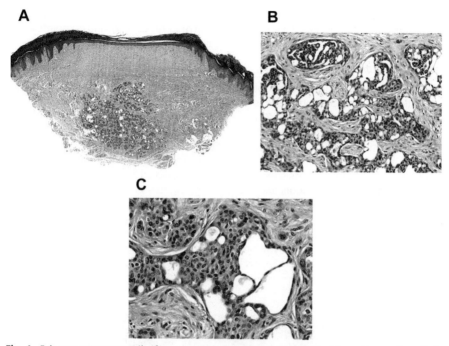

Fig. 1. Primary cutaneous cribriform apocrine carcinoma. This dermal-based tumor is well circumscribed but unencapsulated (*A*, HE, original magnification ×20). It is composed of interconnecting epithelial nests and strands separated by a loose fibrous stroma. Florid duct differentiation gives rise to its cribriform appearance (*B*, HE, original magnification ×200). Tumor cells are medium-sized cuboidal lacking cytologic atypia (*C*, HE, original magnification ×400).

Tubular adenoma shows significant morphologic overlap. It is, however, defined by its tubular growth pattern with preserved myoepithelilal cell differentiation.

Key features: primary cutaneous cribriform apocrine carcinoma

- Rare and possible underrecognized entity
- Distinctive and reproducible histologic features
- Benign behavior with as yet no reported recurrence, metastasis, or mortality
- Perhaps best regarded as adenoma rather than carcinoma

ENDOCRINE MUCIN-PRODUCING SWEAT GLAND CARCINOMA

EMPSGC was originally reported on 1997.[4] It is a rare, poorly documented, and likely underreported entity, closely related to solid papillary carcinoma of the breast or endocrine ductal carcinoma in situ.[4,5] It is characterized by distinctive histologic features, a narrow anatomic distribution, and indolent clinical behavior with favorable prognosis. The tumors may arise in association with mucinous carcinoma and likely represent a precursor.[5]

Clinical Presentation

EMPSGC presents as a solitary, slowly growing swelling or cystic lesion in the periorbital region and the cheek, with a strong predilection for the eyelids.[5] It is debatable whether similar tumors at other body sites truly represent this entity.[6,7] The patients are elderly adults (median, 70 years) with a female predilection (female/male ratio, 2:1).[5] The clinical behavior is indolent with only rare local recurrence following complete excision.[8] No metastases or disease-related mortality has been documented.

Histologic Features

EMPSGC is a well-circumscribed lobulated tumor with solid, cystic, and papillary differentiation in varying proportions. It is located in the dermis and shows no connection with the overlying epidermis (**Fig. 2**A). The solid tumor lobules are composed of uniform, medium-sized ovoid cells with moderate amounts of pale eosinophilic cytoplasm and centrally placed nuclei with a stippled chromatin pattern (see **Fig. 2**B). Cytologic atypia is limited and nuclear pleomorphism is rare. Occasional mitotic activity is present but tumor necrosis is uncommon. Occasional cells contain intracellular mucin. Extracellular mucin pools are also noted giving rise to a cribriform architecture with pseudocysts (see **Fig. 2**B). True cystic spaces are admixed. They may show decapitation secretion and papillary or micropapillary growth (see **Fig. 2**C). Although the tumor nodules show no evidence of myoepithelial differentiation by immunohistochemistry, the tumor rarely involves pre-existing benign structures suggestive of an in situ component and further support of its primary cutaneous origin. A subset of

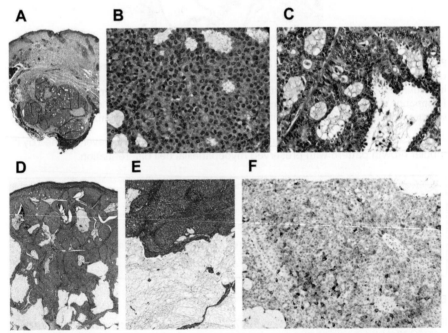

Fig. 2. Endocrine mucin-producing sweat gland carcinoma. The tumor is based within deep dermis and shows a well-demarcated multinodular growth pattern (A, HE, original magnification ×20). The tumor cells are medium sized with eosinophilic cytoplasm and centrally placed nuclei with inconspicuous nucleoli. They show a sheet-like growth pattern with mucin-filled pseudocysts (B, HE, original magnification ×200). True cyst differentiation with apocrine decapitation secretion is also noted (C, HE, original magnification ×200). Endocrine mucin-producing sweat gland carcinoma with transition to mucinous carcinoma characterized by large mucin pools separated by delicate fibrous bands and containing scattered epithelial strands (D [HE, original magnification ×10], E [HE, original magnification ×40]). The tumor expresses the neuroendocrine marker synaptophysin (F, synaptophysin, original magnification ×100).

tumors shows transition to invasive mucinous carcinoma with small tumor islands suspended in large mucin lakes (see **Fig. 2**D, E). EMPSGC may therefore be regarded as a precursor lesion to invasive mucinous carcinoma.

Immunohistochemistry

The tumor cells of EMPSGC are positive for at least one neuroendocrine marker (synaptophysin, chromogranin, neuron-specific enolase, CD57) and low-molecular cytokeratins (Cam5.2 and CK7) (see **Fig. 2**F). EMA highlights luminal differentiation and the tumor cells express estrogen and progesterone receptors. The tumor cells are consistently negative for cytokeratin 20 (CK20) and S100 protein.[5]

Differential Diagnosis

Primary cutaneous mucinous carcinoma is less well demarcated with invasion of deeper tissue. It is characterized by large mucin-filled lakes containing scattered epithelial islands, cords, and strands. Cutaneous metastasis from a visceral primary, particularly of breast origin, is an important consideration. The location on the eyelid and demonstration of a focal in situ component argues in favor of a primary cutaneous tumor. In most instances clinical correlation and investigation for a visceral primary is, however, necessary. Periocular sebaceous carcinoma enters the differential diagnosis because of its basaloid differentiation and location on the eyelids. These tumors show more pronounced cytologic atypia and lack mucin production and cyst differentiation. A connection with the overlying epidermis is often noted and epidermal ulceration and pagetoid spread of tumor cells may be additional findings. The hallmark feature of sebaceous carcinoma is the presence of lipidized cells with a vacuolated cytoplasm and indented nuclei as highlighted by EMA and adipophilin immunohistochemistry. Adenoid cystic carcinoma shows a more infiltrative growth pattern of variable-sized tumor nests, and perineural invasion is almost invariably present. By immunohistochemistry it shows myoepithelial differentiation with expression of SMA and S100 in addition to cytokeratins. Cribriform apocrine carcinoma lacks the solid areas and the mucin production characteristic of EMPSGC. The adenoid-cystic variant of basal cell carcinoma is characterized by more pronounced cytologic atypia with a peripheral palisade and a cleft artifact with the surrounding fibrotic stroma. It lacks true cyst differentiation. Merkel cell carcinoma is characterized by a sheet-like architecture and infiltrative growth. It lacks mucin and cyst differentiation and expresses CK20 by immunohistochemistry.

Key features: endocrine mucin-producing sweat gland carcinoma

- Rare but possibly underrecognized entity related to solid papillary carcinoma of the breast
- Narrow anatomic distribution with strong predilection for eyelids
- Nodular tumors with mucinous pseudocysts, duct differentiation, and bland cytology with neuroendocrine features
- Rare local recurrence but no documented metastases or mortality
- Precursor to primary cutaneous mucinous carcinoma

PRIMARY CUTANEOUS MUCINOUS CARCINOMA

Mucinous carcinoma arising primarily in the skin is a rare sweat gland tumor of low-grade malignancy. It must be separated from cutaneous metastases of mucinous adenocarcinoma of visceral sites, especially the breast, ovary, gastrointestinal, and genitourinary tract.

Clinical Presentation

Primary cutaneous mucinous carcinoma affects the scalp and face of elderly adults (median, 76 years) with a female predominance.[9] There is a particular predilection for the eyelids. Presentation outside the head and neck area is distinctly unusual and should raise suspicion for a cutaneous metastasis of a visceral primary.[9] The tumors are solitary and slowly growing, often showing an erythematous to bluish discoloration. They are of low-grade malignant potential with high local recurrence rates (20%–26%) but only rare metastases, mainly to locoregional lymph nodes.[9] Local excision is the treatment of choice with Mohs micrographic surgery offering particular benefits to minimize local recurrence. A diagnosis of mucinous carcinoma of the skin should also prompt an investigation for a possible underlying primary visceral adenocarcinoma.

Histologic Features

The tumors are characterized by a lobular growth within dermis and subcutaneous fat (**Fig. 3**A). The individual tumor lobules are separated by delicate fibrous bands (see **Fig. 3**B). They are composed of abundant mucin-containing irregularly shaped epithelial islands and strands (see **Fig. 3**B). The tumor cells are cuboidal with varying amounts of eosinophilic cytoplasm that may also contain mucin droplets (see **Fig. 3**C). Nuclear pleomorphism varies. Areas of cribriform and more solid growth patterns may be found in the tumors and glandular structures with papillary projections and decapitation secretion (see **Fig. 3**D). The demonstration of an in situ component by the presence of a layer of actin-positive myoepithelial cells is a helpful clue to the primary cutaneous origin (see **Fig. 3**D). This is a rare finding.

Immunohistochemistry

The tumor cells are positive for cytokeratins AE1/AE3 and Cam5.2. They also express CK7, EMA, CEA, and estrogen and progesterone receptors, but they are consistently negative for CK20 and there is no amplification of Her2/neu by fluorescence in situ hybridization.[9,10] Neuroendocrine markers are expressed in a small number of cases. These may represent tumors arising in the context of EMPSGC, as discussed previously.

Differential Diagnosis

Most importantly, primary cutaneous mucinous carcinoma needs to be distinguished from cutaneous metastases from internal primaries. The presence of so-called "dirty necrosis" and the immunohistochemical expression of CK20 favors an underlying colorectal primary tumor.[9] Exclusion of metastasis from a mammary primary requires clinical work-up.

Key features: primary cutaneous mucinous carcinoma

- Predilection for the head, in particular the scalp and eyelids
- Identical morphologic features to mucinous carcinomas of visceral organs
- Low-grade malignant potential with local recurrence and metastases to lymph nodes, but rare distant metastasis
- Cutaneous metastases from visceral primaries need to be excluded clinically

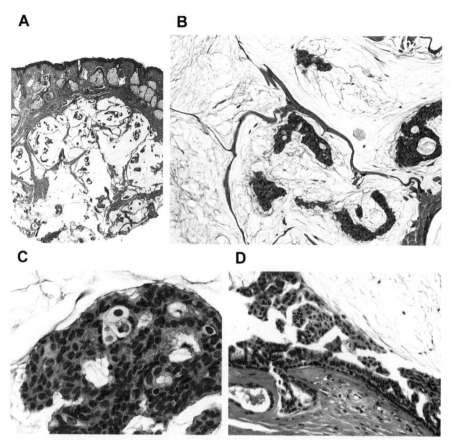

Fig. 3. Primary cutaneous mucinous carcinoma. This large lobulated tumor is centered within dermis with invasion of deeper structures (*A*, HE, original magnification ×10). It is composed of large mucinous pools separated by thin fibrous bands. Irregularly shaped epithelial strands and islands are embedded within the mucin (*B*, HE, original magnification ×40). Tumor cells are polygonal with eosinophilic and focally mucin-filled cytoplasm. Cytologic atypia is variable (*C*, HE, original magnification ×400). Focal cyst formation with micropapillary projections. Also note the second myoepithelial cell layer, a finding in favor of primary cutaneous origin (*D*, HE, original magnification ×200).

PRIMARY CUTANEOUS ADENOID CYSTIC CARCINOMA

Adenoid cystic carcinoma is a distinctive tumor that characteristically affects visceral organs, in particular the salivary glands. Primary cutaneous tumors are rare. They are morphologically identically to their visceral counterparts but show a less aggressive disease course. Awareness and recognition of these tumors and separation from direct extension or cutaneous metastases from underlying visceral primaries is therefore important.

Clinical Presentation

Primary cutaneous adenoid cystic carcinoma affects middle-aged to elderly adults (median, 62 years) without significant gender bias.[11,12] It presents as slowly growing nodules or indurated plaques affecting the head and neck area, especially the scalp. The anatomic distribution is wide and the extremities, the trunk, and the genital areas, in particular the vulva, may also be involved. The primary cutaneous tumors are characterized by potential for local recurrence but distant metastasis and associated mortality is rare.[11,12] In contrast, primary vulvar adenoid cystic carcinoma seems to behave more aggressively with potential for disseminated disease.[11,13]

Histologic Features

The tumor is poorly demarcated and located within the dermis. It shows a diffusely infiltrative growth often with additional invasion of subcutaneous adipose tissue (**Fig. 4**A). The tumor is composed of multiple separate basaloid lobules and islands of varying shapes and sizes containing densely packed epithelioid cells with little cytoplasm and hyperchromatic nuclei (see **Fig. 4**B, C). Mitoses are infrequent and tumor necrosis is rare. The individual tumor islands contain aggregates of stromal mucin, forming pseudocysts and giving rise to a cribriform appearance. They may be surrounded by thickened eosinophilic basement membrane material, which is highlighted

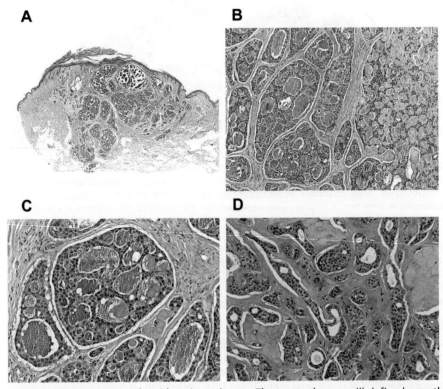

Fig. 4. Primary cutaneous adenoid cystic carcinoma. The tumor shows an ill-defined growth within dermis with invasion of subcutaneous adipose tissue (*A*, HE, original magnification ×20). It is composed of variable-sized nests and islands separated by a fibrous stroma (*B*, HE, original magnification ×200). The epithelioid tumor cells are medium sized without significant nuclear pleomorphism. The formation of the mucin-filled pseudocyst is a hallmark feature, giving rise to the cribriform architecture (*C*, HE, original magnification ×400). Ductal structures are present within the tumor in varying amounts (*D*, HE, original magnification ×200).

by periodic acid–Schiff staining or collagen IV immunohistochemistry. The surrounding tumor stroma appears loose or mucinous. Ductal differentiation is present in the tumor and is highlighted by EMA or CEA immunohistochemistry (see **Fig. 4**D). Perineural infiltration is typically present.

Immunohistochemistry and Genetics

Primary cutaneous adenoid cystic carcinoma expresses cytokeratins AE1/3 and Cam5.2. Myoepithelial differentiation is demonstrated by SMA, SOX10, and S100 staining. Most tumors show positivity for CD117. Ductal structures are highlighted by CEA and EMA.[11]

Analogous to the visceral tumors, the t(6;9) (q22–23;p23–24) translocation leading to the *MYB-NFIB* fusion gene and resulting in MYB overexpression has also been demonstrated in primary cutaneous tumors. Fluorescence in situ hybridization for the *MYB* gene rearrangement or immunohistochemistry for MYB overexpression are helpful diagnostic tools.[14,15]

Differential Diagnosis

Most importantly, primary cutaneous adenoid cystic carcinoma needs to be distinguished from cutaneous extension or metastasis from visceral primary adenoid cystic carcinoma. Because these tumors are indistinguishable from each other on morphology clinical correlation is necessary.

Adenoid cystic basal cell carcinoma shares many similarities with primary cutaneous adenoid cystic carcinoma. It is separated from it by the presence of the peripheral palisade of tumor cells, the stromal cleft artifact, the fibrotic stroma, and lack of duct differentiation.

Key features: primary cutaneous adenoid cystic carcinoma

- Primary cutaneous tumors are morphologically, immunohistochemically, and genetically indistinguishable from adenoid cystic carcinomas at visceral sites
- Primary cutaneous tumors have a more favorable prognosis with local recurrence but only rare metastatic potential
- A cutaneous metastasis needs to be excluded clinically

SPIRADENOCARCINOMA

Spiradenocarcinomas are rare tumors. They are closely related to cylindrocarcinoma and spiradenocylindrocarcinoma and likely represent part of a disease spectrum. Recent studies have shown that morphology is predictive of outcome and recognition of the benign precursor lesion is necessary for the diagnosis.

Clinical Presentation

Spiradenocarcinoma presents as solitary long-standing cutaneous nodules, measuring 3 cm to 4 cm in median, with a history of recent enlargement.[16–19] Its anatomic distribution is wide but there is a predilection for the head and neck area. The patients are elderly and the sexes are affected equally. Most tumors present sporadic, but rarely spiradenocarcinoma may complicate the Brooke-Spiegler syndrome.[18] Histologically, spiradenocarcinomas are divided into morphologically low- and high-grade tumors. This classification also impacts behavior. Morphologically low-grade carcinomas have a 20% local recurrence rate but the risk for metastasis and disease-related mortality is negligible.[19] In contrast, high-grade tumors show significant metastatic potential to lymph nodes, liver, and lung with associated mortality.[16–19]

Histologic Features

Spiradenocarcinomas are multinodular tumors located in the deep dermis and subcutis. Occasionally they may show diffusely infiltrative borders. Recognition of an unequivocal pre-existing spiradenoma is essential for the diagnosis. Morphologically low-grade malignant tumors show an expansile or pushing growth, merging with a pre-existing spiradenoma. On low-power magnification, the malignant component retains many of the architectural characteristics of a spiradenoma (**Fig. 5**A). A hallmark feature is the absence of the dual cell population, typical of spiradenoma. The tumor cells are monotonous and basaloid with mild to moderate atypia and increased mitotic activity (see **Fig. 5**B). Additional features are clear cell change and the formation of

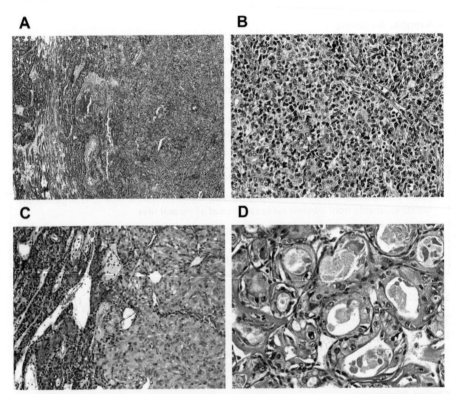

Fig. 5. Spiradenocarcinoma. Morphologically low-grade tumors are characterized by an expansile nodular growth (*right*) merging with a pre-existing benign spiradenoma (*left*). On low-power examination the patterned organization appears similar to spiradenoma (*A*, HE, original magnification ×20). Higher magnification reveals a monotonous proliferation of basaloid epithelial cells with mild to moderate degrees of cytologic atypia. The dual cell population, characteristic of spiradenomas, is lost (*B*, HE, original magnification ×200). Recognition of morphologically high-grade tumors depends on visualization of the preexisting spiradenoma (*C*, HE, original magnification ×100). The malignant component shows features of a poorly differentiated adenocarcinoma (*C*) or adenocarcinoma, not otherwise specified (*D*, HE, original magnification ×200).

squamoid morules. Tumor necrosis and ulceration may also be seen. Morphologically high-grade tumors are characterized by a wide range of histologic features. The malignant aspect resembles poorly differentiated carcinoma or adenocarcinoma, not otherwise specified arising adjacent to a pre-existing spiradenoma (see **Fig. 5**C, D). Sarcomatoid differentiation is rare but seems to be associated with more favorable prognosis.

Immunohistochemistry

The tumor cells express cytokeratins, and duct differentiation is highlighted by EMA or CEA staining. MYB expression is seen in benign spiradenomas and is used as a surrogate marker for the underlying t(6;9) translocation similar to adenoid cystic carcinoma. MYB expression is lost, however, at least in the morphologically low-grade tumors.[19] It serves as a helpful diagnostic marker to distinguish these tumors from benign spiradenoma.

Differential Diagnosis

The separation of morphologically low-grade spiradenocarcinoma from benign spiradenoma is particularly challenging. It requires careful examination with recognition of loss of the dual cell population, the presence of cytologic atypia, and mitotic activity. Immunohistochemistry for MYB is helpful in this setting. High-grade tumors resemble metastases from visceral primaries. The presence of a pre-existing benign spiradenoma is necessary for the correct diagnosis. This may require careful examination and tissue sampling.

Key features: spiradenocarcinoma

- The diagnosis requires the presence of a pre-existing benign spiradenoma
- Morphology is a good predictor of outcome
- Morphologically low-grade tumors have potential for local recurrence
- Distant metastasis and mortality is largely limited to morphologically high-grade tumors

---

DIGITAL PAPILLARY ADENOCARCINOMA

Digital papillary adenocarcinoma is a distinctive but rare sweat gland tumor with a wide morphologic spectrum, ranging from bland, innocuous histologic appearances to those more classical associated with high-grade malignancies. According to their histologic appearances the tumors were initially separated into adenomas and adenocarcinoma.[20] With longer-term follow-up it has become evident that all tumors show potential for malignant behavior independent of their morphology, and they are all regarded as adenocarcinoma.[21,22]

Clinical Presentation

Digital papillary adenocarcinoma has a narrow anatomic distribution with a strong predilection for the distal ends of the digits.[20–23] The palms and soles may also be involved. It presents as small erythematous, brown or skin-colored nodules, measuring from a few millimeters up to multiple centimeters. The patients are mainly middle-aged adults with a strong male predominance.[20–23] The age range is wide and presentation in children and adolescents is not uncommon. The clinical behavior is characterized by high local recurrence (20%–40%) and metastatic rates (15%), mainly to lymph nodes and lung.[21,22] Although disease-related mortality has been

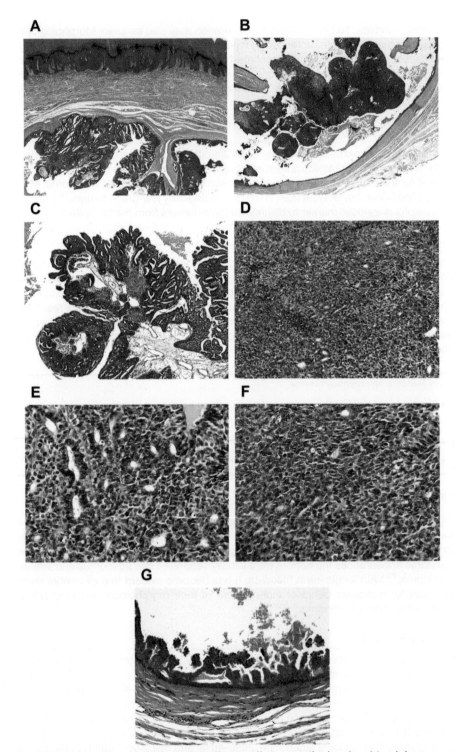

Fig. 6. Digital papillary adenocarcinoma. These well-circumscribed and multinodular tumors show a solid and cystic growth within deep dermis (*A*, *B*, HE, original magnificaiton ×10).

documented, it seems low. The disease course is protracted and long-term follow-up is necessary. Wide local excision or amputation is the recommended treatment because it reduces local recurrence and even distant metastatic rates.[22]

Histologic Features

Digital papillary adenocarcinoma is located in the deep dermis and superficial subcutaneous fat as a well-circumscribed multinodular tumor (**Fig. 6**A, B). The tumor nodules are solid and cystic and show a papillary growth pattern (see **Fig. 6**C–E). They are composed of cuboidal basaloid cells with varying nuclear atypia ranging from mild to severe. Mitotic figures are typically present (see **Fig. 6**F). Additional features include a tubular growth pattern, clear cell change, and squamoid morules. Micropapillary projections are often noted in the cystic elements and a second myoepithelial cell layer can be seen (see **Fig. 6**G). Tumor necrosis and more infiltrative growth in deeper structures may be noted in the morphologically higher-grade tumors.

Immunohistochemistry

Tumor cells express cytokeratins. The luminal differentiation is highlighted by EMA and CEA staining. S100, p63, podoplanin, SMA, and calponin staining demonstrates a second myoepithelial cell layer.

Differential Diagnosis

The tumors may be bland and innocuous on histology. They are easily mistaken for benign skin adnexal tumors, especially apocrine cystadenoma.[23] Apocrine cystadenomas most commonly present on the cheek and digital presentation is distinctly unusual. Reported cases of apocrine cystadenoma on the digits may indeed represent the morphologically low-grade end of the spectrum of digital papillary adenocarcinoma.[23] Careful examination and sampling of these tumors is necessary to identify areas of cytologic atypia and increased mitotic activity. Tubular adenoma may show significant morphologic overlap with papillary digital adenocarcinoma, and it may arise on the distal extremities. In contrast to papillary digital adenocarcinoma it shows a growth pattern of individual tubules separated by a fibrous stroma. Hidradenoma also enters the differential diagnosis. It shows a nodular growth pattern with solid, tubular, and occasionally cystic changes. Clear cell change and squamoid differentiation are additional findings. The tumors rarely affect the distal extremities. At this anatomic location, their diagnosis requires great care. Any degree of cytologic atypia and more overt papillary differentiation should be regarded with caution because these tumors may represent digital papillary adenocarcinomas. Finally, metastases from papillary adenocarcinomas of visceral origin also need to be considered. The demonstration of myoepithelial differentiation in papillary digital adenocarcinoma excludes this possibility.

Prominent papilla formation is a characteristic feature (*C*, HE, original magnification ×40). In areas, the tumor shows a solid, sheet-like growth pattern (*D*, HE, original magnification ×100). Tubular differentiation is an additional feature (*E*, HE, original magnification ×200). The tumor cells are basaloid and show moderate cytologic atypia. Mitotic figures are readily identified (*F*, HE, original magnification ×200). Intraluminal micropapillary projections are present in the cystic areas. Also note the presence of a second myoepithelial cell layer (*G*, HE, original magnification ×100).

> **Key features: digital papillary adenocarcinoma**
>
> - Narrow anatomic distribution with strong predilection for the digits
> - High local recurrence rate and metastatic potential
> - Protracted disease course
> - Histology not predictive of outcome
> - Tumors may easily be mistaken for apocrine cystadenoma or hidradenoma and these diagnosis should be made with great care on the distal extremities
> - Demonstration of myoepithelial differentiation excludes cutaneous metastases

SUMMARY

A confident diagnosis of the entities discussed is possible in most cases. It largely depends on awareness, an index of suspicion, adequate sampling with careful examination of the histologic features, judicious use of immunohistochemistry, and interpretation of the findings in the clinical context.

REFERENCES

1. Rutten A, Kutzner H, Mentzel T, et al. Primary cutaneous cribriform apocrine carcinoma: a clinicopathologic and immunohistochemical study of 26 cases of an under-recognized cutaneous adnexal neoplasm. J Am Acad Dermatol 2009; 61(4):644–51.
2. Adamski H, Le Lan J, Chevrier S, et al. Primary cutaneous cribriform carcinoma: a rare apocrine tumour. J Cutan Pathol 2005;32(8):577–80.
3. Arps DP, Chan MP, Patel RM, et al. Primary cutaneous cribriform carcinoma: report of six cases with clinicopathologic data and immunohistochemical profile. J Cutan Pathol 2015;42(6):379–87.
4. Flieder A, Koerner FC, Pilch BZ, et al. Endocrine mucin-producing sweat gland carcinoma: a cutaneous neoplasm analogous to solid papillary carcinoma of breast. Am J Surg Pathol 1997;21(12):1501–6.
5. Zembowicz A, Garcia CF, Tannous ZS, et al. Endocrine mucin-producing sweat gland carcinoma: twelve new cases suggest that it is a precursor of some invasive mucinous carcinomas. Am J Surg Pathol 2005;29(10):1330–9.
6. Fernandez-Flores A. Considerations before accepting an extra-facial location of endocrine mucin-producing sweat gland carcinoma. J Cutan Pathol 2015; 42(4):297–8.
7. Tsai JH, Hsiao TL, Chen YY, et al. Endocrine mucin-producing sweat gland carcinoma occurring on extra-facial site: a case report. J Cutan Pathol 2014;41(6): 544–7.
8. Koike T, Mikami T, Maegawa J, et al. Recurrent endocrine mucin-producing sweat gland carcinoma in the eyelid. Australas J Dermatol 2013;54(2):e46–9.
9. Kazakov DV, Suster S, LeBoit PE, et al. Mucinous carcinoma of the skin, primary, and secondary: a clinicopathologic study of 63 cases with emphasis on the morphologic spectrum of primary cutaneous forms: homologies with mucinous lesions in the breast. Am J Surg Pathol 2005;29(6):764–82.
10. Levy G, Finkelstein A, McNiff JM. Immunohistochemical techniques to compare primary vs. metastatic mucinous carcinoma of the skin. J Cutan Pathol 2010; 37(4):411–5.

11. Ramakrishnan R, Chaudhry IH, Ramdial P, et al. Primary cutaneous adenoid cystic carcinoma: a clinicopathologic and immunohistochemical study of 27 cases. Am J Surg Pathol 2013;37(10):1603–11.
12. Seab JA, Graham JH. Primary cutaneous adenoid cystic carcinoma. J Am Acad Dermatol 1987;17(1):113–8.
13. Chapman GW Jr, Benda J, Lifshitz S. Adenoid cystic carcinoma of the vulva with lung metastases. A case report. J Reprod Med 1985;30(3):217–20.
14. North JP, McCalmont TH, Fehr A, et al. Detection of MYB alterations and other immunohistochemical markers in primary cutaneous adenoid cystic carcinoma. Am J Surg Pathol 2015;39(10):1347–56.
15. Prieto-Granada CN, Zhang L, Antonescu CR, et al. Primary cutaneous adenoid cystic carcinoma with MYB aberrations: report of three cases and comprehensive review of the literature. J Cutan Pathol 2017;44(2):201–9.
16. Dai B, Kong YY, Cai X, et al. Spiradenocarcinoma, cylindrocarcinoma and spiradenocylindrocarcinoma: a clinicopathological study of nine cases. Histopathology 2014;65(5):658–66.
17. Granter SR, Seeger K, Calonje E, et al. Malignant eccrine spiradenoma (spiradenocarcinoma): a clinicopathologic study of 12 cases. Am J Dermatopathol 2000; 22(2):97–103.
18. Kazakov DV, Zelger B, Rutten A, et al. Morphologic diversity of malignant neoplasms arising in preexisting spiradenoma, cylindroma, and spiradenocylindroma based on the study of 24 cases, sporadic or occurring in the setting of Brooke-Spiegler syndrome. Am J Surg Pathol 2009;33(5):705–19.
19. van der Horst MP, Marusic Z, Hornick JL, et al. Morphologically low-grade spiradenocarcinoma: a clinicopathologic study of 19 cases with emphasis on outcome and MYB expression. Mod Pathol 2015;28(7):944–53.
20. Kao GF, Helwig EB, Graham JH. Aggressive digital papillary adenoma and adenocarcinoma. A clinicopathological study of 57 patients, with histochemical, immunopathological, and ultrastructural observations. J Cutan Pathol 1987; 14(3):129–46.
21. Duke WH, Sherrod TT, Lupton GP. Aggressive digital papillary adenocarcinoma (aggressive digital papillary adenoma and adenocarcinoma revisited). Am J Surg Pathol 2000;24(6):775–84.
22. Suchak R, Wang WL, Prieto VG, et al. Cutaneous digital papillary adenocarcinoma: a clinicopathologic study of 31 cases of a rare neoplasm with new observations. Am J Surg Pathol 2012;36(12):1883–91.
23. Molina-Ruiz AM, Llamas-Velasco M, Rutten A, et al. "Apocrine hidrocystoma and cystadenoma"-like tumor of the digits or toes: a potential diagnostic pitfall of digital papillary adenocarcinoma. Am J Surg Pathol 2016;40(3):410–8.

Fibrohistiocytic Tumors

Ryan C. Romano, DO[a], Karen J. Fritchie, MD[b],*

KEYWORDS

- Fibrohistiocytic • Histiocytes • Fibrous histiocytoma • Xanthogranuloma
- Dermatofibrosarcoma protuberans

KEY POINTS

- Fibrohistiocytic tumors, some of which are common and others of which are rarely encountered, present significant challenges to the dermatopathologist owing to clinical and histopathologic overlap.
- The "fibrohistiocytic" designation does not necessarily denote lineage differentiation in all cases but rather may be used for lesions in which tumor cells resemble histiocytes and/or fibroblasts.
- Most fibrohistiocytic lesions are best diagnosed by careful histologic examination; immunohistochemistry and molecular studies play a limited role in the workup of this family of tumors.

OVERVIEW

Fibrohistiocytic tumors represent a diverse group of mesenchymal neoplasms with widely variable presentations. The "fibrohistiocytic" designation does not necessarily denote lineage differentiation in all cases, but rather may also be used for lesions in which tumor cells resemble histiocytes and/or fibroblasts. These lesions exhibit a range of clinical behavior ranging from reactive (xanthoma) to benign (fibrous histiocytoma and its variants) to tumors with significant local recurrence potential (dermatofibrosarcoma protuberans). This review highlights key morphologic features of these entities, as well as potential diagnostic pitfalls and histologic mimics. Although immunohistochemistry may be helpful in excluding other diagnoses, immunostains play a relatively limited role in the workup of the majority of lesions in this family. A subset of fibrohistiocytic neoplasms, including dermatofibrosarcoma protuberans and angiomatoid fibrous histiocytoma, have unique genetic aberrations, and the use of cytogenetic/molecular studies in these tumors as an adjunct to microscopic examination is discussed.

The authors have nothing to disclose.
[a] Department of Dermatology, Mayo Clinic, Gonda 16, 200 First Street Southwest, Rochester, MN 55905, USA; [b] Division of Anatomic Pathology, Department of Laboratory Medicine and Pathology, Mayo Clinic College of Medicine, Mayo Clinic, Hilton 11, 200 First Street Southwest, Rochester, MN 55905, USA
* Corresponding author.
E-mail address: fritchie.karen@mayo.edu

Clin Lab Med 37 (2017) 603–631
http://dx.doi.org/10.1016/j.cll.2017.05.007
0272-2712/17/© 2017 Elsevier Inc. All rights reserved.

FIBROUS HISTIOCYTOMA AND VARIANTS
Epidemiology and Clinical Features

Fibrous histiocytoma (dermatofibroma) is typically diagnosed in young to middle-aged adults with a female predominance and shows a strong predilection for involving the extremities.[1,2] Most patients present with a single, asymptomatic, long-standing lesion, although multiplicity has been associated with immune suppression.[2,3] The aneurysmal variant may exhibit the clinical appearance of rapid growth secondary to intratumoral hemorrhage.[4] There has been debate as to whether fibrous histiocytoma represents a reactive, inflammatory process or a clonal neoplasm, but the prevailing opinion favors a neoplastic process.[5–7]

Gross Features

The majority of lesions measure less than 2.0 cm and are well-circumscribed (**Fig. 1**A). Cystic change or hemorrhage may be seen.

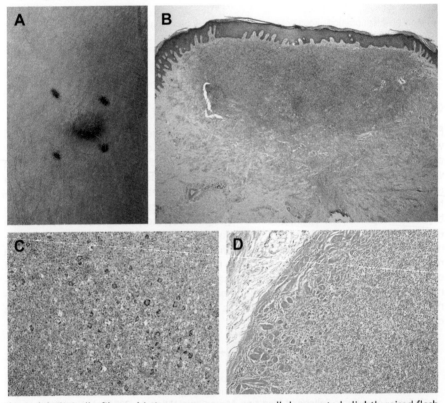

Fig. 1. (A) Clinically, fibrous histiocytoma appears as a well-demarcated, slightly raised flesh-colored to tan-pink papule. Low-power examination (B, H&E, original magnification ×40) shows a circumscribed, dermal-based lesion with a pushing border and lack of significant extension into the subcutis. Closer inspection (C, H&E, original magnification ×100) reveals a polymorphous proliferation of multinucleated giant cells, foamy histocytes, and bland mononuclear cells. The peripheral border shows prominent collagen entrapment (D, H&E, original magnification ×100).

Microscopic Features

Fibrous histiocytomas are characterized by a polymorphous dermal infiltrate of multi-nucleated giant cells, foamy histiocytes, hemosiderin-laden macrophages, and bland spindled cells (**Fig. 1**B, C). In the conventional variant, lesional cells occasionally extend into the superficial aspects of subcutaneous fat, whereas deep fibrous histio-cytomas arise in subcutaneous soft tissue. Examination of the periphery reveals a pushing border with cells enveloping collagen bundles ("collagen trapping") (**Fig. 1**D). Overlying epidermal changes include hyperkeratosis, acanthosis, basilar hyperpigmentation, and a "grenz zone" of normal intervening dermis between the lesion and the epidermis.[2] Numerous histopathologic variants have been described (**Figs. 2–6, Table 1**), and features of multiple variants may coexist within the same lesion.[2,8]

Although fibrous histiocytoma expresses a combination of histiocytic markers including factor XIIIa, CD68, and CD163, careful morphologic examination is often suf-ficient for diagnosis.[9] Myoid marker expression, particularly smooth muscle actin, may be present, and CD34 staining can be appreciated in a small subset of cases, espe-cially at the lesion's periphery.[9,10] Epithelioid fibrous histiocytomas seem to be a distinct subset. They are composed of epithelioid cells, often have a dilated capillary vasculature and an epidermal collarette, and usually lack prominent collagen trap-ping. They are also immunoreactive for EMA and ALK, unlike conventional fibrous histiocytoma.[11–14]

Molecular and Cytogenetic Characteristics

Recurrent gene fusions involving protein kinase C genes (*PRKCB*, *PRKCD*, and *PRKCA*) have been identified in a subset of fibrous histiocytomas.[15,16] *ALK* gene rear-rangement with associated protein overexpression by immunohistochemistry has been shown consistently in epithelioid fibrous histiocytoma.[11–14,17]

Differential Diagnosis

Although the diagnosis of conventional fibrous histiocytoma is generally straightfor-ward, the cellular variant may be difficult to distinguish from nodular fasciitis,

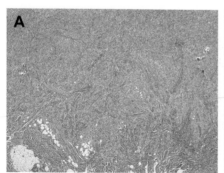
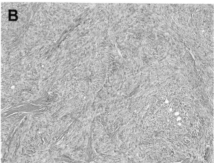

Fig. 2. Cellular fibrous histiocytoma showing a monotonous population of spindled cells with envelopment of collagen fibers at the periphery (*A*, H&E, original magnification ×100). High-power examination (*B*, H&E, original magnification ×200) yields bland cells arranged in short fascicles without significant cytologic atypia. Notice the lack of second-ary elements (foamy histiocytes, hemosiderin-laden macrophages, multinucleated giant cells).

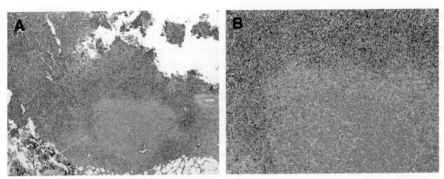

Fig. 3. The aneurysmal variant of fibrous histiocytoma shows cystic spaces filled with blood and hemorrhage (*A*, H&E, original magnification ×100). Abundant hemosiderin-laden macrophages (*B*, H&E, original magnification ×200) can be appreciated adjacent to foci of hemorrhage.

especially on biopsy specimens. The presence of collagen entrapment favors the former, whereas demonstration of *USP6* gene rearrangement supports the latter.[18] The differential diagnosis for cellular fibrous histiocytoma also includes dermatofibrosarcoma protuberans. Dermatofibrosarcoma protuberans shows an extensively infiltrative margin, which contrasts with the pushing border of fibrous histiocytoma. Furthermore, dermatofibrosarcoma protuberans typically shows strong and diffuse CD34 immunoreactivity, and the majority harbor *COL1A1-PDGFB* fusion.

Prognosis

Fibrous histiocytoma are benign lesions with an excellent prognosis. Certain histologic variants, namely the cellular, atypical, and aneurysmal subtypes, have been associated with increased risk of local recurrence (>20%), and conservative but complete excision of these lesions is recommended.[9,10] Rarely, fibrous histiocytoma, including those with conventional morphology may metastasize.[10,19–21] Although there are no morphologic features that reliably predict behavior, recent work by Charli-Joseph

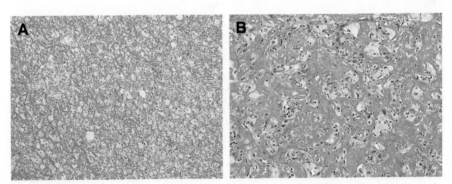

Fig. 4. Lipidized fibrous histiocytomas contain predominantly foamy histiocytes in a sclerotic background (*A*, H&E, original magnification ×200). High-power view (*B*, H&E, original magnification ×400) of the stroma reveals densely eosinophilic material mimicking osteoid.

and colleagues suggests that increased copy number alterations may correlate with more adverse outcome.[22,23]

Key features

1. Conventional variant characterized by dermal-based polymorphous proliferation containing multinucleated giant cells, foamy histiocytes, hemosiderin-laden macrophages and bland mononuclear cells.

2. Smooth contoured border with prominent collagen entrapment at the periphery.

Pitfalls

1. Variants of fibrous histiocytoma may show increased cellularity, nuclear pleomorphism, and mitotic activity.

2. CD34 expression may be observed in a subset of lesional cells, especially toward the periphery of the mass.

3. Epithelioid fibrous histiocytoma expresses EMA and ALK.

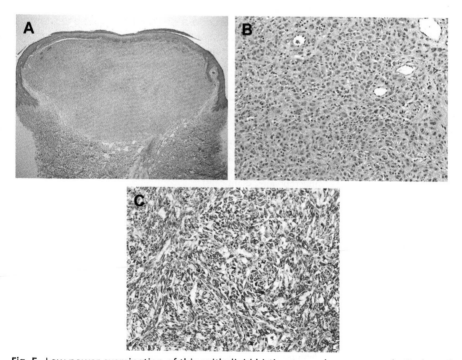

Fig. 5. Low-power examination of this epithelioid histiocytoma shows an exophytic dermal lesion with an epidermal collarette (*A*, H&E, original magnification ×40). The majority of the lesional cells (*B*, H&E, original magnification ×400) are large and epithelioid with eosinophilic or amphophilic cytoplasm. Small capillary-sized blood vessels are readily identifiable. The cells show diffuse expression of ALK (*C*, H&E, original magnification ×400).

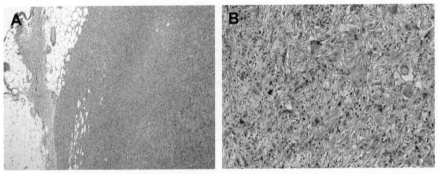

Fig. 6. Atypical fibrous histiocytoma exhibits features of the conventional variant including a circumscribed border with collagen entrapment (A, H&E, original magnification ×100). However, focally, bizarre atypia and atypical mitoses are appreciated (B, H&E, original magnification ×400).

CELLULAR NEUROTHEKEOMA
Epidemiology and Clinical Features

Cellular neurothekeoma primarily affects young to middle-aged adults and demonstrates a slight female predominance.[9,24,25] The head and neck and upper extremities are most commonly affected.[24] Although most cases present as a painless, firm slow-growing nodule, tenderness and pruritus have also been described.[24] Although the term neurothekeoma was introduced to describe a group of dermal-based tumors thought to be of neural origin (classic myxoid neurothekeoma and cellular neurothekeoma), further study revealed that the cellular variant of neurothekeoma lacked immunoreactivity for S100 protein, arguing against nerve sheath derivation.[26–28]

Table 1
Variants of fibrous histiocytoma

Variant	Key Morphologic Features
Cellular fibrous histiocytoma	Monomorphic population of spindle cells Lacks secondary elements (foamy histiocytes, hemosiderin-laden macrophages, giant cells) May show increased mitotic rate May show necrosis
Aneurysmal fibrous histiocytoma	Pseudovascular spaces with red blood cell extravasation and hemosiderin deposition Mitotic figures may be easily appreciated adjacent to the hemorrhagic foci
Lipidized fibrous histiocytoma	Abundant foamy histiocytes in a densely hyalinized stroma Stroma may mimic osteoid matrix
Epithelioid fibrous histiocytoma	Epithelioid to polygonal cells with abundant cytoplasm Distinct epidermal "collarette" Rich vascular network Generally lacks foamy histiocytes, multinucleated giant cells, lymphocytes, and peripheral collagen trapping
Atypical fibrous histiocytoma	Background features resembling conventional fibrous histiocytoma Numerous pleomorphic cells with enlarged hyperchromatic and bizarre nuclei Increased mitotic activity, including atypical mitotic figures

Subsequent gene expression profiling by Sheth and colleagues[29] further validated this hypothesis, suggesting that cellular neurothekeomas demonstrate evidence of fibrohistiocytic lineage.

Gross Features

Cellular neurothekeomas measure less than 3 cm.[24,25] On cut section, the tumor may be composed of multiple discrete nodules or a well-demarcated single mass.[24,25]

Microscopic Features

Histologic examination shows dermal-based nests of spindled to epithelioid cells with a histiocytoid appearance separated by bands of collagen in a lobular or nodular low power configuration (**Fig. 7**). Plexiform architecture, sheetlike growth, myxoid change, or stromal hyalinization may be observed.[9,24] It is not uncommon to see osteoclast-like multinucleated cells distributed throughout the mass.[24] Severe cytologic atypia is rare, but mild cytologic atypia is encountered frequently in the form of nucleoli and nuclear variablility.[24] When mitotic activity is present, it is often low (<5 mitotic figures per 10 high-power fields).[9,30] Vascular invasion, perineural invasion, and necrosis are uncommon findings.[24,30] Immunohistochemically, cellular neurothekeoma expresses a constellation of relatively nonspecific markers, including NKI/C3, MiTF, CD10, CD68, and smooth muscle actin.[25,30–32] Immunoreactivity for NKI/C3 and CD10 is more consistent than immunoreactivity for MiTF, CD68, and smooth muscle actin. Importantly, S100 protein immunoreactivity is absent.[28]

Differential Diagnosis

The primary differential considerations of cellular neurothekeoma include dermal nerve sheath myxoma, spindled melanocytic tumors, fibrous histiocytoma, and plexiform fibrohistiocytic tumor. Dermal nerve sheath myxoma displays S100 immunoreactivity and more extensive myxoid matrix than cellular neurothekeoma. Spitz nevi can be distinguished from cellular neurothekeoma by the presence of a junctional component and expression of S100 protein and melanocyte-specific markers. Fibrous histiocytomas, especially epithelioid fibrous histiocytoma, may mimic cellular neurothekeoma, but these tumors generally lack a nested architecture. Finally, cellular neurothekeomas, which deeply infiltrate the subcutis, may be confused for plexiform fibrohistiocytic tumor. However, cellular neurothekeomas consist of a more monotonous population of histiocytoid cells, lacking the biphasic appearance of plexiform fibrohistiocytic tumor. Recent work by Fox and colleagues[33] has shown frequent MiTF expression in cellular neurothekeomas but not plexiform fibrohistiocytic tumor, suggesting that this may be a helpful ancillary tool in small biopsy samples.

Prognosis

Cellular neurothekeomas are benign but do harbor the potential for local recurrence, especially those that are incompletely excised or involve the head and neck region.[24] Morphologic features such as cytologic atypia, mitotic rate and atypical mitotic figures have not been shown to correlate with adverse outcome.[30]

Key features

1. Histiocytoid spindled and epithelioid cells in a nested configuration.

2. S100 negative.

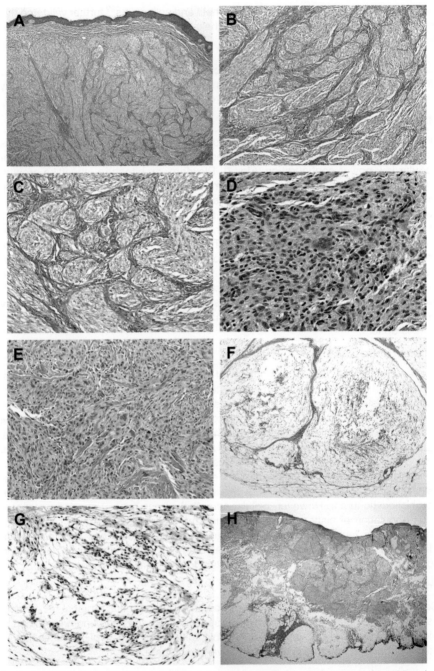

Fig. 7. Dermal-based cellular neurothekeoma with a nested growth pattern (*A*, H&E, original magnification ×40). The lesional cells are partitioned by bands of collagen into small nests and nodules with a vague whorling growth pattern (*B*, H&E, original magnification ×100). High-power examination (*C*, H&E, original magnification ×200) reveals a histiocytoid appearance with pale eosinophilic cytoplasm. Osteoclast-like giant cells (*D*, H&E, original magnification ×400) are not an uncommon finding. Occasionally, cellular

SOLITARY XANTHOGRANULOMA
Epidemiology and Clinical Features

Solitary xanthogranuloma (juvenile xanthogranuloma), the most common form of non-Langerhans cell histiocytosis, typically presents in infants and children with a male predominance.[34] It is noted at birth in approximately one-quarter of cases, and up to 70% of cases present within the first year of life.[34,35] Lesions involve the head and neck region in approximately 50% of cases, followed by the trunk and then extremities.[34,36] Rarely, cutaneous disease may coexist with involvement of deep soft tissue or viscera, and the eye is the most common extracutaneous site of disease.[9]

Gross Features

Lesions measure from millimeters to centimeters in size and vary from red-pink (early) to brown-yellow (fully developed) in color (**Fig. 8A**).[9,36]

Microscopic Features

Solitary xanthogranulomas are composed of sheets of uniform, plump, polygonal histiocytes involving the dermis and abutting the epidermis (**Fig. 8B**). Early lesions tend to have slightly eosinophilic and mostly nonlipidized cytoplasm (**Fig. 8C**), and as lesions age, the cells tend to become lipidized and foamy (**Fig. 8D**).[9] Occasionally, tumors may contain a predominant population of spindled cells with little to no cytoplasmic lipidization.[37] Multinucleated giant cells, including those with Touton features, are characteristic. The background milieu often contains inflammatory cells, including eosinophils, as well as fibrosis. Mitotic activity is generally low. The lesional cells express factor XIIIa, CD163, and CD11c, whereas stains for S100 protein and CD1a are negative.[9,35,37]

Differential Diagnosis

Although Langerhans cell histiocytosis shares clinical and morphologic features with solitary xanthogranuloma, the former shows more eosinophils and fewer Touton giant cells. Furthermore, the cells of Langerhans cell histiocytosis will mark for S100 and CD1a. Xanthomas are composed of a monomorphic population of foamy histiocytes, lacking both eosinophils and Touton giant cells. Finally, fibrous histiocytomas usually affect adults and demonstrate prominent peripheral collagen entrapment without a significant eosinophilic infiltrate.

Prognosis

Lesions tend to flatten and diminish over time, even when multiple.[35] Complete surgical excision is the mainstay of treatment, except in the systemic form, for which chemotherapeutic regimens may be used.[35]

---

neurothekeomas may show an increased mitotic rate and cytologic atypia (*E*, H&E, original magnification ×400). Low-power (*F*, H&E, original magnification ×100) and high-power (*G*, H&E, original magnification ×200) examination of a tumor with significant myxoid change. Closer inspection reveals similar cytologic features to the conventional variant. An example of a cellular neurothekeoma with plexiform architecture (*H*, H&E, original magnification ×40).

Key features

1. Yellow-hued papules or nodules arising most commonly in the head and neck regions within the first 2 years of life.

2. Superficial dermal infiltrate of polygonal histiocytes admixed with multinucleated giant cells, Touton giant cells, and inflammatory cells.

3. CD1a and S100 negative.

Pitfall

Inflammatory background may mimic Langerhans cell histiocytosis.

XANTHOMA
Epidemiology and Clinical Features

Xanthoma is a slow-growing, reactive process formed from aggregates of lipid-laden histiocytes.[38–42] These lesions are classified based on numerous factors, including gross or clinical appearance, anatomic location (such as eyelid or tendon sheath), and the lipoprotein phenotypic profile of the patient (**Table 2**).[9,43–45]

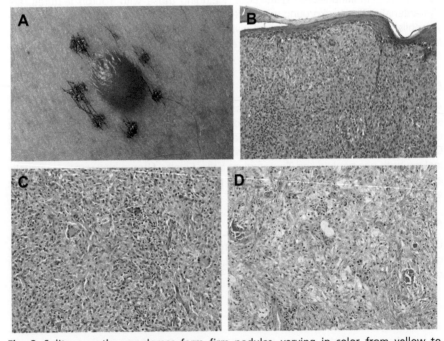

Fig. 8. Solitary xanthogranulomas form firm nodules, varying in color from yellow to erythematous to flesh colored (*A*). Microscopic examination shows a sheetlike proliferation of histiocytes and multinucleated giant cells (*B*, H&E, original magnification ×100). In this example, the giant cells have Touton features. Early lesions are typically nonlipidized (*C*, H&E, original magnification ×200), whereas older lesions show a greater number of lipid-laden histiocytes (*D*, H&E, original magnification ×200).

Table 2
Clinicopathologic features of xanthomas

Type of Xanthoma	Anatomic Sites Affected	Histology
Eruptive	Buttocks, shoulders, extensor surfaces of extremities	Foamy and nonfoamy histiocytes
Tendinous	Tendons	Foamy histiocytes, cholesterol deposits, fibrosis, inflammatory cells
Tuberous	Extensor surfaces of elbows, buttocks, knees	Foamy histiocytes, cholesterol deposits, fibrosis, inflammatory cells
Planar	Skin creases of palms and fingers	Foamy histiocytes
Xanthelasma	Eyelids	Foamy histiocytes

Hypercholesterolemia is not a prerequisite, but the development of xanthomas has been associated with dyslipidemias, hematologic disorders, and visceral malignancies. The presence of multiple lesions should prompt clinical evaluation to exclude systemic disease.[9,46]

Gross Features

Xanthomas are well-circumscribed deep dermal or subcutaneous nodules (**Fig. 9**A) that are variably yellow or tan depending on the amount of lipid, hemorrhage, and fibrosis.[9]

Microscopic Features

Although all subtypes contain a component of foamy histiocytes, the presence of cholesterol deposits, inflammation, and fibrosis are more common in tendinous and tuberous xanthomas (**Figs. 9**B–E and see **Table 2**).

Differential Diagnosis

Cutaneous xanthomas seldom present diagnostic difficulty. However, those attached to the tendon sheath may be confused with localized tenosynovial giant cell tumor (giant cell tumor of tendon sheath). Xanthomas lack the cellular heterogeneity of tenosynovial giant cell tumors. Evidence of hypercholesterolemia, hyperlipidemia, or the presence of multiple lesions favors xanthoma.

Prognosis

Conservative treatment is preferred. Surgical resection is generally reserved for large or symptomatic lesions.[9]

Pitfall

Deep lesions, especially those attached to tendons, may mimic tenosynovial giant cell tumor.

DERMATOFIBROSARCOMA PROTUBERANS
Epidemiology and Clinical Features

Dermatofibrosarcoma protuberans, considered to be a fibrohistiocytic tumor of intermediate malignant potential, most commonly affects the trunk or proximal extremities with a male predominance.[47] These tumors tend to be persistently slow growing (**Fig. 10**A).[47]

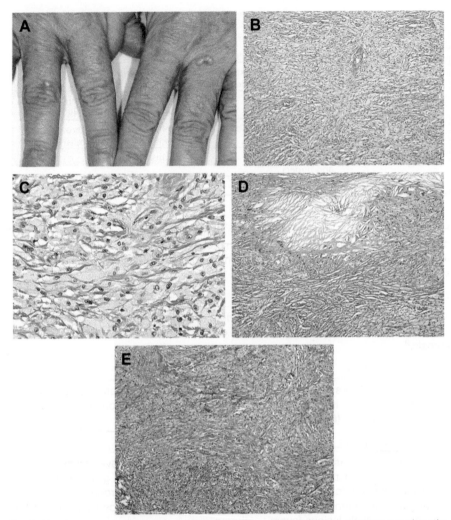

Fig. 9. Xanthomas are yellow-tan to erythematous in color and may present as papules, plaques, or nodules (A). This tuberous xanthoma shows abundant foamy histiocytes (B, H&E, original magnification ×100) with finely vacuolated cytoplasm (C, H&E, original magnification ×400). Cholesterol clefts (D, H&E, original magnification ×100) and variable amounts of fibrosis (E, H&E, original magnification ×100) are also common in the tuberous and tendinous subtypes.

Gross Features

The median size of these tumors is approximately 5.0 cm, although some may measure greater than 10 cm.[47] Sectioning often reveals involvement of both the dermis and subcutis.[47]

Microscopic Features

Conventional dermatofibrosarcoma protuberans consists of uniform slender spindle cells arranged in a whorled or storiform pattern that occupy the dermis with extensive infiltration into subcutaneous fat (**Fig. 10**B–D). Within the subcutis, a "honeycomb"

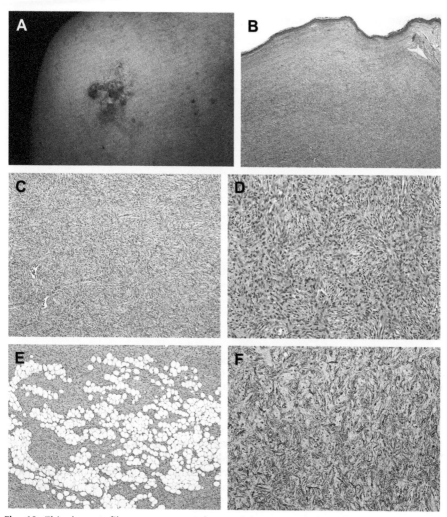

Fig. 10. This dermatofibrosarcoma protuberans (A) presented clinically as a multinodular plaque that developed slowly over a period of approximately 14 years. Examination of the superficial component of dermatofibrosarcoma protuberans shows a cellular spindle cell neoplasm extensively involving the dermis (B, H&E, original magnification ×40). The neoplastic cells (C, H&E, original magnification ×100) are slender with tapered nuclei and arranged in a distinct storiform pattern. High-power view demonstrates lack of significant nuclear atypia (D, H&E, original magnification ×200). The deep aspect of the tumor shows diffuse infiltration through subcutaneous adipose tissue (E, H&E, original magnification ×100). CD34 (F, original magnification ×200) shows strong and diffuse staining.

pattern may be appreciated as tumor cells encase individual fat lobules and extend along fibrous septa (**Fig. 10**E). Myxoid change may be present (**Fig. 11**), and delicate branching vessels are often prominent in these foci.[48] Occasionally, myoid nodules, representing perivascular proliferations of smooth muscle or myofibroblasts around intratumoral vessels, may be noted.[49,50] The mitotic rate in the conventional variant is typically less than 5 mitotic figures per 10 high-power fields.

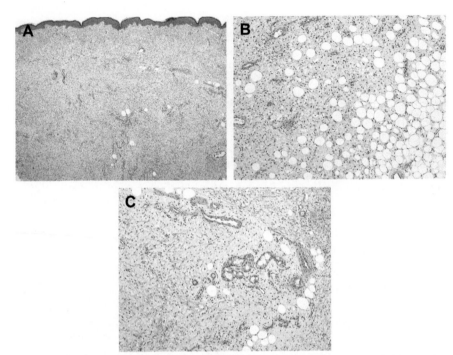

Fig. 11. Myxoid dermatofibrosarcoma protuberans (*A*, H&E, original magnification ×100) with extension through subcutaneous fat (*B*, H&E, original magnification ×200) and around adnexal structures (*C*, H&E, original magnification ×200).

Shmookler and Enzinger first described giant cell fibroblastoma in 1982, hypothesizing that it represented a pediatric variant of dermatofibrosarcoma protuberans. This theory was later confirmed by cytogenetic studies showing similar findings in both entities.[51,52] Although sharing many morphologic features with classic dermatofibrosarcoma protuberans, giant cell fibroblastoma contains distinct pseudovascular spaces lined by multinucleated giant cells (**Fig. 12**).

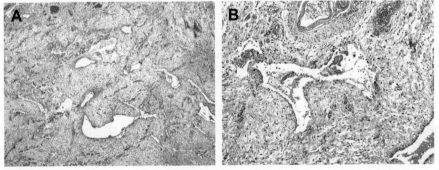

Fig. 12. Giant cell fibroblastoma with prominent pseudovascular spaces (*A*, H&E, original magnification ×100) lined by hyperchromatic giant cells (*B*, H&E, original magnification ×200).

Pigmented dermatofibrosarcoma protuberans (Bednar tumor) is essentially identical to the conventional form, but also harbors varying numbers of pigmented dendritic cells (**Fig. 13**).[53]

Fibrosarcomatous dermatofibrosarcoma protuberans (dermatofibrosarcoma protuberans with fibrosarcomatous change) shows areas displaying herringbone/fascicular architecture with increased mitotic activity (>5 mitotic figures per 10 high-power fields) (**Fig. 14**).[54] It is generally accepted that these areas should represent more than 5% to 10% of the tumor volume to warrant the fibrosarcomatous designation.[9] Dermatofibrosarcoma protuberans shows strong and diffuse expression of CD34 (**Fig. 10F**) except in cases with fibrosarcomatous change which may lose CD34 immunoreactivity.[55]

Molecular and Cytogenetic Characteristics

Dermatofibrosarcoma protuberans and its variants contain either ring chromosomes or linear translocation derivatives resulting in the fusion of COL1A-1 (collagen type 1 alpha 1) from chromosome 17 with PDGFB (platelet-derived growth factor β) on chromosome 22.[56–61] Consequently, PDGFB is placed under control of the COL1A-1 promoter, leading to autocrine stimulation.

Differential Diagnosis

Helpful clues to distinguish fibrous histiocytoma from dermatofibrosarcoma protuberans include the former's circumscription, peripheral collagen entrapment, and polymorphous cellular composition. However, these features may not be appreciated on a limited biopsy, and secondary elements are lacking in the cellular variant of fibrous histiocytoma. Dermatofibrosarcoma protuberans exhibits strong and diffuse CD34 staining in contrast to absent or focal peripheral staining observed in fibrous histiocytomas.

Benign peripheral nerve sheath tumors, particularly the diffuse subtype of neurofibroma, may mimic dermatofibrosarcoma protuberans. Although both show a similar infiltrative growth pattern, dermatofibrosarcoma protuberans lacks S100 immunoreactivity. Diffuse-type neurofibromas will also often contain Meissner-like corpuscles. Neurofibromas may show immunoreactivity for CD34.

Lipofibromatosis-like neural tumor, a rare and recently described mesenchymal neoplasm with recurrent NTRK1 gene fusions, shows clinical and morphologic overlap with dermatofibrosarcoma protuberans.[62] Both are common in children and young

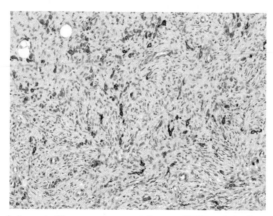

Fig. 13. Pigmented dermatofibrosarcoma protuberans (H&E, original magnification ×200).

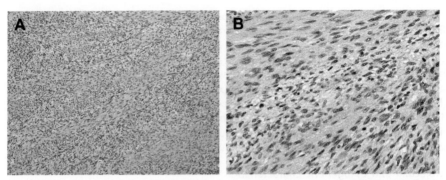

Fig. 14. Fibrosarcomatous transformation in dermatofibrosarcoma is characterized by fascicular/herringbone architecture rather than storiform growth (*A*, H&E, original magnification ×100). Mitotic figures (*B*, H&E, original magnification ×400) are readily identifiable in tumors with fibrosarcomatous change.

adults and express CD34; however, lipofibromatosis-like neural tumor shows consistent S100 expression and lacks aberrations of *PDGFB*.

Finally, cases of dermatofibrosarcoma protuberans with fibrosarcomatous transformation need to be differentiated from other sarcomas with herringbone or fascicular architecture, including synovial sarcoma and malignant peripheral nerve sheath tumor. Synovial sarcoma is usually deep seated, lacks CD34 staining, and is characterized by *SS18 (SYT)* fusions.[63] Malignant peripheral nerve sheath tumor is exceedingly rare at cutaneous sites and, when presenting in the skin, typically has an associated precursor neurofibroma.

Prognosis

Dermatofibrosarcoma protuberans is a locally aggressive tumor with a tendency for local recurrence ranging from 20% to 50%.[47,64,65] Although the true biologic behavior of tumors showing fibrosarcomatous change remains uncertain, there is evidence to suggest that these cases are at increased risk for local recurrence and distant metastasis.[55,66–69] Regardless, all variants of dermatofibrosarcoma protuberans should be treated with wide excision (2- to 3-cm margins). Because these tumors are characterized by autocrine stimulation secondary to overproduction of PDGFB, tyrosine kinase inhibitors may play a role in nonresectable and/or metastatic lesions.[70,71]

Key features

1. Slow-growing dermal nodule or plaque presenting in children or young adults.
2. Storiform proliferation of uniform spindle cells with diffuse infiltration into subcutaneous adipose tissue.
3. CD34 positive.

Pitfall

Fibrosarcomatous dermatofibrosarcoma protuberans may lose CD34 expression.

ANGIOMATOID FIBROUS HISTIOCYTOMA
Epidemiology and Clinical Features

Angiomatoid fibrous histiocytoma (previously known as angiomatoid malignant fibrous histiocytoma) can occur at any age, although children and young adults are most commonly affected. It has a predilection for the extremities.[72–74] Rarely, patients may present with systemic symptoms including anemia, pyrexia, and weight loss.[75,76]

Gross Features

These tumors are often circumscribed and pseudoencapsulated, multinodular or multicystic, and show varying degrees of hemorrhage.[74] The median size is approximately 2 cm, but cases exceeding 10 cm have been reported.[72,74]

Microscopic Features

Angiomatoid fibrous histiocytoma demonstrates a constellation of distinct morphologic features, including a dense fibrous pseudocapsule (**Fig. 15**A), peripheral lymphocyte cuff (**Fig. 15**B), and blood-filled cystic spaces lacking an endothelial lining (**Fig. 15**C). The lesional cells are spindled to ovoid in shape and show a bland histiocytoid appearance (**Fig. 15**D) with syncytial architecture. Less common morphologies include a prominent myxoid background, tumoral giant cells, and small cell pattern.[77–79] The mitotic rate is generally low, but occasional cases show marked nuclear pleomorphism, a finding of uncertain clinical significance.[72,80] Angiomatoid fibrous histiocytoma shows an unusual and unique immunophenotype, expressing the triad of desmin, EMA, and CD68 in approximately one-half of cases (**Fig. 15**E–G).[73,81] Although not diagnostically significant, it is important to recognize that angiomatoid fibrous histiocytoma may express CD99.

Molecular and Cytogenetic Characteristics

Three recurrent translocations have been identified: t(2;22) (q34;q12) (*EWSR1-CREB1*, >90% of cases), t(12;22) (q13;q12) (*EWSR1-ATF1*), and t(12;16) (q13;p11) (*FUS-ATF1*).[82–84]

Differential Diagnosis

The differential diagnosis of angiomatoid fibrous histiocytoma is broad, but the main considerations include aneurysmal fibrous histiocytoma, nodal metastasis, and Ewing sarcoma. Although aneurysmal fibrous histiocytoma often causes diagnostic confusion owing to similarities in name, this entity displays peripheral collagen entrapment rather than pseudoencapsulation with a lymphoid cuff. Furthermore, the cellular composition of aneurysmal fibrous histiocytoma is generally more heterogeneous, containing foamy histiocytes and multinucleated giant cells. The presence of a lymphoid cuff may raise the possibility of metastatic tumor deposits in a lymph node. Angiomatoid fibrous histiocytoma, however, lacks true nodal architecture, including subcapsular and medullary sinuses. Additionally, angiomatoid fibrous histiocytoma occurs most commonly in an age group in which metastatic disease would be unusual. Last, tumors with small cell morphology may mimic Ewing sarcoma. This differential is further complicated by the fact that both tumors may express CD99 and harbor rearrangements of *EWSR1*. Attention to the presence of fibrous pseudocapsule, lymphoid cuff, and cystic change may provide helpful clues. Because Ewing sarcoma most commonly shows *EWSR1-FLI* or *EWSR1-ERG* fusions, reverse transcription polymerase chain reaction can be used to identify specific fusion transcripts to differentiate these 2 entities on biopsy specimens.

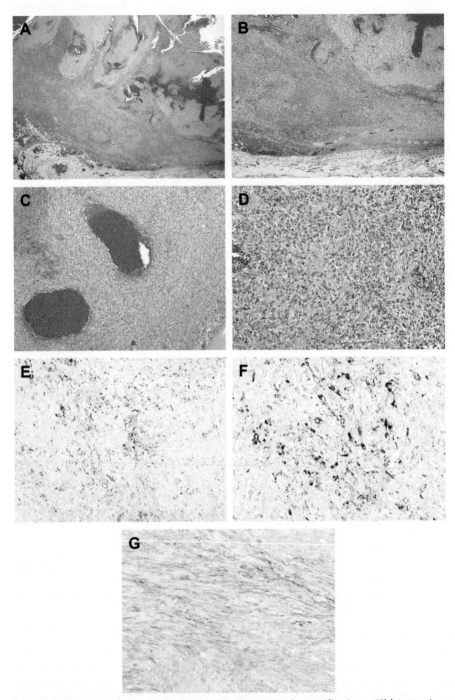

Fig. 15. Angiomatoid fibrous histiocytoma (*A*, H&E, original magnification ×40) has a unique low power appearance with a central cystic change, fibrous pseudocapsule and dense lymphoid cuff (*B*, H&E, original magnification ×100). Cystic hemorrhage in angiomatoid fibrous histiocytoma (*C*, H&E, original magnification ×200). The tumor cells (*D*, H&E, original magnification ×400) show histiocytoid morphology with pale eosinophilic cytoplasm and ovoid nuclei. Angiomatoid fibrous histiocytomas generally show focal staining with desmin (*E*, original magnification ×400), CD68 (*F*, original magnification ×400) and EMA (*G*, original magnification ×400).

Prognosis

Although Enzinger initially considered this tumor to be a variant of malignant fibrous histiocytoma in his initial description in 1979, subsequent work has shown a local recurrence rate of approximately 10% to 15% with only rare cases of metastatic disease.[72,74] To date, no clinical or histologic features, nor the presence of any specific genetic abnormality, as outlined, have been able to predict clinical behavior. Wide local excision with close clinical surveillance remains the treatment of choice.

Key features

1. Patients may exhibit systemic symptoms including fever and weight loss.
2. Characteristic appearance includes fibrous pseudocapsule, lymphoid cuff, and cystic change.
3. Approximately 50% of cases express triad of desmin, EMA, and CD68.
4. *EWSR1-CREB1* is the most common gene fusion.

Pitfalls

1. May mimic nodal lymph node metastasis.
2. Cases with small cell pattern may be mistaken for Ewing sarcoma given the presence of CD99 staining and *EWSR1* rearrangement.

PLEXIFORM FIBROHISTIOCYTIC TUMOR
Epidemiology and Clinical Features

Plexiform fibrohistiocytic tumor is a locally aggressive and rarely metastasizing mesenchymal tumor that most often arises in children, adolescents and young adults, with the majority of cases presenting in the first 2 decades of life.[85,86] Lesions show a predilection for the upper extremities, particularly distal, and are described as solitary, progressively enlarging masses.[85,86]

Gross Features

Lesions are poorly circumscribed, multilobulated or multinodular, and often seated in the subcutaneous fat or deep dermis, although extension into the upper dermis or skeletal muscle may be observed.[85,86]

Microscopic Features

Plexiform fibrohistiocytic tumor is a poorly circumscribed biphasic neoplasm composed of balls of mononuclear histiocytoid cells, osteoclast-like multinucleated giant cells, and bland spindled cells surrounded by interlacing fascicles of fibroblasts (**Fig. 16**).[85,86] These 2 components are found in variable proportions with approximately 40% showing classic bimorphic histology. The mononuclear cells resemble histiocytes with pale, eosinophilic cytoplasm with round-to-oval centrally placed nuclei. Mitotic activity and cytologic atypia tend to be minimal.[85,86] Immunohistochemically, CD68 is variably expressed, and smooth muscle actin is often positive in the spindled cells with a "tram-track" appearance.[86,87]

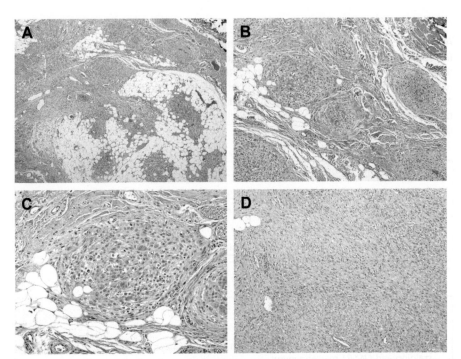

Fig. 16. Low-power examination of plexiform fibrohistiocytic tumor (*A*, H&E, original magnification ×100) reveals a poorly circumscribed proliferation of giant cell–rich nodules (*B*, H&E, original magnification ×200) linked by fibroblastic fascicles. The nodules are composed of osteoclast-type giant cells and histiocytoid mononuclear cells (*C*, H&E, original magnification ×400). The intervening fascicles (*D*, H&E, original magnification ×200) harbor bland spindle cells devoid of giant cells and histiocytes.

Differential Diagnosis

The differential diagnosis includes other mesenchymal neoplasms, such as giant cell tumor of soft tissue, cellular neurothekeoma, and fibrous hamartoma of infancy. Both giant cell tumor of soft tissue and cellular neurothekeoma lack the biphasic appearance of plexiform fibrohistiocytic tumor. Furthermore, giant cell tumor of soft tissue usually affects adults and does not exhibit an infiltrative growth pattern. Cellular neurothekeomas show a predilection for the head and neck region, exhibit a nested arrangement of histiocytoid cells separated by bands of collagen, and lack ramifying fibroblastic fascicles. Fibrous hamartoma of infancy usually presents in the first 2 years of life and demonstrates triphasic morphology, including whorls of primitive-appearing spindled cells.

Plexiform fibrohistiocytic tumor must also be differentiated from granulomatous inflammation. The presence of a fibroblastic component and lack of an associated inflammatory infiltrate are helpful morphologic clues that support the diagnosis of plexiform fibrohistiocytic tumor.

Prognosis

The local recurrence rate of plexiform fibrohistiocytic tumor reaches 40%.[86] Rare cases with regional lymph node metastasis and pulmonary metastasis have been reported.[85–88]

Key features

1. Poorly circumscribed biphasic neoplasm most commonly arising in the upper extremities of children and young adults.

2. Small nodules of mononuclear histiocytoid cells, osteoclast-type giant cells, and fibroblasts admixed with short and ramifying fascicles of fibroblasts.

Pitfall

Plexiform fibrohistiocytic tumor may mimic granulomatous inflammation.

ATYPICAL FIBROXANTHOMA
Epidemiology and Clinical Features

Atypical fibroxanthoma is a superficial undifferentiated tumor which has a predilection for sun-exposed sites of older individuals.[89,90] The term 'atypical fibroxanthoma' should be reserved for lesions measuring less than 2 cm and lacking the following: (1) significant involvement of the subcutis, (2) necrosis, and (3) vascular invasion. Tumors with any of these features should be classified as pleomorphic dermal sarcoma. Lesions tend to grow rapidly, and present as pink or erythematous nodules or plaques with central ulceration or scaling, often leading to confusion with squamous cell carcinoma or basal cell carcinoma on the basis of clinical examination. Risk factors include solar or therapeutic radiation and immunosuppression.[91–95] Although immunohistochemical techniques often fail to identify a line of differentiation for these tumors, there is ultrastructural evidence that these tumors exhibit fibroblastic/myofibroblastic features.[96,97]

Gross Features

Gross findings include a solitary nodule or polypoid masses, which may show ulceration and measures less than 2 cm (**Fig. 17A**).

Microscopic Features

Atypical fibroxanthoma is characterized by a fascicular or storiform pattern of atypical spindled or epithelioid cells within the dermis often abutting the epidermis (**Fig. 17B–C**). The deep margin may be pushing or infiltrative, but significant extension into subcutaneous adipose tissue is not allowed. The mitotic rate is variable, but may be brisk with atypical mitoses (**Fig. 17D**). Other morphologic findings may include multinucleated giant cells, myxoid stromal change (**Fig. 17E**), and admixed inflammation. Vascular invasion and necrosis are absent.

Immunohistochemical analysis is critical for the diagnosis of atypical fibroxanthoma, because this is ultimately a diagnosis of exclusion. Although there are rare case reports of keratin immunoreactivity in atypical fibroxanthoma, these tumors generally lack staining for cytokeratins and p63, as well as S100 and other melanocytic markers.[98–100] Because there is evidence that this entity may have fibroblastic or myofibroblastic derivation, smooth muscle actin expression may be appreciated; however, significant desmin staining is absent. Immunohistochemical stains such as CD10, CD68, CD163, and CD99 are nonspecific and uninformative in this setting.[101–104]

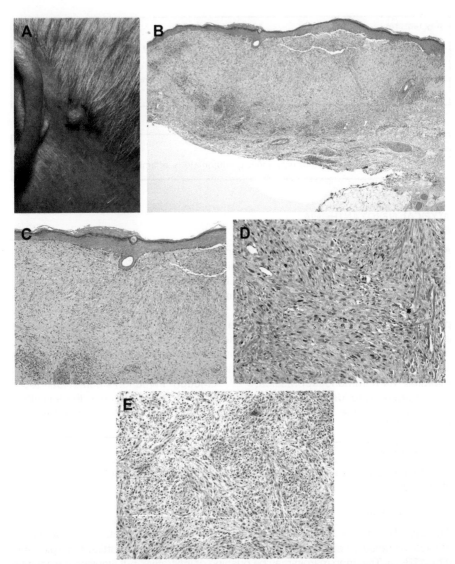

Fig. 17. Atypical fibroxanthoma presenting as a firm raised erythematous nodule (*A*). Atypical fibroxanthoma showing involvement limited to the dermis (*B*, H&E, original magnification ×40). The tumor cells are predominantly spindled with cytologic atypia (*C*, H&E, original magnification ×100). The overlying epidermis is unremarkable. High-power examination (*D*, H&E, original magnification ×200) reveals nuclear hyperchromasia and a brisk mitotic rate. The background stroma can show myxoid features (*E*, H&E, original magnification ×100).

Differential Diagnosis

The histologic differential diagnosis is vast and includes poorly differentiated malignancies, such as sarcomatoid carcinoma, spindle cell or desmoplastic melanoma, and specific sarcomas such as leiomyosarcoma, rhabdomyosarcoma, and angiosarcoma. As such, the initial evaluation should include pancytokeratin, high-molecular-weight cytokeratin, and S100. Additional melanocytic markers should be used when there is a high degree of suspicion for melanoma. Various myogenic markers, including smooth muscle actin, desmin, myogenin, and myoD1, are helpful to exclude leiomyosarcoma and rhabdomyosarcoma. Finally, angiosarcoma frequently presents as an ulcerated lesion on sun-damaged skin, and endothelial markers such as CD31, FLI-1, and ERG are critical to rule out this possibility.

Although immunostains are critical in the diagnosis of atypical fibroxanthoma, it is critical to not overlook important morphologic clues. Careful examination of the epidermis, if present, may yield an in situ or junctional component, and this finding may be more valuable than an extensive immunohistochemical workup. In superficially sampled lesions where it is not possible to distinguish between atypical fibroxanthoma and pleomorphic dermal sarcoma, it is best to render a descriptive diagnosis of pleomorphic dermal neoplasm with a recommendation to completely excise the lesion with negative margins for complete assessment of the lesion.

Prognosis

The prognosis for atypical fibroxanthoma when strictly defined by the criteria listed previously is excellent. The local recurrence rate seems to be less than 10%, with some series reporting rates as low as 0% to 1%.[90,105,106] Multiple large series have failed to show metastatic potential.[90,105,106] Wide local excision or Mohs micrographic surgery are the preferred treatments.[107,108] Pleomorphic dermal sarcomas, in contrast, have a significant risk of local recurrence and metastasis.[109,110]

Key features

1. Localized to the dermis with minimal, if any, involvement of the subcutis.

2. Less than 2 cm.

3. No necrosis.

4. No vascular invasion.

5. If there is infiltration into subcutis, necrosis, perineural, or lymphatic invasion, consider a diagnosis of pleomorphic dermal sarcoma.

Pitfall

Atypical fibroxanthoma may contain S100-positive dendritic cells and CD31-positive histiocytes.

ACKNOWLEDGMENTS

We kindly thank G. Frank Holmes, III, MD, Pathology Associates, Valley View Hospital, Glenwood Springs, Colorado, for his facilitation of our use of clinical and pathologic material.

REFERENCES

1. Gonzalez S, Duarte I. Benign fibrous histiocytoma of the skin. A morphologic study of 290 cases. Pathol Res Pract 1982;174:379–91.

2. Han TY, Chang HS, Lee JH, et al. A clinical and histopathological study of 122 cases of dermatofibroma (benign fibrous histiocytoma). Ann Dermatol 2011;23:185–92.

3. Newman DM, Walter JB. Multiple dermatofibromas in patients with systemic lupus erythematosus on immunosuppressive therapy. N Engl J Med 1973;289: 842–3.
4. Santa Cruz DJ, Kyriakos M. Aneurysmal ("angiomatoid") fibrous histiocytoma of the skin. Cancer 1981;47:2053–61.
5. Vanni R, Fletcher CD, Sciot R, et al. Cytogenetic evidence of clonality in cutaneous benign fibrous histiocytomas: a report of the CHAMP study group. Histopathology 2000;37:212–7.
6. Vanni R, Marras S, Faa G, et al. Cellular fibrous histiocytoma of the skin: evidence of a clonal process with different karyotype from dermatofibrosarcoma. Genes Chromosomes Cancer 1997;18:314–7.
7. Chen TC, Kuo T, Chan HL. Dermatofibroma is a clonal proliferative disease. J Cutan Pathol 2000;27:36–9.
8. Zelger BG, Sidoroff A, Zelger B. Combined dermatofibroma: co-existence of two or more variant patterns in a single lesion. Histopathology 2000;36:529–39.
9. Goldblum John R, Folpe Andrew L, Weiss Sharon W, et al. Enzinger and Weiss's soft tissue tumors. 6th edition. Philadelphia: Saunders/Elsevier; 2014.
10. Gleason BC, Fletcher CD. Deep "benign" fibrous histiocytoma: clinicopathologic analysis of 69 cases of a rare tumor indicating occasional metastatic potential. Am J Surg Pathol 2008;32:354–62.
11. Doyle LA, Fletcher CD. EMA positivity in epithelioid fibrous histiocytoma: a potential diagnostic pitfall. J Cutan Pathol 2011;38:697–703.
12. Doyle LA, Marino-Enriquez A, Fletcher CD, et al. ALK rearrangement and overexpression in epithelioid fibrous histiocytoma. Mod Pathol 2015;28:904–12.
13. Jedrych J, Nikiforova M, Kennedy TF, et al. Epithelioid cell histiocytoma of the skin with clonal ALK gene rearrangement resulting in VCL-ALK and SQSTM1-ALK gene fusions. Br J Dermatol 2015;172:1427–9.
14. Szablewski V, Laurent-Roussel S, Rethers L, et al. Atypical fibrous histiocytoma of the skin with CD30 and p80/ALK1 positivity and ALK gene rearrangement. J Cutan Pathol 2014;41:715–9.
15. Plaszczyca A, Nilsson J, Magnusson L, et al. Fusions involving protein kinase C and membrane-associated proteins in benign fibrous histiocytoma. Int J Biochem Cell Biol 2014;53:475–81.
16. Walther C, Hofvander J, Nilsson J, et al. Gene fusion detection in formalin-fixed paraffin-embedded benign fibrous histiocytomas using fluorescence in situ hybridization and RNA sequencing. Lab Invest 2015;95:1071–6.
17. Creytens D, Ferdinande L, Van Dorpe J. ALK rearrangement and overexpression in an unusual cutaneous epithelioid tumor with a peculiar whorled "Perineurioma-like" growth pattern: epithelioid fibrous histiocytoma. Appl Immunohistochem Mol Morphol 2016. [Epub ahead of print].
18. Erickson-Johnson MR, Chou MM, Evers BR, et al. Nodular fasciitis: a novel model of transient neoplasia induced by MYH9-USP6 gene fusion. Lab Invest 2011;91:1427–33.
19. Colome-Grimmer MI, Evans HL. Metastasizing cellular dermatofibroma. A report of two cases. Am J Surg Pathol 1996;20:1361–7.
20. Guillou L, Gebhard S, Salmeron M, et al. Metastasizing fibrous histiocytoma of the skin: a clinicopathologic and immunohistochemical analysis of three cases. Mod Pathol 2000;13:654–60.
21. Lodewick E, Avermaete A, Blom WA, et al. Fatal case of metastatic cellular fibrous histiocytoma: case report and review of literature. Am J Dermatopathol 2014;36:e156–62.

22. Charli-Joseph Y, Saggini A, Doyle LA, et al. DNA copy number changes in tumors within the spectrum of cellular, atypical, and metastasizing fibrous histiocytoma. J Am Acad Dermatol 2014;71:256–63.
23. Doyle LA, Fletcher CD. Metastasizing "benign" cutaneous fibrous histiocytoma: a clinicopathologic analysis of 16 cases. Am J Surg Pathol 2013;37:484–95.
24. Hornick JL, Fletcher CD. Cellular neurothekeoma: detailed characterization in a series of 133 cases. Am J Surg Pathol 2007;31:329–40.
25. Fetsch JF, Laskin WB, Hallman JR, et al. Neurothekeoma: an analysis of 178 tumors with detailed immunohistochemical data and long-term patient follow-up information. Am J Surg Pathol 2007;31:1103–14.
26. Gallager RL, Helwig EB. Neurothekeoma–a benign cutaneous tumor of neural origin. Am J Clin Pathol 1980;74:759–64.
27. Rosati LA, Fratamico FC, Eusebi V. Cellular neurothekeoma. Appl Pathol 1986;4: 186–91.
28. Laskin WB, Fetsch JF, Miettinen M. The "neurothekeoma": immunohistochemical analysis distinguishes the true nerve sheath myxoma from its mimics. Hum Pathol 2000;31:1230–41.
29. Sheth S, Li X, Binder S, et al. Differential gene expression profiles of neurothekeomas and nerve sheath myxomas by microarray analysis. Mod Pathol 2011; 24:343–54.
30. Stratton J, Billings SD. Cellular neurothekeoma: analysis of 37 cases emphasizing atypical histologic features. Mod Pathol 2014;27:701–10.
31. Han TY, Han B, Lee YC, et al. A rare case of atypical myxoid cellular neurothekeoma in a 6-year-old girl. Pediatr Dermatol 2016;33:e123–4.
32. Kaddu S, Leinweber B. Podoplanin expression in fibrous histiocytomas and cellular neurothekeomas. Am J Dermatopathol 2009;31:137–9.
33. Fox MD, Billings SD, Gleason BC, et al. Expression of MiTF may be helpful in differentiating cellular neurothekeoma from plexiform fibrohistiocytic tumor (histiocytoid predominant) in a partial biopsy specimen. Am J Dermatopathol 2012; 34:157–60.
34. Dehner LP. Juvenile xanthogranulomas in the first two decades of life: a clinicopathologic study of 174 cases with cutaneous and extracutaneous manifestations. Am J Surg Pathol 2003;27:579–93.
35. Janssen D, Harms D. Juvenile xanthogranuloma in childhood and adolescence: a clinicopathologic study of 129 patients from the kiel pediatric tumor registry. Am J Surg Pathol 2005;29:21–8.
36. Ringel E, Moschella S. Primary histiocytic dermatoses. Arch Dermatol 1985;121: 1531–41.
37. Sandell RF, Carter JM, Folpe AL. Solitary (juvenile) xanthogranuloma: a comprehensive immunohistochemical study emphasizing recently developed markers of histiocytic lineage. Hum Pathol 2015;46:1390–7.
38. Crocker AC. Skin xanthomas in childhood. Pediatrics 1951;8:573–97.
39. Fredrickson DS, Lees RS. A system for phenotyping hyperlipoproteinemia. Circulation 1965;31:321–7.
40. Marcoval J, Moreno A, Bordas X, et al. Diffuse plane xanthoma: clinicopathologic study of 8 cases. J Am Acad Dermatol 1998;39:439–42.
41. Wilkes LL. Tendon xanthoma in type IV hyperlipoproteinemia. South Med J 1977; 70:254–5.
42. Wilson DE, Floweres CM, Hershgold EJ, et al. Multiple myeloma, cryoglobulinemia and xanthomatosis. Distinct clinical and biochemical syndromes in two patients. Am J Med 1975;59:721–9.

43. Parker F. Xanthomas and hyperlipidemias. J Am Acad Dermatol 1985;13:1–30.
44. Cruz PD Jr, East C, Bergstresser PR. Dermal, subcutaneous, and tendon xanthomas: diagnostic markers for specific lipoprotein disorders. J Am Acad Dermatol 1988;19:95–111.
45. Brewer HB Jr, Zech LA, Gregg RE, et al. NIH conference. Type III hyperlipoproteinemia: diagnosis, molecular defects, pathology, and treatment. Ann Intern Med 1983;98:623–40.
46. Broeshart JH, Prens EP, Habets WJ, et al. Normolipemic plane xanthoma associated with adenocarcinoma and severe itch. J Am Acad Dermatol 2003;49:119–22.
47. Taylor HB, Helwig EB. Dermatofibrosarcoma protuberans. A study of 115 cases. Cancer 1962;15:717–25.
48. Fletcher CD, Evans BJ, MacArtney JC, et al. Dermatofibrosarcoma protuberans: a clinicopathological and immunohistochemical study with a review of the literature. Histopathology 1985;9:921–38.
49. Sanz-Trelles A, Ayala-Carbonero A, Rodrigo-Fernandez I, et al. Leiomyomatous nodules and bundles of vascular origin in the fibrosarcomatous variant of dermatofibrosarcoma protuberans. J Cutan Pathol 1998;25:44–9.
50. Morimitsu Y, Hisaoka M, Okamoto S, et al. Dermatofibrosarcoma protuberans and its fibrosarcomatous variant with areas of myoid differentiation: a report of three cases. Histopathology 1998;32:547–51.
51. Shmookler BM, Enzinger FM, Weiss SW. Giant cell fibroblastoma. A juvenile form of dermatofibrosarcoma protuberans. Cancer 1989;64:2154–61.
52. Dal Cin P, Sciot R, de Wever I, et al. Cytogenetic and immunohistochemical evidence that giant cell fibroblastoma is related to dermatofibrosarcoma protuberans. Genes Chromosomes Cancer 1996;15:73–5.
53. Ding JA, Hashimoto H, Sugimoto T, et al. Bednar tumor (pigmented dermatofibrosarcoma protuberans). An analysis of six cases. Acta Pathol Jpn 1990;40:744–54.
54. Wrotnowski U, Cooper PH, Shmookler BM. Fibrosarcomatous change in dermatofibrosarcoma protuberans. Am J Surg Pathol 1988;12:287–93.
55. Mentzel T, Beham A, Katenkamp D, et al. Fibrosarcomatous ("high-grade") dermatofibrosarcoma protuberans: clinicopathologic and immunohistochemical study of a series of 41 cases with emphasis on prognostic significance. Am J Surg Pathol 1998;22:576–87.
56. Sirvent N, Maire G, Pedeutour F. Genetics of dermatofibrosarcoma protuberans family of tumors: from ring chromosomes to tyrosine kinase inhibitor treatment. Genes Chromosomes Cancer 2003;37:1–19.
57. Simon MP, Pedeutour F, Sirvent N, et al. Deregulation of the platelet-derived growth factor B-chain gene via fusion with collagen gene COL1A1 in dermatofibrosarcoma protuberans and giant-cell fibroblastoma. Nat Genet 1997;15:95–8.
58. Mandahl N, Heim S, Willen H, et al. Supernumerary ring chromosome as the sole cytogenetic abnormality in a dermatofibrosarcoma protuberans. Cancer Genet Cytogenet 1990;49:273–5.
59. Nishio J, Iwasaki H, Ohjimi Y, et al. Supernumerary ring chromosomes in dermatofibrosarcoma protuberans may contain sequences from 8q11.2-qter and 17q21-qter: a combined cytogenetic and comparative genomic hybridization study. Cancer Genet Cytogenet 2001;129:102–6.
60. O'Brien KP, Seroussi E, Dal Cin P, et al. Various regions within the alpha-helical domain of the COL1A1 gene are fused to the second exon of the PDGFB gene

in dermatofibrosarcomas and giant-cell fibroblastomas. Genes Chromosomes Cancer 1998;23:187–93.

61. Shimizu A, O'Brien KP, Sjoblom T, et al. The dermatofibrosarcoma protuberans-associated collagen type Ialpha1/platelet-derived growth factor (PDGF) B-chain fusion gene generates a transforming protein that is processed to functional PDGF-BB. Cancer Res 1999;59:3719–23.

62. Agaram NP, Zhang L, Sung YS, et al. Recurrent NTRK1 gene fusions define a novel subset of locally aggressive lipofibromatosis-like neural tumors. Am J Surg Pathol 2016;40:1407–16.

63. Fletcher CDM, Bridge JA, Hogendoorn PCW, et al, editors. WHO classification of tumors of soft tissue and bone. 4th edition. Lyon (France): International Agency for Research on Cancer; 2013.

64. McPeak CJ, Cruz T, Nicastri AD. Dermatofibrosarcoma protuberans: an analysis of 86 cases–five with metastasis. Ann Surg 1967;166:803–16.

65. Fiore M, Miceli R, Mussi C, et al. Dermatofibrosarcoma protuberans treated at a single institution: a surgical disease with a high cure rate. J Clin Oncol 2005;23: 7669–75.

66. Connelly JH, Evans HL. Dermatofibrosarcoma protuberans. A clinicopathologic review with emphasis on fibrosarcomatous areas. Am J Surg Pathol 1992,16: 921–5.

67. Diaz-Cascajo C, Weyers W, Borrego L, et al. Dermatofibrosarcoma protuberans with fibrosarcomatous areas: a clinico-pathologic and immunohistochemic study in four cases. Am J Dermatopathol 1997;19:562–7.

68. Hisaoka M, Okamoto S, Morimitsu Y, et al. Dermatofibrosarcoma protuberans with fibrosarcomatous areas. Molecular abnormalities of the p53 pathway in fibrosarcomatous transformation of dermatofibrosarcoma protuberans. Virchows Arch 1998;433:323–9.

69. Bowne WB, Antonescu CR, Leung DH, et al. Dermatofibrosarcoma protuberans: a clinicopathologic analysis of patients treated and followed at a single institution. Cancer 2000;88:2711–20.

70. Sjoblom T, Shimizu A, O'Brien KP, et al. Growth inhibition of dermatofibrosarcoma protuberans tumors by the platelet-derived growth factor receptor antagonist STI571 through induction of apoptosis. Cancer Res 2001;61:5778–83.

71. Rubin BP, Schuetze SM, Eary JF, et al. Molecular targeting of platelet-derived growth factor B by imatinib mesylate in a patient with metastatic dermatofibrosarcoma protuberans. J Clin Oncol 2002;20:3586–91.

72. Costa MJ, Weiss SW. Angiomatoid malignant fibrous histiocytoma. A follow-up study of 108 cases with evaluation of possible histologic predictors of outcome. Am J Surg Pathol 1990;14:1126–32.

73. Fanburg-Smith JC, Miettinen M. Angiomatoid "malignant" fibrous histiocytoma: a clinicopathologic study of 158 cases and further exploration of the myoid phenotype. Hum Pathol 1999;30:1336–43.

74. Enzinger FM. Angiomatoid malignant fibrous histiocytoma: a distinct fibrohistiocytic tumor of children and young adults simulating a vascular neoplasm. Cancer 1979;44:2147–57.

75. Pettinato G, Manivel JC, De Rosa G, et al. Angiomatoid malignant fibrous histiocytoma: cytologic, immunohistochemical, ultrastructural, and flow cytometric study of 20 cases. Mod Pathol 1990;3:479–87.

76. Davies KA, Cope AP, Schofield JB, et al. A rare mediastinal tumour presenting with systemic effects due to IL-6 and tumour necrosis factor (TNF) production. Clin Exp Immunol 1995;99:117–23.

77. Schaefer IM, Fletcher CD. Myxoid variant of so-called angiomatoid "malignant fibrous histiocytoma": clinicopathologic characterization in a series of 21 cases. Am J Surg Pathol 2014;38:816–23.

78. Moura RD, Wang X, Lonzo ML, et al. Reticular angiomatoid "malignant" fibrous histiocytoma–a case report with cytogenetics and molecular genetic analyses. Hum Pathol 2011;42:1359–63.

79. Chen G, Folpe AL, Colby TV, et al. Angiomatoid fibrous histiocytoma: unusual sites and unusual morphology. Mod Pathol 2011;24:1560–70.

80. Weinreb I, Rubin BP, Goldblum JR. Pleomorphic angiomatoid fibrous histiocytoma: a case confirmed by fluorescence in situ hybridization analysis for EWSR1 rearrangement. J Cutan Pathol 2008;35:855–60.

81. Fletcher CD. Angiomatoid "malignant fibrous histiocytoma": an immunohistochemical study indicative of myoid differentiation. Hum Pathol 1991;22:563–8.

82. Waters BL, Panagopoulos I, Allen EF. Genetic characterization of angiomatoid fibrous histiocytoma identifies fusion of the FUS and ATF-1 genes induced by a chromosomal translocation involving bands 12q13 and 16p11. Cancer Genet Cytogenet 2000;121:109–16.

83. Rossi S, Szuhai K, Ijszenga M, et al. EWSR1-CREB1 and EWSR1-ATF1 fusion genes in angiomatoid fibrous histiocytoma. Clin Cancer Res 2007;13:7322–8.

84. Antonescu CR, Dal Cin P, Nafa K, et al. EWSR1-CREB1 is the predominant gene fusion in angiomatoid fibrous histiocytoma. Genes Chromosomes Cancer 2007; 46:1051–60.

85. Enzinger FM, Zhang RY. Plexiform fibrohistiocytic tumor presenting in children and young adults. An analysis of 65 cases. Am J Surg Pathol 1988;12:818–26.

86. Remstein ED, Arndt CA, Nascimento AG. Plexiform fibrohistiocytic tumor: clinicopathologic analysis of 22 cases. Am J Surg Pathol 1999;23:662–70.

87. Moosavi C, Jha P, Fanburg-Smith JC. An update on plexiform fibrohistiocytic tumor and addition of 66 new cases from the Armed Forces Institute of Pathology, in honor of Franz M. Enzinger, MD. Ann Diagn Pathol 2007;11:313–9.

88. Salomao DR, Nascimento AG. Plexiform fibrohistiocytic tumor with systemic metastases: a case report. Am J Surg Pathol 1997;21:469–76.

89. Dahl I. Atypical fibroxanthoma of the skin. A clinico-pathological study of 57 cases. Acta Pathol Microbiol Scand A 1976;84:183–97.

90. Fretzin DF, Helwig EB. Atypical fibroxanthoma of the skin. A clinicopathologic study of 140 cases. Cancer 1973;31:1541–52.

91. Dei Tos AP, Maestro R, Doglioni C, et al. Ultraviolet-induced p53 mutations in atypical fibroxanthoma. Am J Pathol 1994;145:11–7.

92. Sakamoto A. Atypical fibroxanthoma. Clin Med Oncol 2008;2:117–27.

93. Sakamoto A, Oda Y, Itakura E, et al. Immunoexpression of ultraviolet photoproducts and p53 mutation analysis in atypical fibroxanthoma and superficial malignant fibrous histiocytoma. Mod Pathol 2001;14:581–8.

94. Perrett CM, Macedo C, Francis N, et al. Atypical fibroxanthoma in an HIV-infected individual. J Cutan Pathol 2011;38:357–9.

95. Ferri E, Iaderosa GA, Armato E. Atypical fibroxanthoma of the external ear in a cardiac transplant recipient: case report and the causal role of the immunosuppressive therapy. Auris Nasus Larynx 2008;35:260–3.

96. Ito A, Yamada N, Yoshida Y, et al. Myofibroblastic differentiation in atypical fibroxanthomas occurring on sun-exposed skin and in a burn scar: an ultrastructural and immunohistochemical study. J Cutan Pathol 2011;38:670–6.

97. Barr RJ, Wuerker RB, Graham JH. Ultrastructure of atypical fibroxanthoma. Cancer 1977;40:736–43.

98. Bansal C, Sinkre P, Stewart D, et al. Two cases of cytokeratin positivity in atypical fibroxanthoma. J Clin Pathol 2007;60:716–7.
99. Gleason BC, Calder KB, Cibull TL, et al. Utility of p63 in the differential diagnosis of atypical fibroxanthoma and spindle cell squamous cell carcinoma. J Cutan Pathol 2009;36:543–7.
100. Suarez-Vilela D, Izquierdo FM, Escobar-Stein J, et al. Atypical fibroxanthoma with T-cytotoxic inflammatory infiltrate and aberrant expression of cytokeratin. J Cutan Pathol 2011;38:930–2.
101. de Feraudy S, Mar N, McCalmont TH. Evaluation of CD10 and procollagen 1 expression in atypical fibroxanthoma and dermatofibroma. Am J Surg Pathol 2008;32:1111–22.
102. Kanner WA, Brill LB 2nd, Patterson JW, et al. CD10, p63 and CD99 expression in the differential diagnosis of atypical fibroxanthoma, spindle cell squamous cell carcinoma and desmoplastic melanoma. J Cutan Pathol 2010;37:744–50.
103. Nakamura Y, Abe Y, Ichimiya M, et al. Atypical fibroxanthoma presenting immunoreactivity against CD10 and CD99. J Dermatol 2010;37:387–9.
104. Pouryazdanparast P, Yu L, Cutlan JE, et al. Diagnostic value of CD163 in cutaneous spindle cell lesions. J Cutan Pathol 2009;36:859–64.
105. Mirza B, Weedon D. Atypical fibroxanthoma: a clinicopathological study of 89 cases. Australas J Dermatol 2005;46:235–8.
106. Beer TW, Drury P, Heenan PJ. Atypical fibroxanthoma: a histological and immunohistochemical review of 171 cases. Am J Dermatopathol 2010;32:533–40.
107. Ang GC, Roenigk RK, Otley CC, et al. More than 2 decades of treating atypical fibroxanthoma at Mayo Clinic: what have we learned from 91 patients? Dermatol Surg 2009;35:765–72.
108. Wollina U, Schonlebe J, Koch A, et al. Atypical fibroxanthoma: a series of 25 cases. J Eur Acad Dermatol Venereol 2010;24:943–6.
109. Miller K, Goodlad JR, Brenn T. Pleomorphic dermal sarcoma: adverse histologic features predict aggressive behavior and allow distinction from atypical fibroxanthoma. Am J Surg Pathol 2012;36:1317–26.
110. Tardío JC, Pinedo F, Aramburu JA, et al. Leomorphic dermal sarcoma: a more aggressive neoplasm than previously estimated. J Cutan Pathol 2016;43:101–12.

Cutaneous Malignant Vascular Neoplasms

Wonwoo Shon, DO[a],*, Steven D. Billings, MD[b]

KEYWORDS

- Angiosarcoma • Atypical vascular lesion • Epithelioid hemangioendothelioma
- Cutaneous vascular tumors • Molecular pathology

KEY POINTS

- Angiosarcoma may be sporadic or may arise in the setting of chronic lymphedema (eg, Stewart-Treves syndrome) or secondary to radiation therapy.
- The increased use of adjuvant radiation therapy to treat various cancer types led to the awareness of radiation-induced atypical vascular lesion.
- Differentiating radiation-induced atypical vascular lesion and early evolving angiosarcoma requires precise microscopic evaluation in conjunction with clinicopathologic correlation and ancillary studies.
- Epithelioid hemangioendothelioma is a malignant vascular tumor that generally behaves in a less aggressive fashion than conventional angiosarcoma.
- Newer molecular techniques provide more accurate classification of cutaneous malignant vascular tumors.

CUTANEOUS ANGIOSARCOMA
Overview

Cutaneous angiosarcoma is a rare malignant vascular neoplasm that can develop in practically any body site. It is typically divided into 3 distinct groups: (1) primary sporadic angiosarcoma, (2) postradiation angiosarcoma, and (3) chronic lymphedema-associated angiosarcoma. Many examples of angiosarcoma frequently exhibit both vascular and lymphatic differentiation. Therefore, the historical terms, *hemangiosarcoma* and *lymphangiosarcoma*, are no longer applicable.

Clinical Features

Primary sporadic cutaneous angiosarcoma typically affects elderly adults, most commonly occurring in sun-damaged skin of the head and neck region. The

[a] Department of Pathology and Laboratory Medicine, Cedars-Sinai Medical Center, 8700 Beverly Boulevard, Room 8612, Los Angeles, CA 90048, USA; [b] Department of Pathology, Cleveland Clinic Lerner College of Medicine, Cleveland Clinic, 9500 Euclid Avenue, L25, Cleveland, OH 44195, USA
* Corresponding author.
E-mail address: wonwoo.shon@cshs.org

Clin Lab Med 37 (2017) 633–646
http://dx.doi.org/10.1016/j.cll.2017.06.004
0272-2712/17/© 2017 Elsevier Inc. All rights reserved.

labmed.theclinics.com

demographic suggest an etiologic role for ultraviolet exposure, but this concept is still debatable, as the presence of *TERT* promoter mutation (ultraviolet light-signature mutation) was not detected in a recent study.[1] Clinically, the early stage of superficial disease can be very deceptive and often confused with other cutaneous processes (eg, cellulitis or bruise). As the tumor progresses, it transforms into elevated plaques and nodules with or without ulceration. Approximately half of the patients initially present with multifocal satellite lesions that are close to the original tumor. In these cases, clinically determining the extent of the disease process is often difficult; thus, mapping biopsy strategy in the anatomic area of suspicion is recommended.

By definition, postradiation angiosarcoma develops within a prior radiation field. The incidence of postradiation angiosarcoma has increased as breast-conserving surgery with adjuvant radiation therapy has become standard care for those patients with early breast cancer. Although the usual antecedent malignancies are breast or gynecologic malignancies, it can occur in patients with a wide range of benign and malignant disorders, such as eczema, sinusitis, hemangiomas, hematolymphoid malignancies, head and neck and penile squamous cell carcinomas, and rectal carcinomas.[2] In the setting of breast cancer, the mean interval preceding angiosarcoma is shorter than that of other postradiation sarcomas. The mean latency is approximately 5 years and may present as soon as 1 to 2 years after radiation therapy.[3,4] Notably, when the radiation therapy is administered for benign antecedent disorders, which typically receive less irradiation, the median interval preceding angiosarcoma is 22 years (range, 4–40 years).[5]

Chronic lymphedema-associated angiosarcoma typically affects patients who have undergone radical/modified radical mastectomies and axillary lymph node dissection for breast carcinoma (Stewart -Treves syndrome). Most frequently, the lesion begins to develop on the inner aspect of the arm affected by lymphedema. This clinical subtype is decreasing because of the shift toward breast-conserving lumpectomy surgery and sentinel lymph node biopsy, as mentioned previously. Angiosarcoma may also develop in association with chronic congenital, posttraumatic, idiopathic, infectious (eg, filariasis), and obesity-associated lymphedema.[6,7] The average period from the onset of postmastectomy lymphedema to the appearance of angiosarcoma is approximately 10 years. Those lesions arising in the setting of chronic congenital and filariasis lymphedema often have a later onset (>20 years). The affected areas typically show pitting, indurated, or "peau d'orange" skin with violaceous macular, papular, or polypoid tumors.

Histopathologic Features

Regardless of the clinical subtype, cutaneous angiosarcoma has a broad morphologic spectrum.[3,4] Classically, angiosarcoma consists of architecturally complex, anastomosing vessels that dissect through dermal collagen (**Fig. 1**). The vessels are lined by atypical hyperchromatic endothelial cells with multilayering of endothelial cells. In some cases the atypia is subtle and multilayering may be absent or focal. The neoplastic vessels sometimes take on a sinusoidal growth pattern (see **Fig. 1**). Epithelioid angiosarcoma has vasoformative channels lined by tumor cells with enlarged round nuclei and abundant amphophilic cytoplasm or solid sheets of epithelioid tumor cells (**Fig. 2**).[8] Other cases may show solid fascicles of hyperchromatic spindled cells. In cases of a predominantly sheetlike or fascicular pattern, intratumoral hemorrhage is often a clue to consider the possibility of angiosarcoma.[9] Vasoformative areas are often present at the periphery of the tumor (**Fig. 3**). Cases may also have a mix of vasoformative and solid areas. In the setting of postradiation angiosarcoma of the breast, 2 additional patterns have been described. The tumor can be arranged in clusters of

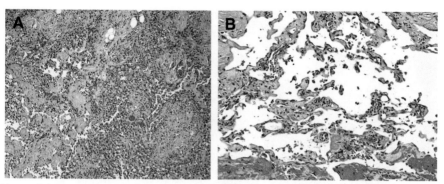

Fig. 1. (*A*) Cutaneous angiosarcoma characterized by neoplastic vessels lined by atypical endothelial cells dissecting between dermal collagen. (*B*) Angiosarcoma with sinusoidal vascular pattern.

atypical vessels somewhat reminiscent of a lobule of capillaries (**Fig. 4**) or as atypical cells lining noncomplex vessels or as single cells in the dermis with hemorrhage superficially resembling radiation dermatitis (**Fig. 5**).[10,11]

Immunohistochemical Features

By immunohistochemistry, the tumor cells express the typical endothelial markers, including CD31, CD34, FLI-1, and ERG (**Fig. 6**) and occasionally, putative lymphatic markers, such as D2-40, vascular endothelial growth factor (VEGF), and Prox1.[12,13] WT1 and Claudin-5 can be expressed, although the actual diagnostic utility of these markers is limited at this point.[14,15] Epithelioid angiosarcomas may also express low-molecular-weight cytokeratin, EMA, and CD30.[8] Actin stains may highlight pericytes in vasoformative areas, but pericytes typically are absent in the solid areas. Finally, some previous studies postulated the usefulness of antibodies specifically directed against members of signal transduction pathways (eg, caveolin), which potentially can help to differentiate benign vascular lesions from angiosarcomas.[16]

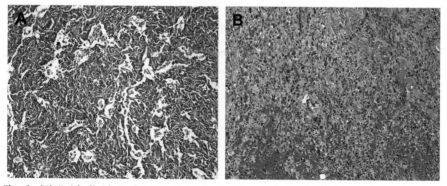

Fig. 2. (*A*) Epithelioid angiosarcoma with vascular channels lined by atypical epithelioid endothelial cells (*B*). Epithelioid angiosarcoma with solid sheets of atypical endothelial cells without obvious vascular channel formation.

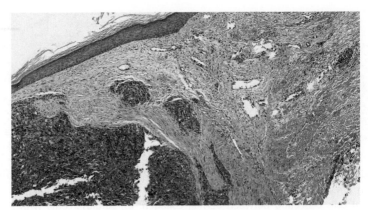

Fig. 3. Angiosarcoma with solid spindle cell areas and focal vasoformative areas at periphery of the tumor.

Genetic Features

Angiosarcoma is characterized by the overexpression of genes for vascular-specific receptor tyrosine kinases, including *TIE1, KDR, TEK*, and *FLT1 (VEGFR1)*.[17] In secondary angiosarcomas (postradiation and chronic lymphedema-associated), *MYC* gene amplification and expression is present in greater than 90% of cases and is presumed to play a key oncogenic role (**Fig. 7**).[18–21] Although gene amplification of *MYC* seems to be a specific genetic event of secondary angiosarcomas, more recent studies found the presence of *MYC* gene amplification and protein overexpression in a small subset of primary (non–radiation-associated) cutaneous and soft tissue angiosarcomas.[22,23] *FLT4* (encoding for VEGF3) co-amplification and recurrent somatic mutations in two angiogenesis-signaling genes, *PTPRB* and *PLCG1,* have also been found in subsets of secondary angiosarcomas.[24] Recently, rare examples

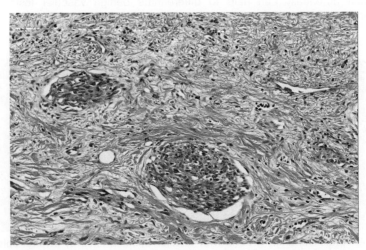

Fig. 4. Capillary lobule pattern of postradiation angiosarcoma with discrete nodules of atypical vessels.

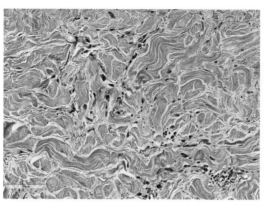

Fig. 5. Radiation dermatitis–like pattern of postradiation angiosarcoma with subtle vascular channels lined by atypical endothelial cells.

of predominantly nonvasoformative primary cutaneous angiosarcoma with epithelioid and spindled morphology have found the presence of *CIC* mutation.[19]

Differential Diagnosis

The primary differential diagnosis is with other vascular neoplasms. Although the infiltrative growth pattern, cytologic atypia, endothelial multilayering, and mitotic activity typically allows for recognition, there are some vascular neoplasms that may be confused with angiosarcoma. Kaposi sarcoma in the patch stage is composed of vessels that dissect through dermal collagen, but the degree of cytologic atypia is less, and multilayering is not typically present. Plaque and nodular Kaposi sarcoma is composed of fascicles of spindled cells with slitlike vascular spaces and can bear some resemblance to spindled forms of angiosarcoma, but the lesional cells of Kaposi sarcoma are less atypical.[9] The clinical setting of Kaposi sarcoma is also different. In problematic cases, immunohistochemical stains for HHV8 latent nuclear antigen will resolve the differential diagnosis, as Kaposi sarcoma is consistently positive, unlike angiosarcoma. Retiform hemangioendothelioma has architecturally complex vessels,

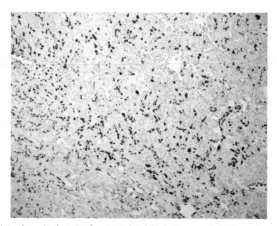

Fig. 6. Immunohistochemical stain for ERG highlighting nuclei of angiosarcoma.

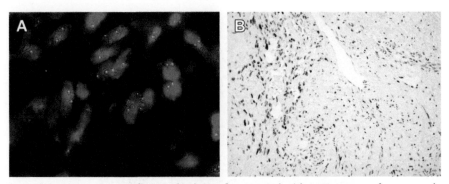

Fig. 7. (A) *MYC* gene amplification (*red signal*) compared with centromere reference probe (*green signal*) in postradiation angiosarcoma demonstrated by fluorescence in situ hybridization. (B) Immunohistochemical stain for MYC shows strong nuclear staining in postradiation angiosarcoma.

but less nuclear pleomorphism, and typically presents in the extremities of younger patients.[25] Spindled angiosarcoma arising in sun-damaged skin of the head and neck needs to be distinguished from atypical fibroxanthoma, pleomorphic dermal sarcoma, sarcomatoid squamous cell carcinoma, and spindle cell melanoma.[26] Immunohistochemistry allows ready distinction if one considers angiosarcoma in the differential diagnosis. An important clue is the presence of intratumoral hemorrhage. One should also carefully examine the periphery of the tumor if available, as vasoformative areas are often focally present. For epithelioid angiosarcoma, the differential diagnosis is broad and may include poorly differentiated carcinoma, melanoma, epithelioid sarcoma, and hematolymphoid tumors, such as anaplastic large cell lymphoma and histiocytic sarcoma.[8] Intratumoral hemorrhage again is a clue in tumors with less obvious vasiformation as is the amphophilic cytoplasm often seen in epithelioid angiosarcoma. Immunohistochemistry for endothelial cell markers is discriminatory. Expression of ERG (N-terminus) and FLI-1 nuclear has been documented in the subsets of epithelioid sarcomas, and granular CD31 immunoreactivity in intratumoral macrophages of nonvascular tumors should be recognized as a critical diagnostic pitfall.[27,28] Postradiation angiosarcoma has significant overlap with postradiation atypical vascular lesion discussed in more detail below. The absence of MYC expression or *MYC* amplification in atypical vascular lesion allows distinction in most problematic cases.[20,21]

Prognosis and Treatment

The prognosis of most angiosarcomas is generally poor, with a 5-year overall disease-specific survival rate of 30% to 50% based on recent studies. Local recurrence is common because of the highly infiltrative growth pattern. This growth pattern often makes it difficult to achieve negative surgical margins. The exact role of histologic grade on prognosis is controversial, and angiosarcomas are not formally graded by the widely accepted National Cancer Institute or French Federation Nationale des Centers de Lutte Contre le Cancer grading systems. In a series of 69 cases of sporadic cutaneous angiosarcoma, age older than 70 years, tumor necrosis, and epithelioid morphologic features were associated with an adverse clinical outcome.[29] The best chance for long-term survival seems to entail radical surgery at the time of the initial diagnosis. Adjuvant radiation therapy and taxane-based chemotherapy are found to have some therapeutic role. Unfortunately, long-term survival is still uncommon.[30]

ATYPICAL VASCULAR LESION
Overview

Although not a malignant vascular neoplasm, atypical vascular lesion is described separately because of the critical need to distinguish it from postradiation angiosarcoma.[31] These lesions are difficult to separate from early-stage angiosarcomas, both clinically and histologically. Atypical vascular lesion has also been described under the rubric of postradiation therapy lymphangioma/lymphangiectasia, benign lymphangiomatous papules, and benign lymphangioendothelioma in previously irradiated skin.[31–34]

Clinical Features

By definition, atypical vascular lesions develop in skin after radiation for various conditions. Most patients are women with a history of mammary carcinoma. The lesions typically appear as single or multiple erythematous papules or ecchymotic plaques months or years after radiation therapy, with a mean latency of 3 years. Most atypical vascular lesions are small (<1 cm) (**Fig. 8**).[31,33,34]

Pathologic Features

Histologically, atypical vascular lesions can exhibit several patterns, and some investigators prefer to separate them into 2 groups, namely, lymphatic-type and vascular-type.[35] Many lymphatic-type atypical vascular lesions are characterized by well-marginated proliferation of dilated and branched vascular spaces, resembling benign lymphangioma (benign lymphangiomatous papule).[31,33–35] These vessels are lined by bland-appearing flat or hobnail endothelial cells with occasional small papillary projections (**Fig. 9**). Some of these vessels can show a more infiltrative and interanastomosing pattern, which often has a notable dermal collagen dissection (lymphangioendotheliomalike pattern).[34] A rare subset of atypical vascular lesions typically resembles hobnail hemangioma or microvenular hemangioma, characterized by a proliferation of small capillary-type vessels with or without nuclear atypia (**Fig. 10**).[35] In some examples, both lymphatic and vascular patterns are seen within the same lesion.

Immunohistochemical Features

The endothelial cells are positive for typical endothelial makers, such as CD31, FLI-1, and ERG protein. Lymphatic-type atypical vascular lesions are positive for

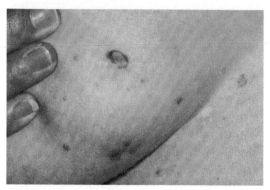

Fig. 8. Atypical vascular lesions presenting as translucent lymphangiomatous papules on previously irradiated breast skin.

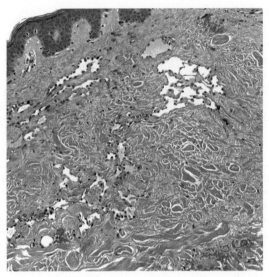

Fig. 9. Lymphatic-type atypical vascular lesion characterized by ectatic vessels lined by hobnail endothelial cells.

podoplanin/D2-40 but may be only focally positive for CD34 and have an incomplete pericyte layer seen with SMA stains.[34] Vascular-type atypical vascular lesions have a complete pericyte layer.[35] Actin stain highlights the pericyte component of the capillary-type vessels in those lesions with a vascular pattern.[35]

Differential Diagnosis

In this clinical context, the main differential diagnosis is postradiation angiosarcoma. Generally speaking, atypical vascular lesions lack the cytologic atypia, multilayering, and mitotic activity of angiosarcoma.[3,4,31] They are also relatively circumscribed and typically confined to the dermis. Nevertheless, distinction can be quite problematic in biopsy specimens, and recategorization of atypical vascular lesions as angiosarcoma is not uncommon in tumors diagnosed only by histologic criteria in limited

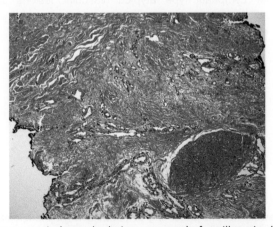

Fig. 10. Vascular-type atypical vascular lesion composed of capillary-sized vessels.

biopsy material.[36] As previously mentioned, greater than 90% of postradiation angiosarcomas have amplification of *MYC* and nuclear expression of MYC, and assessment for *MYC* gene amplification and protein overexpression has rapidly developed into a useful diagnostic tool in distinguishing angiosarcoma from atypical vascular lesion, as atypical vascular lesions do not have *MYC* amplification and only rarely and focally express MYC by immunohistochemistry.[18,20,21] The authors also noticed in the routine evaluation of postirradiation cutaneous vascular lesions that rare MYC immunohistochemistry-positive endothelial cells may be presented in nonangiosarcoma cases. Therefore, fluorescence in situ hybridization to determine *MYC* gene amplification should be considered in problematic cases.[23]

Prognosis and Treatment

At this point, conservative excision of the lesion is recommended for atypical vascular lesions if clinically feasible. Furthermore, rare cases of malignant transformation and coexistence of atypical vascular lesions with angiosarcoma have been reported, indicating that careful follow-up in conjunction with appropriate sampling is critical.[4,35]

EPITHELIOID HEMANGIOENDOTHELIOMA
Overview

Epithelioid hemangioendothelioma was first described by Weiss and Enzinger in 1982.[37] Although it was originally categorized as an intermediate (borderline) malignancy, the current World Health Organization soft tissue tumor classification considers epithelioid hemangioendothelioma to be a low-grade, though fully malignant, vascular tumor, because of its higher metastatic rate and more aggressive behavior than other hemangioendotheliomas.[38]

Clinical Features

Epithelioid hemangioendothelioma can affect patients of all age groups, but it is rare during childhood. Clinically, this tumor typically occurs as a solitary lesion on the extremities. The tumor can involve larger preexisting vessels and may cause ulceration or pain.[37] Cutaneous lesions typically have a nondescript clinical appearance, and a vascular tumor is not usually suspected at the time of biopsy.[8,39] In patients with multiple cutaneous tumor nodules, metastasizing deep soft tissue or osseous epithelioid hemangioendothelioma should be ruled out.

Pathologic Features

Microscopically, epithelioid hemangioendothelioma typically has chains, cords, or lobules of bland-looking epithelioid cells embedded in characteristic myxochondroid or hyalinized stromal matrix (**Fig. 11**).[8,37,39] Spindle or dendritic tumor cells may occasionally be present (**Fig. 12**). Some tumors occur within a preexisting lager vessel and may induce luminal obliteration by the neoplastic cells.[37] Scattered neoplastic cells have cytoplasmic vacuoles containing erythrocytes as a sign of early endothelial differentiation. Although the nuclear atypia is mild and mitotic activity is minimal, a subset of lesions can contain tumor cells with high-grade morphology that has been described as "malignant" epithelioid hemangioendothelioma and can be difficult to distinguish from epithelioid angiosarcoma at times.

Immunohistochemical Features

Immunohistochemically, epithelioid hemangioendotheliomas show a typical endothelial phenotype, expressing CD31, CD34, FLI-1, and ERG protein. Similar to other epithelioid vascular tumors, Keratins (low molecular weight) are often expressed,

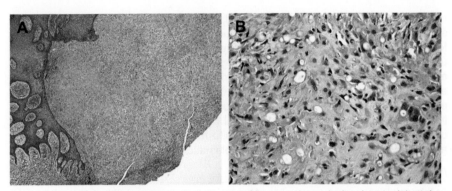

Fig. 11. (*A*) Epithelioid hemangioendothelioma infiltrating through the dermis. (*B*) Higher power image shows relatively bland endothelial cells, many with intracytoplasmic vacuoles, embedded in myxohyaline stroma.

but the tumor cells are typically negative for EMA. As discussed more detail later, epithelioid hemangioendotheliomas have rearrangement of *CAMTA1*.[40] Immunohistochemical stains to detect nuclear CAMTA1 expression are an effective surrogate for molecular studies and are a sensitive and specific test to confirm the diagnosis.[41]

Genetic Features

Almost all cases of epithelioid hemangioendothelioma have a t(1;3)(p36;q23–25) translocation that results in a fusion of *WWTR1* (3q23–24) with *CAMTA1* (1p36).[40] Recently, *YAP1-TFE3* fusions have been described in a subset of epithelioid hemangioendotheliomas with more vasoformative features, but this variant has not yet been described in cutaneous tumors.[42]

Differential Diagnosis

Epithelioid angiosarcoma differs from epithelioid hemangioendothelioma by virtue of its more significant cytologic atypia, diffuse mitotic activity and lack of characteristic myxohyaline matrix. In difficult cases, especially for those tumors with high-grade

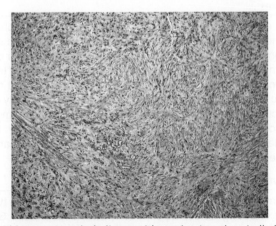

Fig. 12. Epithelioid hemangioendothelioma with predominantly spindled morphology.

morphology, identification of *CAMTA1* rearrangement or nuclear expression of CAMTA1 can aid in this distinction.[40,41]

Other cutaneous vascular tumors with epithelioid morphology, such as pseudo-myogenic/epithelioid sarcoma–like hemangioendothelioma and epithelioid he-mangioma, bear little, if any, resemblance to epithelioid hemangioendothelioma beyond coexpression of keratin and endothelial makers.[8] Moreover, pseudomyo-genic/epithelioid sarcoma–like hemangioendothelioma shows a distinctive immu-nophenotype. Only 50% to 70% of tumors are positive for CD31, and the neoplastic cells are typically negative for CD34. Most pseudomyogenic/epithelioid sarcoma–like hemangioendotheliomas contain a characteristic *SERPINE1-FOSB* fusion derived from t(7;19)(q22;q13).[43] Nuclear expression of FOSB protein was found recently to be a sensitive surrogate marker of this gene rearrangement.[44] Epithelioid hemangioma has more obvious vasoformation and frequently has an associated inflammatory component (angiolymphoid hyperplasia with eosinophilia).[8]

Because the vascular nature of the tumor may not be apparent on routine sections, epithelioid hemangioendothelioma is often confused with nonvascular neoplasms, such as epithelioid sarcoma, metastatic carcinoma, or possibly cutaneous mixed tumor/myoepithelioma. The loss of SMARCB1 (INI-1) protein expression is helpful in distinguishing epithelioid sarcoma from epithelioid hemangioendothelioma.[45] Meta-static breast carcinoma often has a cordlike growth pattern but lacks the myxohyaline stroma and immunoreactivity for vascular markers. Cutaneous mixed tumors and myoepitheliomas have myxohyaline stroma but are negative for vascular markers. Again, it should be remembered that epithelioid hemangioendothelioma may be positive for cytokeratins.

Prognosis and Treatment

As mentioned above, epithelioid hemangioendothelioma is currently classified as a low-grade malignant vascular tumor with a risk of lymph node or distant metastasis of approximately 20% to 30%. It has been suggested that aggressive behavior is more frequent in histologically high-grade variants of epithelioid hemangioendothelioma.[46] A more recent series of 49 soft tissue epithelioid hemangioendothelioma proposed that tumors can be stratified into two risk groups based on mitotic activity (3 mitotic figures per 50 high-power fields) and tumor size (>3 cm).[47] In this study, high-grade histologic features were not predictive of outcome. Compared with deep soft tissue and visceral examples, superficial cutaneous epithelioid hemangioendotheliomas seem to have a better prognosis. The treatment of choice for epithelioid hemangioen-dotheliomas is surgical excision with adequate margins, although one anecdotal report showed that topical application of imiquimod resulted in good response, but this should not be first line therapy.[48]

REFERENCES

1. Liau JY, Tsai JH, Yang CY, et al. Alternative lengthening of telomeres phenotype in malignant vascular tumors is highly associated with loss of ATRX expression and is frequently observed in hepatic angiosarcomas. Hum Pathol 2015;46:1360–6.

2. Edeiken S, Russo DP, Knecht J, et al. Angiosarcoma after tylectomy and radiation therapy for carcioma of the breast. Cancer 1992;70:644–7.

3. Billings SD, McKenney JK, Folpe AL, et al. Cutaneous angiosarcoma following breast-conserving surgery and radiation: an analysis of 27 cases. Am J Surg Pathol 2004;28:781–8.

4. Brenn T, Fletcher CD. Radiation-associated cutaneous atypical vascular lesions and angiosarcoma: clinicopathologic analysis of 42 cases. Am J Surg Pathol 2005;29(8):983–96.

5. Naus DM, Kelsen D, Clark DG. Radiation-induced angiosarcoma. Cancer 1987; 60:777–9.

6. Shon W, Ida CM, Boland-Froemming JM, et al. Cutaneous angiosarcoma arising in massive localized lymphedema of the morbidly obese: a report of five cases and review of the literature. J Cutan Pathol 2011;38:560–4.

7. Shon W, Wada DA, Folpe AL, et al. Angiosarcoma in a patient iwth congenital nonhereditary lymphedema. Cutis 2012;90:248–51.

8. Ko JS, Billings SD. Diagnostically challenging epithelioid vascular tumors. Surg Pathol Clin 2015;8:331–51.

9. Marušić Z, Billings SD. Histopathology of spindle cell vascular tumors. Surg Pathol Clin 2017;10:345–66.

10. Di Tommaso L, Rosai J. The capillary lobule: a deceptively benign feature of post-radiation angiosarcoma of the skin: report of three cases. Am J Dermatopathol 2005;27:301–5.

11. Daniels BH, Ko JS, Rowe JJ, et al. Radiation-associated angiosarcoma in the setting of breast cancer mimicking radiation dermatitis: a diagnostic pitfall. J Cutan Pathol 2017;44:456–61.

12. Miettinen M. Immunohistochemistry of soft tissue tumours - review with emphasis on 10 markers. Histopathology 2014;64:101–18.

13. Miettinen M, Wang ZF, Paetau A, et al. ERG transcription factor as an immunohistochemical marker for vascular endothelial tumors and prostatic carcinoma. Am J Surg Pathol 2011;35:432–41.

14. Timar J, Meszaros L, Orosz Z, et al. WT1 expression in angiogenic tumours of the skin. Histopathology 2005;47:67–73.

15. Miettinen M, Sarlomo-Rikala M, Wang ZF. Claudin-5 as an immunohistochemical marker for angiosarcoma and hemangioendotheliomas. Am J Surg Pathol 2011; 35:1848–56.

16. Morgan MB, Stevens GL, Tannenbaum M, et al. Expression of the caveolins in dermal vascular tumors. J Cutan Pathol 2001;28:24–8.

17. Antonescu CR, Yoshida A, Guo T, et al. KDR activating mutations in human angiosarcomas are sensitive to specific kinase inhibitors. Cancer Res 2009;69:7175–9.

18. Guo T, Zhang L, Chang NE, et al. Consistent MYC and FLT4 gene amplification in radiation-induced angiosarcoma but not in other radiation-associated atypical vascular lesions. Genes Chromosomes Cancer 2011;50:25–33.

19. Huang SC, Zhang L, Sung YS, et al. Recurrent CIC gene abnormalities in angiosarcomas: a molecular study of 120 cases with concurrent investigation of PLCG1, KDR, MYC, and FLT4 gene alterations. Am J Surg Pathol 2016;40: 645–55.

20. Fernandez AP, Sun Y, Tubbs RR, et al. FISH for MYC amplification and anti-MYC immunohistochemistry: useful diagnostic tools in the assessment of secondary angiosarcoma and atypical vascular proliferations. J Cutan Pathol 2012;39: 234–42.

21. Mentzel T, Schildhaus HU, Palmedo G, et al. Postradiation cutaneous angiosarcoma after treatment of breast carcinoma is characterized by MYC amplification in contrast to atypical vascular lesions after radiotherapy and control cases: clinicopathological, immunohistochemical and molecular analysis of 66 cases. Mod Pathol 2012;25:75–85.

22. Italiano A, Thomas R, Breen M, et al. The miR-17-92 cluster and its target THBSI are differently expressed in angiosarcomas dependent on MYC amplification. Genes Chromosomes Cancer 2012;51:569–78.

23. Shon W, Sukov WR, Jenkins SM, et al. MYC amplification and overexpression in primary cutaneous angiosarcoma: a fluorescence in-situ hybridization and immunohistochemical study. Mod Pathol 2014;27:509–15.

24. Behjati S, Tarpey PS, Sheldon H, et al. Recurrent PTPRB and PLCG1 mutations in angiosarcoma. Nat Genet 2014;46:376–9.

25. Calonje E, Fletcher CD, Wilson-Jones E, et al. Retiform hemangioendothelioma. A distinctive form of low-grade angiosarcoma delineated in a series of 15 cases. Am J Surg Pathol 1994;18:115–25.

26. Thum C, Husain EA, Mulholland K, et al. Atypical fibroxanthoma with pseudoangiomatous features: a histological and immunohistochemical mimic of cutaneous angiosarcoma. Ann Diagn Pathol 2013;17:502–7.

27. Stockman DL, Hornick JL, Deavers MT, et al. ERG and FLI1 protein expression in epithelioid sarcoma. Mod Pathol 2014;27:496–501.

28. McKenney JK, Weiss SW, Folpe AL. CD31 exprssion in intratumoral macrophages: a potential diagnostic pitfall. Am J Surg Pathol 2001;25:1167–73.

29. Deyrup AT, McKenney JK, Tighiouart M, et al. Sporadic cutaneous angiosarcomas. a proprosal for risk stratification based on 69 cases. Am J Surg Pathol 2008;32:72–7.

30. Shon W, Jenkins SM, Ross DT, et al. Angiosarcoma: a study of 98 cases with immunohistochemical evaluation of TLE3, a recently described marker of potential taxane responsiveness. J Cutan Pathol 2011;38:961–6.

31. Fineberg S, Rosen PP. Cutaneous angiosarcoma and atypical vascular lesions of the skin and breast after radiation therapy for breast carcinoma. Am J Clin Pathol 1994;102:757–63.

32. Rosso R, Gianelli U, Carnevali L. Acquired progressive lymphangioma of the skin following radiotherapy for breast carcinoma. J Cutan Pathol 1995;22:164–7.

33. Diaz-Cascajo C, Borghi S, Weyers W, et al. Benign lymphangiomatous papules of the skin following radiotherapy: a report of five new cases and review of the literature. Histopathology 1999;35:319–27.

34. Requena L, Kutzner H, Mentzel T, et al. Benign vascular proliferations in irradiated skin. Am J Surg Pathol 2002;26:328–37.

35. Patton KT, Deyrup AT, Weiss SW. Atypical vascular lesions after surgery and radiation of the breast: a clinicopathologic study of 32 cases analyzing histologic heterogeneity and associated with angiosarcoma. Am J Surg Pathol 2008;32:943–50.

36. Mattoch IW, Robbins JB, Kempson RL, et al. Post-radiotherapy vascular proliferations in mammary skin: a clinicopathologic study of 11 cases. J Am Acad Dermatol 2007;57:126–33.

37. Weiss SW, Enzinger FM. Epithelioid hemangioendothelioma: a vascular tumor often mistaken for a carcinoma. Cancer 1982;50(5):970–81.

38. Fletcher CDM, Bridge JA, Hogendoorn PCW, et al. World Health Organization Classification of tumours of soft tissue and bone 2013, in press

39. Quante M, Patel NK, Hill S, et al. Epithelioid hemangioendothelioma presenting in the skin: a clinicopathologic study of eight cases. Am J Dermatopathol 1998;20:541–6.

40. Tanas MR, Sboner A, Oliveira AM, et al. Identification of a disease-defining gene fusion in epithelioid hemangioendothelioma. Sci Transl Med 2011;3:98ra82.

41. Doyle LA, Fletcher CDM, Hornick JL. Nuclear expression of CAMTA1 distinguishes epithelioid hemangioendothelioma from histologic mimics. Am J Surg Pathol 2016;40:94–102.

42. Antonescu CR, Le Loarer F, Mosquera JM, et al. Novel YAP1-TFE3 fusion defines a distinct subset of epithelioid hemangioendothelioma. Genes Chromosomes Cancer 2013;52:775–84.

43. Trombetta D, Magnusson L, von Steyern FV, et al. Translocation t(7;19)(q22;q13)- a recurrent chromosome aberration in pseudomyogenic hemangioendothelioma? Cancer Genet 2011;204:211–5.

44. Huang YP, Fletcher CDM, Hornick JL. FOSB is a useful diagnostic marker for pseudomyogenic hemangioendothelioma. Am J Surg Pathol 2017;41:596–606.

45. Hornick JL, Dal Cin P, Fletcher CD. Loss of INI1 expression is characteristic of both conventional and proximal-type epithelioid sarcoma. Am J Surg Pathol 2009;33:542–50.

46. Weiss SW, Ishak KG, Dail DH, et al. Epithelioid hemangioendothelioma and related lesions. Semin Diagn Pathol 1986;3:259–87.

47. Deyrup AT, Tighiouart M, Montag AG, et al. Epithelioid hemangioendothelioma of soft tissue: a proposal for risk stratification based on 49 cases. Am J Surg Pathol 2008;32:924–7.

48. Sanchez-Carpintero I, Martinez MI, Mihm M, et al. Clinical and histopathologic observations of the action of imiquimod in an epithelioid hemangioendothelioma and Paget's mammary disease. J Am Acad Dermatol 2006;55:75–9.

Soft Tissue Tumors of Uncertain Histogenesis
A Review for Dermatopathologists

Darya Buehler, MD[a],*, Paul Weisman, MD[b]

KEYWORDS

- Epithelioid sarcoma • Clear cell sarcoma • Ossifying fibromyxoid tumor (OFMT)
- PEComa • Pleomorphic hyalinizing angiectatic tumor (PHAT)
- Hemosiderotic fibrolipomatous tumor (HFLT)

KEY POINTS

- Soft tissue tumors of uncertain histogenesis are a diverse group of mesenchymal neoplasms that often arise in the dermis or subcutis.
- These uncommon neoplasms can present a major diagnostic challenge to dermatopathologists because they closely mimic melanoma, carcinoma, fibrous histiocytoma, or granulomatous inflammation.
- Our ability to diagnose these tumors continues to improve with advances in their molecular genetic characterization.

INTRODUCTION

The mesenchymal tumors discussed herein represent a heterogeneous group of neoplasms with distinctive morphologic, immunophenotypic, and molecular genetic features. These tumors often arise in the dermis or subcutis and can pose a major diagnostic challenge because they closely mimic cases routinely encountered in dermatopathology practice such as melanoma, carcinoma, fibrous histiocytoma, schwannoma, or granulomatous inflammation. This article reviews the clinical presentation, histopathology, differential diagnosis, and diagnostic pitfalls of epithelioid sarcoma (ES), clear cell sarcoma (CCS), perivascular epithelioid cell tumor (PEComa), ossifying fibromyxoid tumor (OFMT), pleomorphic hyalinizing angiectatic tumor (PHAT), and hemosiderotic fibrolipomatous tumor (HFLT). Associated molecular genetic findings are also reviewed with an emphasis on their diagnostic usefulness.

The authors have nothing to disclose.
[a] Department of Pathology and Laboratory Medicine, University of Wisconsin School of Medicine and Public Health, 600 Highland Avenue, L5/184 CSC, Madison, WI 53792, USA;
[b] Department of Pathology and Laboratory Medicine, University of Wisconsin School of Medicine and Public Health, 600 Highland Avenue, B1779 WIMR, Madison, WI 53792, USA
* Corresponding author.
E-mail address: buehler2@wisc.edu

Clin Lab Med 37 (2017) 647–671
http://dx.doi.org/10.1016/j.cll.2017.06.005
0272-2712/17/© 2017 Elsevier Inc. All rights reserved.

EPITHELIOID SARCOMA

ES is a distinctive malignant neoplasm with predominantly epithelioid morphology that was first described by Enzinger in 1970[1] followed by an expanded series by Chase and Enzinger in 1985.[2] There are 2 types of ES: the conventional or distal type and the proximal type with a predilection for proximal or axial locations, rhabdoid morphology and more aggressive behavior.[3] Both types are characterized by mutations in the *SMARCB1/hSNF5/INI1* gene on chromosome 22q11.[4,5]

Clinical Features

Distal-type ES presents over a wide age range, with a peak in the second to third decades[2,6]; it may occur in young children comprising up to 7% to 8% of nonrhabdomyosarcomatous pediatric sarcomas.[7] Distal-type ES manifests as a firm, slowly growing subcutaneous mass, plaque, or nonhealing ulcer in the distal extremities, especially the fingers, hands, and forearm.[2] It is not uncommon to see a patient with a long-standing history of recurrent "inflammation," "warts," or "ulcers" on the fingers. Distal-type ES tends to grow along nerve trunks, fascial planes, and tendons,[1,2] accounting for the high rate of local recurrence (80%–90%).[2,8] Late metastases occur in up to 50% of patients and most commonly involve the lymph nodes and lung, and less commonly bones and skin (especially the scalp).[2]

Proximal-type ES, first described by Guillou and colleagues[3] in 1997, typically occurs as a deep-seated mass in a relatively older population, usually the fourth decade and above.[3,9,10] Common sites include the proximal limbs and limb girdles as well as the pelvis, perineum, genital areas, head and neck, and mediastinum. In contrast with the slow, indolent course of distal-type ES, proximal-type ES pursues a more aggressive clinical course with rapid progression to systemic metastases.[3]

Histologic Features

Distal-type ES usually presents as an infiltrative dermal or subcutaneous nodule or nodules with ill-defined margins. The nodules often surround a zone of central geographic necrosis or fibrosis around which the tumor cells show a palisaded arrangement, imparting a pseudogranulomatous appearance (**Fig. 1**A). Cytologically, the tumor is composed of relatively uniform epithelioid or spindled cells arranged in nests, cords, or single files. The cells have round to oval nuclei, vesicular chromatin, inconspicuous nucleoli, and eosinophilic cytoplasm, and can resemble histiocytes (see **Fig. 1**B). Nuclear atypia ranges from mild to severe, but many examples of this lesion are deceptively bland. Although mitotic activity is usually low (<5/10 high-power fields [HPF]), perineural and vascular invasion are common and are helpful in establishing the diagnosis in cytologically bland cases (see **Fig. 1**C). Variable amounts of chronic inflammation and fibrosis are present and can cause distal-type ES to be mistaken for nonspecific inflammatory change (see **Fig. 1**D). Of a particular importance is the pseudogranulomatous appearance of distal-type ES, which can lead to misdiagnosis as a palisading granulomatous dermatitis. Other reported morphologic features include hemorrhage, necrosis, angiomatoid change, calcifications, osseous or cartilaginous metaplasia, and a predominantly spindle cell variant that can masquerade as a benign fibroblastic or fibrohistiocytic lesion.[1,2,9]

Proximal-type ES is a large, subcutaneous, or deep-seated mass composed of sheets of large, overtly atypical and mitotically active epithelioid cells with round nuclei, prominent nucleoli, and dense eosinophilic cytoplasm (**Fig. 2**A, B). A frequent, although not invariable finding, is the presence of a perinuclear hyaline eosinophilic

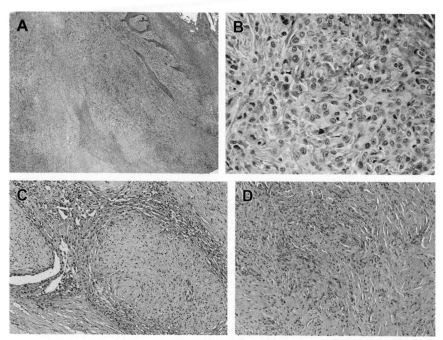

Fig. 1. Distal-type epithelioid sarcoma. (*A*) Ill-defined dermal nodule with tumor cells coalescing around a zone of central geographic necrosis imparting a pseudogranulomatous appearance (H&E, original magnification ×40). (*B*) Uniform epithelioid to spindled cells with oval nuclei, vesicular chromatin, inconspicuous nucleoli and dense eosinophilic cytoplasm; mild nuclear atypia and occasional mitotic figures are present (H&E, original magnification ×400). (*C*) Perineural invasion in epithelioid sarcoma (H&E, original magnification ×100). (*D*) Prominent fibrosis and chronic inflammation in distal-type epithelioid sarcoma, which can be mistaken for nonspecific inflammatory change (H&E, original magnification ×100).

rhabdoid inclusion (see **Fig. 2**C). Ultrastructurally, this inclusion is usually composed of cytokeratin.[3]

Immunohistochemistry and Molecular and Genetic Findings

By immunohistochemistry (IHC), most distal and proximal-type ES express low- and high-molecular-weight cytokeratins and epithelial membrane antigen (EMA). Approximately 60% are positive for CD34.[9,11,12] Smooth muscle actin (SMA) and S100 protein are occasionally positive.[12] Both types of ES are characterized by inactivation of the *SMARCB1/hSNF5/INI-1* gene on chromosome 22q11, which encodes a subunit of SWI/SNF chromatin remodeling complex. This results in loss of nuclear expression of INI1 (SMARCB1) by IHC in approximately 90% of cases.[5,12] Because INI1 is ubiquitously expressed in normal tissues and most neoplasms, loss of expression is a very helpful diagnostic feature (see **Fig. 2**D).

Differential Diagnosis

The most important mimickers of distal-type ES are granulomatous inflammatory processes (granuloma annulare, rheumatoid nodule, and necrobiosis lipoidica), infectious granulomas, and benign fibrohistiocytic tumors. Benign histiocytes and fibroblasts in these entities lack cytologic atypia, which is usually at least focally present in distal ES. By IHC, the histiocytes in granulomatous proliferations and fibrous histiocytomas

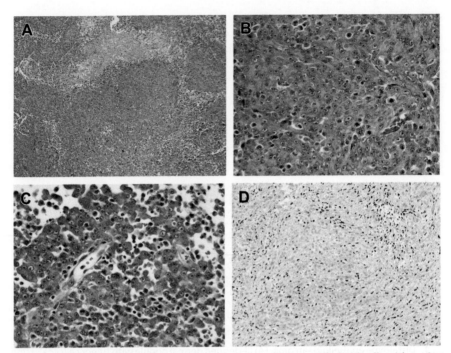

Fig. 2. Proximal-type epithelioid sarcoma. (*A*) Sheets of large epithelioid cells with eosinophilic cytoplasm and areas of necrosis (H&E, original magnification ×40). (*B*) The tumor cells have round nuclei with overt atypia, prominent nucleoli and mitotic activity (H&E, original magnification ×400). (*C*) Rhabdoid morphology with perinuclear hyaline eosinophilic inclusion (H&E, original magnification ×400). (*D*) Loss of INI1 expression in the tumor nuclei; background stromal fibroblasts and vasculature retain INI1 expression (INI1 immunostain, original magnification ×100).

express CD68 and CD163, lack cytokeratin and EMA immunoreactivity, and retain INI1 expression. Finally, a high index of suspicion for ES should be maintained in any distal extremity lesion from a young patient, especially in a long-standing, recurrent or otherwise unusual process.

Distal-type ES with more overt cytologic atypia can resemble cutaneous adnexal carcinoma or squamous cell carcinoma, which have substantial immunohistochemical overlap with distal-type ES. However, carcinomas usually lack geographic necrosis with peripheral palisading. Moreover, adnexal and squamous cell carcinomas are negative for CD34, have retained INI1 expression, and are usually positive for CK5/6, unlike distal-type ES.[9,13]

Pseudomyogenic or ES-like hemangioendothelioma[14,15] is a distinctive epithelioid vascular neoplasm of intermediate malignancy that also affects distal extremities of young adults and presents as a multifocal disease. The aptly named tumor is composed of sheets or fascicles of plump, cytokeratin-positive epithelioid, or spindled cells with abundant eosinophilic cytoplasm, mild nuclear atypia, and low mitotic activity, all of which may be seen in distal-type ES. Pseudomyogenic hemangioendothelioma can be distinguished based on its more prominent fascicular myoid component, the lack of a nodular growth pattern, and geographic necrosis and the expression of cytokeratins, retained INI1 expression and expression of vascular markers CD31, ERG (C-terminus), and Fli-1. In contrast with ES, EMA and CD34 are consistently negative in pseudomyogenic hemangioendothelioma. Recently, a pathognomonic *SERPINE1/FOSB* rearrangement has been described in pseudomyogenic hemangioendothelioma and molecular studies to detect *FOSB* rearrangements and IHC to detect nuclear expression of FOSB can be of use in challenging cases.[16,17]

In contrast with distal-type ES, proximal-type ES is readily recognizable as a high-grade malignancy. However, it can closely mimic other malignant cutaneous tumors with epithelioid morphology. Amelanotic melanoma can be distinguished from proximal-type ES by expression of melanocytic markers, lack of cytokeratin and CD34 expression, and retained INI1 expression. Epithelioid angiosarcoma may express both cytokeratins and CD34, but consistently expresses a variety of true vascular markers and shows retained INI1 expression. Epithelioid malignant peripheral nerve sheath tumor (MPNST) may be associated with a nerve and has prominent myxoid stroma, a feature not usually seen in proximal-type ES. Epithelioid MPNST is strongly and diffusely positive for S100 and is usually negative for cytokeratins. However, INI1 IHC may not be helpful in this context, because approximately 70% of epithelioid MPNSTs show loss of nuclear expression.[18] Perhaps the most difficult epithelioid tumor to distinguish from proximal-type ES is myoepithelial carcinoma (malignant myoepithelioma). Myoepithelial carcinoma is a more morphologically heterogenous tumor that typically coexpresses cytokeratins and markers of myoepithelial differentiation (p63, SMA, GFAP, and/or S100) and is negative for CD34. Approximately 50% of cases show rearrangement of *EWSR1* gene.[19] A potential pitfall is that myoepithelial carcinoma also shows loss of INI1 expression in approximately 50% of cases.[20]

Prognosis and Treatment

Distal-type ES has a protracted clinical course characterized by a very high rate of local recurrence (80%–90%) and a significant rate of late metastasis (up to 50%) to lymph nodes and distant sites.[2,21] The 5-year overall survival is 65% to 78%[6] and up to 92% in the pediatric population.[7] Conversely, proximal-type ES is associated with an aggressive clinical course and early metastases in 54% to 75% of patients.[3,10] Radical excision is the treatment of choice for both types.[6] Although sometimes performed, there are no uniform guidelines regarding lymph node dissection or sentinel lymph node biopsy in ES.[22–24] A recent study reported a better overall survival in patients with resectable ES and negative lymph nodes compared with those with positive lymph nodes or those in whom the lymph node status was not evaluated.[24] Key features of ES are summarized in **Box 1**.

CLEAR CELL SARCOMA

CCS is a rare soft tissue sarcoma with true melanocytic differentiation, first described by Enzinger as a deep-seated soft tissue tumor primarily involving tendons and aponeuroses.[25] CCS bears close morphologic, immunophenotypic, and ultrastructural resemblance to melanoma, which is reflected in its former name "malignant melanoma of soft parts."[26] However, CCS is biologically and genetically distinct from melanoma. CCS is characterized by a balanced t(12;22) (q13;q12) or t(2;22) (q34;q12) translocation resulting in *EWSR1/ATF1* or *EWSR1/CREB1* fusion transcripts, respectively.[27–31] The resultant proteins are thought to constitutively activate *MITF*, which drives the tumor's melanocytic phenotype (discussed elsewhere in this article).

Clinical Features

CCS usually presents in young adults in the second to fourth decades, although a wide age range may be affected. CCS shows a predilection for the distal limbs, especially

---

Box 1
Key features: epithelioid sarcoma

Distal-type epithelioid sarcoma

- Epidemiology: young individuals in their 20s and 30s
- Clinical presentation: distal extremities - most common sarcoma of hands; subtle presentation as a nonhealing ulcer or a slowly growing subcutaneous mass
- Grows along nerve trunks and fascial planes; new nodules occur more proximally
- Histology: nodular growth pattern surrounding a geographic zone of central necrosis with palisading of tumor cells, mimicking granulomatous inflammation
- Uniform epithelioid to spindled cells that can resemble histiocytes
- Nuclear atypia can be very mild, especially in cases with predominantly spindle cell morphology; mitotic activity is usually low (<5/10 high-power fields)
- Perineural and vascular invasion are common
- Diagnostic mimickers: granuloma annulare, rheumatoid nodule, necrobiosis lipoidica, infectious granulomas, benign fibrohistiocytic tumors, epithelioid sarcoma-like/ pseudomyogenic hemangioendothelioma
- Prognosis: indolent clinical course with high rate of local recurrence and late metastases to lymph nodes, lung, bone, and skin

Proximal-type epithelioid sarcoma

- Epidemiology: older adults with a predilection for proximal limbs, trunk, head and neck, genital areas, pelvis, and perineum
- Clinical presentation: large, overtly malignant soft tissue mass
- Histology: sheets of large epithelioid cells with round nuclei, prominent nucleoli and dense eosinophilic cytoplasm; marked nuclear atypia and mitotic activity
- Perinuclear hyaline "rhabdoid" inclusions
- Diagnostic mimickers: epithelioid angiosarcoma, epithelioid malignant peripheral nerve sheath tumor, myoepithelial carcinoma
- Prognosis: aggressive sarcoma with rapid progression to systemic metastasis
- Both types of epithelioid sarcoma express cytokeratins, EMA, CD34 (60%) and demonstrate loss of SMARCB1/INI1 nuclear expression (90%)

---

the ankle and foot, and presents as a slowly growing, deep soft tissue mass with an attachment to tendons, aponeuroses, or fasciae.[25,26,30–33] Cutaneous involvement occurs either as a secondary extension from the underlying soft tissue tumor or as a primary dermal neoplasm, which may involve the subcutis[34–38] (**Fig. 3**A). Like their more deeply seated counterparts, cutaneous CCS also tend to occur in the distal extremities and less frequently on the trunk, proximal limbs, or head and neck. They are usually small, less than 2 cm in size. Rarely, they are grossly pigmented.[26]

Histologic Features

CCS is composed of nests and fascicles of uniform spindled to fusiform cells separated by fibrous bands (see **Fig. 3**B). The overlying dermis is usually uninvolved and the epidermis is intact,[26] but in cutaneous CCS, the epidermis may be ulcerated. Most cutaneous cases are dermal-based tumors. However, nests of tumor cells at the dermal–epidermal junction mimicking the junctional component of a melanoma,

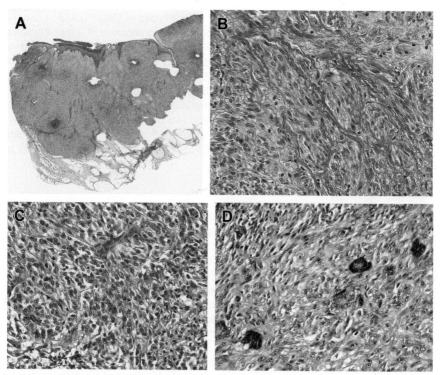

Fig. 3. Clear cell sarcoma. (*A*) Cutaneous clear cell sarcoma with involvement of the subcutis (H&E, original magnification ×10). (*B*) Nests and fascicles of uniform spindled to fusiform cells separated by delicate fibrous bands (H&E, original magnification ×200). (*C*) The tumor cells show overt nuclear atypia with prominent nucleoli, and palely eosinophilic granular cytoplasm (H&E, original magnification ×200). (*D*) Distinctive wreathlike multinucleated tumor giant cells in clear cell sarcoma (H&E, original magnification ×200).

as well as intraepidermal pagetoid spread, have been documented.[34,36,38] The cytoplasmic clearing occurs owing to accumulation of glycogen,[26] but truly optically clear cytoplasm is uncommon in CCSs; more often, the cytoplasm is palely eosinophilic and finely granular, resembling that of a cellular blue nevus or melanoma (see **Fig. 3**C). In most cases, the cells are overtly atypical with large vesicular nuclei and prominent nucleoli, but marked nuclear pleomorphism is not characteristic and the mitotic rate is highly variable. The stroma is usually sclerotic. Multinucleated wreathlike tumor giant cells are a very helpful feature, but are not present consistently (see **Fig. 3**D). Melanin pigment can be demonstrated by light microscopic examination in a minority of cases and in up to 70% of cases with histochemical stains.[26,30,34] Less common morphologic variations include rhabdoid features, bizarre pleomorphic cells, alveolar architecture, and seminoma-like patterns.[30] Metastatic CCS may acquire a more epithelioid or pleomorphic appearance reminiscent of melanoma or carcinoma.[26]

Immunohistochemistry and Molecular and Genetic Findings

CCSs diffusely express S100 protein and, in most cases, coexpress the melanocytic markers Melan-A, HMB45, SOX10, MiTF, and NKI/C3. Synaptophysin, CD57, EMA, CD34, and CD117 (c-KIT) expression have been observed in a minority of cases.[30] Cytokeratins, desmin, and SMA stains are usually negative. The hallmark of CCS is a balanced t(12;22)(q13;q12) translocation resulting in fusion of *EWSR1* with the cAMP-regulated transcription factor *ATF1*.[27–31] Four types of *EWSR1/ATF1* chimeric transcripts have been identified[27] without prognostic significance.[29] A less common t(2;22)(q34;q12) rearrangement with *EWSR1/CREB1* fusion, primarily found in gastrointestinal CCS,[39] has also been found in soft tissue and cutaneous examples.[30,31] The downstream effect of the *EWSR/ATF1* fusion in CCS is constitutive activation of the melanocyte-specific MITF (MITF-M) promoter,[28,40] resulting in aberrant MITF expression that drives the melanocytic phenotype and c-Met oncogenic signaling.[41] The fusion transcripts can be detected by reverse transcriptase polymerase chain reaction in more than 90% of cases.[27–29,31] Fluorescence in situ hybridization (FISH) testing can detect the *EWSR1* gene rearrangement in 70% to 100% of cases.[31,42,43]

Differential Diagnosis

It is essential to distinguish CCS from other neoplasms with melanocytic differentiation. The most problematic tumor in this regard is cutaneous or metastatic spindle cell melanoma, which can be virtually identical in terms of its morphology and immunophenotype. The monotonous appearance of the tumor nests (in contrast with more heterogenous appearance in spindle cell melanomas) and the presence of wreathlike giant cells favor CCS.[34,35] A junctional or lentiginous component is more typical of melanoma. However, as mentioned, rare cases of CCS with epidermal involvement have all been observed.[34,36,38] Molecular testing allows distinction, because melanomas are negative for *EWSR1* gene rearrangements[42] and often harbor *BRAF* mutations, which are rare in CCS.[33,44]

Amelanotic cellular blue nevus can resemble CCS because of the increased cellularity, nested arrangement of uniform spindle cells surrounded by fibrous bands, and scattered multinucleated giant cells. Cutaneous CCS that secondarily involve the subcutis can mimic the dumbbell-shaped extension seen in cellular blue nevi. The presence of a second population of slender dendritic melanocytes, similar to those seen in common blue nevi, helps to distinguish cellular blue nevus from CCS.[45] Most cellular blue nevi also lack the cytologic atypia and mitotic activity. Atypical and so-called malignant cellular blue nevi (blue nevus–like melanomas) may have a conventional blue nevus component and lack *EWSR1* rearrangements.

Cutaneous CCS with predominantly clear cytoplasm may have to be distinguished from cutaneous PEComas. The delicate capillary vasculature surrounding the nests of tumor cells in PEComas is not characteristic of CCS. Cutaneous PEComas coexpress markers of melanocytic and smooth muscle differentiation (SMA, desmin, and caldesmon), the latter of which are consistently negative in CCS.[30] PEComas lack *EWSR1* rearrangements.

Prognosis and Treatment

CCS has a protracted clinical course but ultimately behaves aggressively, with a propensity for local recurrence (up to 40%) and a high rate of lymph node and systemic metastases, most often to the lungs and bone. The 5-year overall survival is 40% to 60%.[26,29,30,32,33,46] Adverse prognostic features include size, necrosis, local recurrence, and lymph node metastasis.[24] The behavior of cutaneous examples seems to be similar to their soft tissue counterparts.[38] Radical surgery remains the treatment of choice. There are no uniform guidelines regarding lymph node dissection or sentinel lymph node biopsy in CCS.[22–24,47] Conventional chemotherapy is of little benefit in CCS,[29,33,46] but candidate therapeutic targets have been proposed, including c-Met.[41] The key features of CCS are summarized in **Box 2**.

Box 2
Key features: clear cell sarcoma

- Epidemiology: young adults in their 20s, 30s, and 40s
- Clinical presentation: slow-growing tumor in distal extremities (especially ankle or foot)
- Cutaneous examples occur via secondary extension from a deeply seated tumor or as a primary cutaneous tumor
- Histology: nests of uniform spindled to fusiform cells, separated by fibrous bands
- Atypical cells with large vesicular nuclei and prominent nucleoli but marked nuclear pleomorphism is not characteristic
- Usually lack involvement of the epidermal/dermal junction or epidermis, although rare cases have been reported
- Multinucleated wreathlike tumor giant cells are a very helpful feature
- Positive for all melanocytic markers
- Molecular: harbor *EWSR1/ATF1* or *EWSR1/CREB1* rearrangements
- Diagnostic mimickers: spindle cell malignant melanoma, amelanotic cellular blue nevus and cutaneous perivascular epithelioid cell tumor; these lack the characteristic *EWSR1* rearrangements

---

CUTANEOUS PERIVASCULAR EPITHELIOID CELL TUMOR

PEComas are a diverse family of mesenchymal neoplasms characterized by unusual epithelioid perivascular cells that coexpress smooth muscle and melanocytic markers.[48–50] PEComas occurs at various anatomic sites, including the skin, soft tissue, bone, viscera, and related structures, such as pelvic ligaments.[51,52] The PEComa family also includes distinctive visceral tumors, such as lymphangioleiomyomatosis, renal angiomyolipoma, and clear cell "sugar" tumor of the lung, and shows an association with tuberous sclerosis complex.[51,52] Primary cutaneous PEComas were first reported in 2005[53,54] and several case reports and series followed.[38,55–58] Cutaneous examples account for 8% of all PEComas in one expert consultation practice.[56] Cutaneous PEComas seem to be clinically and genetically distinct from their visceral and soft tissue counterparts (discussed elsewhere in this article).

Clinical Features

Primary cutaneous PEComa typically affect adults in the fourth decade, with a striking female predilection.[54,56] Cutaneous tumors usually affect the legs, arms, or trunk and present as firm, tan, or pink-colored small (<2 cm) cutaneous nodules or plaques.

Histologic Features

Cutaneous PEComas are centered on the dermis (**Fig. 4**A) and are composed of irregular dermal nests, sheets, or cords of epithelioid to spindled cells with clear or granular eosinophilic cytoplasm surrounded delicate capillary vessels (see **Fig. 4**B, C). The cells at the periphery of the lesion intermingle with dermal collagen in a pattern reminiscent of benign fibrous histiocytoma (see **Fig. 4**D). The overlying epidermis is usually uninvolved, but the subcutis can be involved with either a pushing or infiltrative margin.[56] The cells have round, vesicular nuclei with small but very distinct nucleoli. A mild degree of pleomorphism and multinucleated giant cells with peripherally located nuclei can be seen.[56] The mitotic count is typically low (<1/10 HPF).

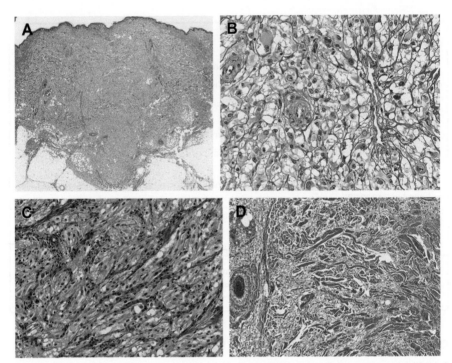

Fig. 4. Cutaneous perivascular epithelioid cell tumor (PEComa). (*A*) Irregular dermal-based neoplasm with intact overlying epidermis (H&E, original magnification ×10). (*B, C*) Nests and sheets of tightly packed epithelioid or spindled cells with clear or granular eosinophilic neoplasm surrounded by delicate branching capillary vessels (H&E, original magnifications ×400 and ×200, respectively). (*D*) The cells at the periphery of the lesion intermingle with dermal collagen resembling fibrous histiocytoma (H&E, original magnification ×100).

Immunohistochemistry and Molecular and Genetic Findings

PEComas demonstrate variable coexpression of melanocytic markers (MITF, NKI/C3, HMB45, Melan A, and S100) and markers of smooth muscle differentiation (desmin, SMA, caldesmon, and calponin).[54,56,58] HMB45 and MITF are the most sensitive melanocytic markers in cutaneous PEComas, whereas focal S100 protein expression is seen in a minority of cases. Of the muscle markers, desmin seems to be the most sensitive, but cases with SMA expression in the absence of desmin expression occur.[56] Cytokeratins and EMA are negative in PEComa.[58]

Visceral and soft tissue PEComas may be associated with *TSC1/TSC2* mutations and tuberous sclerosis complex with downstream activation of the mammalian target of rapamycin pathway.[52] A subset of PEComas show transcription factor E3 (*TFE3*) gene rearrangements, which may drive the myomelanocytic phenotype in these tumors.[52] However, reported primary cutaneous PEComas do not seem to be associated with either *TSC* mutations or *TFE3* rearrangements.[59]

Differential Diagnosis

A variety of tumors are in the differential diagnosis. Benign fibrous histiocytoma with clear cell change (referred to as clear cell fibrous histiocytoma[60]) can be confused with PEComa. Fibrous histiocytoma can be distinguished from PEComa by the presence of overlying epidermal hyperplasia, a conventional short spindle cell component with irregular nuclei, the lack of a distinctive capillary vasculature, and the absence of melanocytic differentiation. Granular cell tumor can be distinguished based on a syncytial arrangement and absence of prominent vasculature. An uncommon clear cell variant of granular cell tumor described by Zedek and colleagues[61] can be more difficult to distinguish from PEComa, because it is has very similar cytologic characteristics. However, both conventional and clear cell granular cell tumors are negative for HMB45, Melan A, desmin, and SMA, and are uniformly strongly positive for S100 protein. Cutaneous myoepitheliomas with clear cell morphology have somewhat overlapping immunophenotype because markers of myoepithelial differentiation S100, SOX10, SMA, and calponin can also be expressed in cutaneous PEComas. However, myoepithelial tumors can be ready distinguished from PEComas by coexpression of cytokeratins, EMA, and a lack of HMB-45 or MiTF immunoreactivity.

Of the malignant tumors with clear cytoplasm, metastatic carcinomas and melanoma with balloon cell change are the most important entities to exclude. Metastatic renal cell and hepatocellular carcinoma can be separated from PEComa based on cytokeratin immunoreactivity and lack of melanocytic and smooth muscle marker expression. Balloon cell melanoma and balloon cell nevi can resemble cutaneous PEComa.[62] Helpful distinguishing features include the presence of a junctional melanocytic component, peripheral inflammatory infiltrates, and lack of prominent capillary vasculature. By IHC, balloon cell nevi and melanoma diffusely express S100 protein and lack expression of smooth muscle markers. The differential diagnosis with CCS is discussed elsewhere in this article.

Prognosis and Treatment

Visceral and soft tissue PEComas demonstrate a spectrum of biological behavior ranging from benign to overtly malignant.[50,63] Histologic criteria for malignancy in PEComas were proposed by Folpe and colleagues.[50] In their study, size greater than 5 cm, an infiltrative growth pattern, high nuclear grade, mitotic activity greater than 1/50 HPF, necrosis, and vascular invasion were associated with local recurrence and metastases. The authors proposed that PEComas lacking any of these features be classified as benign, those with 2 or more features as malignant, and those with only nuclear pleomorphism/giant cells (so-called symplastic PEComas) or size greater than 5 cm as having uncertain malignant potential. In contrast with their visceral and soft tissue counterparts, cutaneous PEComas almost always behave in a benign fashion and rarely recur.[54–58] Very few malignant cutaneous and subcutaneous PEComa have been reported[38,64,65] and additional studies are necessary to determine if this prognostication system is applicable to cutaneous tumors. Key features of cutaneous PEComa are summarized in **Box 3**.

OSSIFYING FIBROMYXOID TUMOR

OFMT is a mesenchymal neoplasm of uncertain differentiation with a predilection for the superficial soft tissue of the extremities and diverse histologic appearances that classically include a distinctive peripheral shell of bone. Although earlier immunohistochemical and ultrastructural studies suggested nerve sheath, myoepithelial, smooth muscle, cartilaginous, and even osteogenic differentiation for this tumor,[66–71] recent genetic analyses indicate that OFMT is a translocation-associated tumor, with rearrangements most commonly involving *PHF1*.[72–75] Most behave in a benign fashion with a small but definite risk of local recurrence (approximately 20%) and low risk of metastasis (<5%). However, a small proportion of cases, particularly those with atypical histologic features, have higher rates of local recurrence and potential for metastasis.[71,76,77]

Box 3
Key features: cutaneous perivascular epithelioid cell tumor

- Epidemiology: affects adults in their 40s, usually females
- Clinical presentation: typically affects the legs, arms, or trunk
- Clinically small (<2 cm) and may resemble fibrous histiocytoma
- Histology: nests of clear to eosinophilic epithelioid or spindle cells separated by delicate vascular septae, with perivascular condensation
- Round, vesicular nuclei with small but very distinct nucleoli and mild cellular pleomorphism; mitotic count is very low (<1/10 high-power fields)
- Multinucleated giant cells with peripherally located nuclei
- Coexpress melanocytic and smooth muscle markers
- Molecular: cutaneous perivascular epithelioid cell tumors lack the *TFE-3* rearrangements and the association with tuberous sclerosis complex seen in extracutaneous tumors
- Diagnostic mimickers: malignant: metastatic carcinomas (renal cell, hepatocellular), melanocytic tumors with clear cell or balloon cell change and clear cell sarcoma; benign: fibrous histiocytoma, granular cell tumor
- Prognosis: predominantly benign with only rare reports of malignant cases; it is unclear if established criteria for malignancy in extracutaneous perivascular epithelioid cell tumors apply to cutaneous tumors

---

Clinical Features

OFMT most commonly presents in middle-aged adults without a gender predilection. Most are solitary, well-circumscribed masses involving the lower limbs, but may present anywhere, including skeletal muscle, mediastinum, retroperitoneum, thyroid gland, and breast.[78] The average size is 3 to 4 cm.[71–73,79,80]

Histologic Features

OFMT is circumscribed with a fibrous pseudocapsule centered in the subcutis, with only rare dermal involvement. Focal infiltrative growth and microscopic satellite nodules may be seen.[71,79] The classic histologic feature is the peripheral shell of mature lamellar bone (**Fig. 5**A); however, this feature is only present in 40% to 85% of cases[71,73,79,80] with the remaining case representing the so-called nonossifying variant of OFMT. Both variants are variably cellular and are composed of epithelioid or spindled cells arranged in corded, nested, trabecular, or sheet-like patterns; the stroma shows variable proportions of myxoid, fibrous, densely hyalinized, and chondroid zones (see **Fig. 5**B–E), and may show deposits of woven bone. Many cases show prominent curved vessels. Microcystic changes (see **Fig. 5**F), spindle cell areas with or without fascicle formation (see **Fig. 5**G), and rhabdoid-like morphology[74] can occur. This morphologic diversity may occasionally be present within a single case. Irrespective of the growth pattern, all OFMTs show strikingly similar, uniform oval nuclei with fine chromatin and delicate pinpoint nucleoli (see **Fig. 5**H). These nuclear features are one of the most helpful clues in identifying OFMT. In most cases, the nuclei are banal, and there is virtually no mitotic activity.

More worrisome histologic features, including nuclear atypia, high cellularity, necrosis, or increased mitotic activity, can be associated with aggressive behavior.[76,77] An outcomes-based risk stratification system divided OFMTs into typical, atypical, and malignant forms.[71] Malignant OFMT is defined as having high nuclear grade (**Fig. 6**A) or a combination of high cellularity and a mitotic count of greater than 2

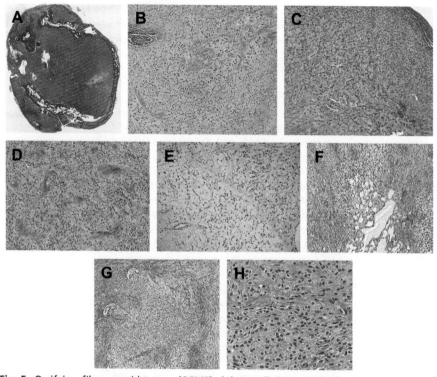

Fig. 5. Ossifying fibromyxoid tumor (OFMT). (*A*) A well-circumscribed cellular mass with a characteristic peripheral shell of lamellar bone (H&E, original magnification ×10). (*B–G*) Growth patterns in OFMT: nested (*B*), corded (*C*), sheetlike, and (*D*) with collagenous stroma, trabecular with myxoid stroma (*E*), microcystic change (*F*), and fascicular pattern (*G*) (H&E, original magnification ×100). (*H*) Very uniform oval nuclei with fine chromatin and delicate pinpoint nucleoli in typical OFMT (H&E, original magnification ×400).

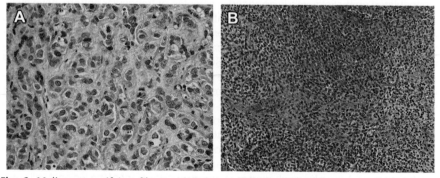

Fig. 6. Malignant ossifying fibromyxoid tumor (OFMT). (*A*) Malignant OFMT with high-grade nuclear atypia and mitotic activity (H&E, original magnification ×400). (*B*) Malignant OFMT with increased cellularity and mitotic activity greater than 2 per 50 high-power fields (H&E, original magnification ×100).

per 50 HPF (see **Fig. 6**B). Cases fulfilling at least 1 atypical feature such as a mitotic count of greater than 2 per 50 HPF alone or high cellularity or moderate nuclear atypia with a mitotic count of 2 or more per 50 HPF are considered atypical OFMTs. Although some cases of malignant OFMT arise de novo,[73] areas reminiscent of benign OFMT are usually present in malignant OFMT.[71,80]

Immunohistochemistry and Molecular and Genetic Findings

OFMTs express S100 protein in approximately 70% to 90% of cases, but expression can be focal. Desmin is expressed in 10% to 40% of cases.[72,74,80,81] OFMTs show inconsistent immunoreactivity for SMA, p63, GFAP, and CD10. EMA and cytokeratins may show focal expression, although only in a minority and more often in malignant OFMT. OFMTs are negative for melanocytic markers, CD34, and CD31. Approximately one-quarter of cases are focally positive for MUC4.[82]

More than 80% of OFMTs have recurrent gene rearrangements, most commonly involving *PHF1* on 6p21 with fusion partners including *EP400*, *MEAF6*, and *EPC1*.[72–74] Novel variant fusions include *ZC3H7B-BCOR*, *CREBBP-BCOR1*, and *KDMA2-WWTR1*.[74,75] Most of these genes participate in epigenetic regulation and histone modification.[75] FISH for *PHF1* rearrangements is a useful diagnostic test in difficult cases.

Differential Diagnosis

Given the variety of growth patterns and the lack of a peripheral shell of bone in many cases, it is not surprising that OFMTs often are mistaken for other mesenchymal neoplasms. The most difficult differential diagnosis in our opinion is with cutaneous myoepithelioma and myoepithelial carcinoma. Similar to OFMT, cutaneous myoepithelioma consists of epithelioid or spindled cells arranged in various combinations of reticular, trabecular, and nested patterns, within a fibromyxoid stroma.[83] Cartilaginous and osseous differentiation may occur in myoepithelial tumors, although it rarely takes the form of a peripheral rim of mature lamellar bone as seen in OFMT. Markers of myoepithelial differentiation such as p63, SMA, and particularly S100 protein are of limited value because they are also expressed in OFMT. However, strong diffuse expression of keratins and EMA would favor a myoepithelial tumor because these epithelial markers are expressed in only a small percentage of OFMT and usually focally.[71,79,81] *PHF1* rearrangement has not been observed in myoepithelial tumors which, in contrast, may demonstrate rearrangements of either *EWSR1* (approximately 50% of cases)[19,84] or *PLAG1*.[85]

Epithelioid schwannomas resemble OFMT, because they are also composed of encapsulated epithelioid cells in arranged in a nested or trabecular pattern, have hyalinized or myxoid stroma, and often lack Antoni A areas.[86,87] The nuclei in epithelioid schwannomas are more irregular and reniform in appearance. The presence of a conventional schwannoma component, a true capsule with EMA or GLUT-1–positive perineurial cells and immunoreactivity for SOX10 favor epithelioid schwannoma.[88] Malignant OFMT may be confused with the epithelioid MPNST. Although this distinction might be virtually impossible in some cases, epithelioid MPNSTs typically present as a deep-seated soft tissue tumor, lack desmin, and show diffuse, strong S100 expression.[18] INI1 loss is characteristic of epithelioid MPNSTs, whereas INI1 is usually retained or only focally lost in a mosaic pattern in OFMT.[81]

Typical OFMT, particularly cases with a prominent spindle cell component, need to be distinguished from low-grade fibromyxoid sarcoma (LGFMS), which may arise in superficial locations.[89] A prominent whorled or storiform arrangement of the lesional cells and characteristic arcades of vessels in myxoid zones favor LGFMS. OFMTs with particularly densely hyalinized stroma and cordlike arrangement of the lesional cells can be confused with sclerosing epithelioid fibrosarcoma (SEF). By IHC, both LGFMS and

SEF are more often positive for EMA and negative for S100. Immunoreactivity for MUC4, a sensitive and specific marker of both LGFMS and SEF, can be positive in 20% to 30% of OFMT,[81,82] although the staining is usually focal. Diagnostically challenging cases can be resolved by application of FISH testing for *FUS* (rearranged in both LGFMS and SEF).

Although the hallmark feature of OFMT is a well-formed shell of lamellar bone at the tumor periphery, some cases show a more diffuse, lacelike, or random pattern of woven bone deposition.[66] If such cases are associated with atypical or malignant cytology, they may be mistaken for extraskeletal osteosarcoma. Marked atypia and nuclear pleomorphism favor osteosarcoma because these features are not typical of OFMT, even in malignant cases. Clinical history is also very helpful, because most cutaneous or subcutaneous osteosarcomas represent metastases.

Prognosis and Treatment

Although most OFMTs behave in a benign fashion, it is important to remember that even the most cytologically banal OFMT can recur, and there is a small risk of metastasis that can be assessed using the aforementioned 3-tier system developed by Folpe and Weiss.[71] In their study, typical OFMTs had a 12% rate of local recurrence and a 4% rate of metastasis, whereas the rate of both local recurrence and metastasis was increased to 60% for malignant OFMTs. The rates of local recurrence and metastasis in cases with at least 1 atypical feature (classified as atypical OFMT) were similar to those of typical OFMTs, at 13% and 6%, respectively. This prognostic system was retrospectively validated in series by Graham and colleagues[81] and Atanaskova-Mesinkovska and colleagues,[80] who showed that local recurrences and systemic metastases occurred only in cases classified as malignant OFMT; atypical OFMTs in these series did not recur or metastasize. Reported metastatic sites include the lungs, adrenal glands, and soft tissue.[66,71,80,81] Surgical excision is the treatment of choice in OFMT. Key features of OFMT are summarized in **Box 4**.

Box 4
Key features: ossifying fibromyxoid tumor

- Epidemiology: middle-aged adults with no gender predilection
- Clinical presentation: solitary, superficial mass, most commonly in lower limbs, but also upper limbs, trunk, and head and neck
- Histology: well-circumscribed subcutaneous lesion with fibrous pseudocapsule and occasional satellite nodules
- A rim of mature lamellar bone is extremely characteristic, but is only present in 40% to 85% of cases
- Many architectural patterns, but all have uniform, oval nuclei with fine chromatin and pinpoint nucleoli; exceptions are atypical and malignant cases, which may be classified by a system developed by Folpe and Weiss[71]
- Molecular: 85% of cases harbor rearrangements involving *PHF1* gene, regardless of tumor grade; fluorescence in situ hybridization probes are commercially available
- Diagnostic mimickers of typical ossifying fibromyxoid tumor: myoepithelial tumors, epithelioid schwannomas, low-grade fibromyxoid sarcoma, and sclerosing epithelioid fibrosarcoma
- Diagnostic mimickers of malignant ossifying fibromyxoid tumor: epithelioid malignant peripheral nerve sheath tumor, myoepithelial carcinoma, and extraskeletal osteosarcoma
- Prognosis: typical cases may recur and very rarely metastasize; malignant cases show a higher rate of local recurrence and metastasis

PLEOMORPHIC HYALINIZING ANGIECTATIC TUMOR AND HEMOSIDEROTIC FIBROLIPOMATOUS TUMOR

PHAT and HFLT are distinctive subcutaneous neoplasms of adults with the potential for local recurrence and, in rare cases, progression to sarcoma. Although morphologically these tumors may be distinct, cases with features of both have been described,[90] and both tumors are characterized by *TGFBR3* and *MGEA5* rearrangements[91] suggesting that they are related (discussed elsewhere in this article).

Clinical Features

PHAT usually arises in middle-aged adults and has a predilection for the lower extremities, but can also occur at other sites such as the arm, thigh, buttocks, or trunk, and has a median size of approximately 6 cm.[90,92] Because angiectatic vessels are a prominent feature, PHAT may be clinically mistaken for a hematoma or vascular neoplasm. HFLT was initially thought to represent a reactive process possibly related to trauma,[93] but it was subsequently recognized as a true neoplasm.[90,94] HFLT also manifests as a slowly growing subcutaneous mass or plaque, with a female predilection and a tendency to affect the dorsal surface of the ankle, foot, or hand, although other sites may be involved.[93,94]

Histologic Features

The morphologic features of PHAT and HFLT are presented in **Figs. 7** and **8**. PHAT is a vaguely circumscribed mass composed of spindled or pleomorphic cells surrounding

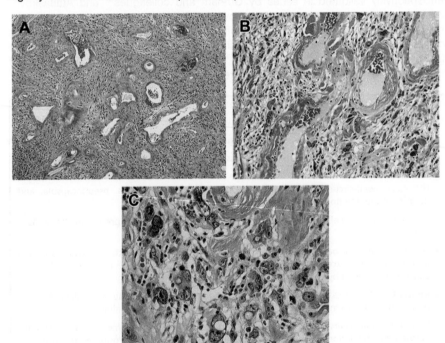

Fig. 7. Pleomorphic hyalinizing angiectatic tumor. (*A*) Sheets of spindled or pleomorphic fibroblasts surrounding clusters of thin-walled, ectatic vessels with subendothelial fibrin deposits and perivascular hyalinization (H&E, original magnification ×100). (*B, C*) Pleomorphic spindle cells with frequent intranuclear inclusions and occasional intracytoplasmic hemosiderin deposits; mitotic figures are absent (H&E, original magnification ×400). ([*A*] *Courtesy of* Dr Karen Fritchie, Department of Laboratory Medicine and Pathology, Mayo Clinic, Rochester, MN.)

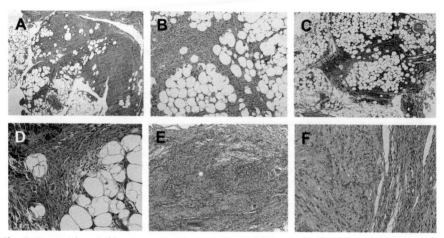

Fig. 8. Hemosiderotic fibrolipomatous tumor. (*A, B*) Cellular neoplasm with ill-defined border composed of fascicular proliferations of bland fibroblasts that percolate through adipose tissue in a streaming or more diffuse honeycomb-like pattern reminiscent of DFSP (H&E, original magnification ×40 and ×100, respectively). (*C*) Another example of HFLT with prominent hemosiderin pigment that can be found in the stroma, in macrophages and in the cytoplasm of spindle cells (H&E, original magnification ×40). (*D*) HFLT is composed of fibroblasts without atypia or mitotic activity (H&E, original magnification ×200). (*E*) HFLT with progression to a more cellular spindle cell neoplasm with myxoid stroma and prominent inflammatory component reminiscent of myxoinflammatory fibroblastic sarcoma (H&E, original magnification ×200). (*F*) HFLT (*star, right*) with progression to a more cellular spindle cell proliferation with prominent nuclear atypia, macronucleoli and increased mitotic activity, consistent with spindle cell sarcoma (H&E, original magnification ×100). ([*A, B*] *Courtesy of* Dr Karen Fritchie, Department of Laboratory Medicine and Pathology, Mayo Clinic, Rochester, MN.)

clusters of thin-walled, ectatic vessels with subendothelial and intraluminal fibrin deposits and perivascular hyalinization (**Fig. 7**A). Although PHAT may seem circumscribed at low power, the margin is usually infiltrative. The lesional cells range from spindled to strikingly pleomorphic and may show frequent intranuclear inclusions (see **Fig. 7**B, C). Mitotic activity in PHAT is very low (<1/50 HPF). Hemosiderin deposits can be seen in macrophages or in the cytoplasm of the lesional cells. Scattered inflammatory cells are usually present.

HFLTs are ill-defined fascicular proliferations of bland fibroblasts that percolate through adipose tissue in a streaming, whorling, nodular, or more diffuse honeycomb-like pattern reminiscent of dermatofibrosarcoma protuberans (DFSP; **Fig. 8**A, B). Hemosiderin is also prominent in HFLT and is variably found in the stroma, in macrophages and in the cytoplasm of spindle cells (see **Fig. 8**C). Myxoid stroma is focally present[90] and usually there is a prominent inflammatory component. Cytologically, HFLT is composed of bland fibroblasts without significant mitotic activity and may contain scattered osteoclast-type giant cells (see **Fig. 8**D). Small ectatic vessels with mural hyalinization or fibrinous thrombi may be present.[90,94] HFLT-like areas can be found at the periphery or admixed with otherwise typical examples of PHAT. This observation led to a hypothesis that HFLT might be a precursor lesion to PHAT.[90]

Rarely, PHAT and HFLT may progress to a sarcoma of variable histologic grade, more often in the setting of recurrences.[91,95–98] The sarcomas associated with PHAT and HFLT often have myxoid stroma and a prominent inflammatory infiltrate and can show morphologic resemblance to myxoinflammatory fibroblastic sarcoma (MIFS). Solid, undifferentiated spindle cell sarcoma-like morphology has also been reported[98] (see **Fig. 8**E, F).

Immunohistochemistry and Genetics

Most PHATs and HFLTs are positive for CD34 and negative for S100, SMA, and desmin.[90–94] HFLT harbors a recurrent t(1;10) (p22;q24) rearrangement involving the TGFBR3 and MGEA5 genes.[95,96] TGFBR3 and MGEA5 gene rearrangements have also been found in tumors showing mixed features of HFLT and PHAT and, less consistently, in classic PHAT,[91,96] findings that further support the view that PHAT and HFLT may be related. FISH for TGFBR3 and MGEA5 rearrangements can be used in diagnostically challenging cases.

More controversial is the relationship of HFLT and PHAT to MIFS, a distinctive low-grade sarcoma that typically involves distal extremities of middle-aged adults. Recent genetic and molecular studies showed that some cases of MIFS also harbor TGFBR3 and MGEA5 rearrangements, including cases with mixed features of HFLT and MIFS.[91,96,98,99] These studies suggest that HFLT, PHAT, and MIFS may represent a morphologic spectrum of related lesions. However, Zreik and colleagues[98] recently showed that TGFBR3 and MGEA5 rearrangements common to hybrid HFLT and MIFS (75%) are quite unusual in pure MIFS that lack an HFLT component (6%). The authors also emphasized that some of the myxoid sarcomas associated with HFLT are histologically high-grade tumors (uncommon in classic examples of MIFS) and lack the typical stromal hyalinization and virocyte (Reed-Sternberg–like) cells that epitomize MIFS. Based on these findings, the authors concluded that myxoid sarcomas that occur in association with HFLT might be unrelated to MIFS, but may rather represent a form of sarcomatous progression in HFLT. The pathogenetic link between these entities continues to be investigated.

Differential Diagnosis

PHAT can closely mimic schwannoma with degenerative ("ancient") change, which often contains clusters of hyalinized vessels, inflammatory aggregates, and pleomorphic Schwann cells. In contrast with PHAT, schwannomas are well-circumscribed and encapsulated lesions without an HFLT-like component at the periphery. S100 protein is diffusely expressed in schwannomas and is consistently negative in PHAT. Owing to the striking degree of nuclear atypia and pleomorphism often seen in PHAT, it can be misdiagnosed as undifferentiated pleomorphic sarcoma; however, a lack of mitotic activity would favor the former. By contrast, identification of a bona fide spindle cell sarcoma with myxoid stroma in association with a classic PHAT may indicate sarcomatous transformation.

Important mimickers of HFLT include DFSP, plexiform fibrohistiocytic tumor, and atypical lipomatous tumor. Like HFLT, plexiform fibrohistiocytic tumor is a slow-growing, infiltrative, subcutaneous neoplasm with similarly bland fibroblastic cells arranged in fascicles.[100] However, in plexiform fibrohistiocytic tumor, these fascicles connect nodules of epithelioid histiocytic cells admixed with osteoclast-type giant cells. This pattern contrasts with the more monotonous appearance of HFLT, which lacks these nodules. The spindle cell component of plexiform fibrohistiocytic tumor expresses SMA in keeping with its myofibroblastic phenotype; SMA is typically negative in HFLT. Separating DFSP and HFLT can be difficult, especially in a small biopsy. DFSP has a more uniform appearance than HFLT and lacks hemosiderin deposits and ectatic hyalinized vessels. FISH for the characteristic PDGFβ rearrangement of DFSP can be used in difficult cases. In both plexiform fibrohistiocytic tumor and DFSP, fatty infiltration occurs at the edge of the tumor whereas in HFLT the adipocytic component is more intimately admixed with the lesional fibroblasts and may dominate the histologic picture.[94] Atypical lipomatous tumor rarely occurs in superficial locations and can be distinguished from HFLT by the presence of hyperchromatic stromal cells and lack of hemosiderin deposits. In the pediatric population, lipofibromatosis[101] may seem to be similar to HFLT and can be distinguished based on the more monotonous appearance of the lesional cells and collections of small, univacuolated cells at the interface between the adipocytic and spindle cell components. Giant cells and hemosiderin deposits are not typical of lipofibromatosis.

Prognosis and Treatment

Because of their infiltrative nature, both PHAT and HFLT are associated with a significant risk (30%–50%) of local recurrence and, therefore, are considered to represent tumors of intermediate malignant potential.[94] Examples of HFLT and PHAT that are associated with transformation to sarcoma acquire metastatic potential although only limited reported cases exist in the literature to date.[97] Key features of PHAT and HFLT are summarized in **Box 5**.

Box 5
Key features: PHAT and HFLT

PHAT

- Epidemiology: middle-aged adults

- Clinical presentation: slow-growing subcutaneous neoplasm with infiltrative border, most common in lower extremities (leg, ankle, and foot)

- Histology: spindled to pleomorphic fibroblasts with frequent intranuclear inclusions surrounding hyalinized, thin-walled ectatic vessels with fibrin deposition

- Hemosiderin (in lesional cells or macrophages) and scattered inflammatory cells

- Marked nuclear atypia and pleomorphism, but low mitotic activity (<1/50 high-power fields)

- Diagnostic mimickers of PHAT: schwannomas (S100+) and pleomorphic sarcomas (high mitotic rate); presence of bona fide sarcomatous areas in an otherwise classic PHAT indicates malignant transformation, which may occur

- Prognosis: recur locally in 30% to 50% of cases; may show malignant transformation

HFLT

- Epidemiology: middle-aged adults with a female predilection

- Clinical presentation: slow-growing subcutaneous mass on the dorsal surface of the ankle, foot, or hand

- Histology: ill-defined lesions with a fascicular, whorling, or honeycomb patterned growth of bland-appearing fibroblasts percolating through adipose tissue

- Hemosiderin pigment is prominent as are inflammatory cells

- Mitotic activity is very low or absent

- May occur at periphery of PHAT

- Diagnostic mimickers of HFLT: dermatofibrosarcoma protuberans (*COL1A1-PDGFB* rearrangement), atypical lipomatous tumor (lacks *TGFBR3* and *MGEA5* gene rearrangements), plexiform fibrohistiocytic tumor (smooth muscle actin positive)

- Prognosis: as in PHAT, HFLT may recur locally in 30% to 50% of cases and may show malignant transformation

- IHC and molecular: most PHAT and HFLT are positive for CD34 and negative for S100, smooth muscle actin, and desmin. Rearrangements in *TGFBR3* and *MGEA5* genes present in HFLT, mixed HFLT/PHAT, and, less commonly, in classic PHAT.

Abbreviations: HFLT, hemosiderotic fibrolipomatous tumor; PHAT, pleomorphic hyalinizing angiectatic tumor.

REFERENCES

1. Enzinger FM. Epithelioid sarcoma. A sarcoma simulating a granuloma or a carcinoma. Cancer 1970;26(5):1029.
2. Chase DR, Enzinger FM. Epithelioid sarcoma. Diagnosis, prognostic indicators, and treatment. Am J Surg Pathol 1985;9(4):241.
3. Guillou L, Wadden C, Coindre JM, et al. "Proximal-type" epithelioid sarcoma, a distinctive aggressive neoplasm showing rhabdoid features. Clinicopathologic, immunohistochemical, and ultrastructural study of a series. Am J Surg Pathol 1997;21(2):130.
4. Modena P, Lualdi E, Facchinetti F, et al. SMARCB1/INI1 tumor suppressor gene is frequently inactivated in epithelioid sarcomas. Cancer Res 2005;65(10):4012.
5. Hornick JL, Dal Cin P, Fletcher CD. Loss of INI1 expression is characteristic of both conventional and proximal-type epithelioid sarcoma. Am J Surg Pathol 2009;33(4):542.
6. Jawad MU, Extein J, Min ES, et al. Prognostic factors for survival in patients with epithelioid sarcoma: 441 cases from the SEER database. Clin Orthop Relat Res 2009;467(11):2939.
7. Casanova M, Ferrari A, Collini P, et al. Epithelioid sarcoma in children and adolescents: a report from the Italian Soft Tissue Sarcoma Committee. Cancer 2006; 106(3):708.
8. Baratti D, Pennacchioli E, Casali PG, et al. Epithelioid sarcoma: prognostic factors and survival in a series of patients treated at a single institution. Ann Surg Oncol 2007;14(12):3542.
9. Miettinen M, Fanburg-Smith JC, Virolainen M, et al. Epithelioid sarcoma: an immunohistochemical analysis of 112 classical and variant cases and a discussion of the differential diagnosis. Hum Pathol 1999;30(8):934.
10. Hasegawa T, Matsuno Y, Shimoda T, et al. Proximal-type epithelioid sarcoma: a clinicopathologic study of 20 cases. Mod Pathol 2001;14(7):655.
11. Laskin WB, Miettinen M. Epithelioid sarcoma: new insights based on an extended immunohistochemical analysis. Arch Pathol Lab Med 2003;127(9): 1161.
12. Chbani L, Guillou L, Terrier P, et al. Epithelioid sarcoma: a clinicopathologic and immunohistochemical analysis of 106 cases from the French Sarcoma Group. Am J Clin Pathol 2009;131(2):222.
13. Lin L, Skacel M, Sigel JE, et al. Epithelioid sarcoma: an immunohistochemical analysis evaluating the utility of cytokeratin 5/6 in distinguishing superficial epithelioid sarcoma from spindled squamous cell carcinoma. J Cutan Pathol 2003;30(2):114.
14. Billings SD, Folpe AL, Weiss SW. Epithelioid sarcoma-like hemangioendothelioma. Am J Surg Pathol 2003;27(1):48.
15. Hornick JL, Fletcher CD. Pseudomyogenic hemangioendothelioma: a distinctive, often multicentric tumor with indolent behavior. Am J Surg Pathol 2011; 35(2):190.
16. Walther C, Tayebwa J, Lilljebjorn H, et al. A novel SERPINE1-FOSB fusion gene results in transcriptional up-regulation of FOSB in pseudomyogenic haemangioendothelioma. J Pathol 2014;232(5):534.
17. Hung YP, Fletcher CD, Hornick JL. FOSB is a useful diagnostic marker for pseudomyogenic hemangioendothelioma. Am J Surg Pathol 2017;41(5):596.
18. Jo VY, Fletcher CD. Epithelioid malignant peripheral nerve sheath tumor: clinicopathologic analysis of 63 cases. Am J Surg Pathol 2015;39(5):673.

19. Antonescu CR, Zhang L, Chang NE, et al. EWSR1-POU5F1 fusion in soft tissue myoepithelial tumors. A molecular analysis of sixty-six cases, including soft tissue, bone, and visceral lesions, showing common involvement of the EWSR1 gene. Genes Chromosomes Cancer 2010;49(12):1114.
20. Thway K, Bown N, Miah A, et al. Rhabdoid variant of myoepithelial carcinoma, with EWSR1 rearrangement: expanding the spectrum of EWSR1-rearranged myoepithelial tumors. Head Neck Pathol 2015;9(2):273.
21. Thway K, Jones RL, Noujaim J, et al. Epithelioid sarcoma: diagnostic features and genetics. Adv Anat Pathol 2016;23(1):41.
22. Maduekwe UN, Hornicek FJ, Springfield DS, et al. Role of sentinel lymph node biopsy in the staging of synovial, epithelioid, and clear cell sarcomas. Ann Surg Oncol 2009;16(5):1356.
23. Sherman KL, Kinnier CV, Farina DA, et al. Examination of national lymph node evaluation practices for adult extremity soft tissue sarcoma. J Surg Oncol 2014;110(6):682.
24. Ecker BL, Peters MG, McMillan MT, et al. Implications of lymph node evaluation in the management of resectable soft tissue sarcoma. Ann Surg Oncol 2017; 24(2):425.
25. Enzinger FM. Clear-cell sarcoma of tendons and aponeuroses. An analysis of 21 cases. Cancer 1965;18:1163.
26. Chung EB, Enzinger FM. Malignant melanoma of soft parts. A reassessment of clear cell sarcoma. Am J Surg Pathol 1983;7(5):405.
27. Panagopoulos I, Mertens F, Debiec-Rychter M, et al. Molecular genetic characterization of the EWS/ATF1 fusion gene in clear cell sarcoma of tendons and aponeuroses. Int J Cancer 2002;99(4):560.
28. Antonescu CR, Tschernyavsky SJ, Woodruff JM, et al. Molecular diagnosis of clear cell sarcoma: detection of EWS-ATF1 and MITF-M transcripts and histopathological and ultrastructural analysis of 12 cases. J Mol Diagn 2002;4(1):44.
29. Coindre JM, Hostein I, Terrier P, et al. Diagnosis of clear cell sarcoma by real-time reverse transcriptase-polymerase chain reaction analysis of paraffin embedded tissues: clinicopathologic and molecular analysis of 44 patients from the French sarcoma group. Cancer 2006;107(5):1055.
30. Hisaoka M, Ishida T, Kuo TT, et al. Clear cell sarcoma of soft tissue: a clinicopathologic, immunohistochemical, and molecular analysis of 33 cases. Am J Surg Pathol 2008;32(3):452.
31. Wang WL, Mayordomo E, Zhang W, et al. Detection and characterization of EWSR1/ATF1 and EWSR1/CREB1 chimeric transcripts in clear cell sarcoma (melanoma of soft parts). Mod Pathol 2009;22(9):1201.
32. Lucas DR, Nascimento AG, Sim FH. Clear cell sarcoma of soft tissues. Mayo Clinic experience with 35 cases. Am J Surg Pathol 1992;16(12):1197.
33. Hocar O, Le Cesne A, Berissi S, et al. Clear cell sarcoma (malignant melanoma) of soft parts: a clinicopathologic study of 52 cases. Dermatol Res Pract 2012; 2012:984096.
34. Hantschke M, Mentzel T, Rutten A, et al. Cutaneous clear cell sarcoma: a clinicopathologic, immunohistochemical, and molecular analysis of 12 cases emphasizing its distinction from dermal melanoma. Am J Surg Pathol 2010; 34(2):216.
35. Falconieri G, Bacchi CE, Luzar B. Cutaneous clear cell sarcoma: report of three cases of a potentially underestimated mimicker of spindle cell melanoma. Am J Dermatopathol 2012;34(6):619.

36. Kiuru M, Hameed M, Busam KJ. Compound clear cell sarcoma misdiagnosed as a Spitz nevus. J Cutan Pathol 2013;40(11):950.
37. Sidiropoulos M, Busam K, Guitart J, et al. Superficial paramucosal clear cell sarcoma of the soft parts resembling melanoma in a 13-year-old boy. J Cutan Pathol 2013;40(2):265.
38. Feasel PC, Cheah AL, Fritchie K, et al. Primary clear cell sarcoma of the head and neck: a case series with review of the literature. J Cutan Pathol 2016; 43(10):838.
39. Antonescu CR, Nafa K, Segal NH, et al. EWS-CREB1: a recurrent variant fusion in clear cell sarcoma–association with gastrointestinal location and absence of melanocytic differentiation. Clin Cancer Res 2006;12(18):5356.
40. Davis IJ, Kim JJ, Ozsolak F, et al. Oncogenic MITF dysregulation in clear cell sarcoma: defining the MiT family of human cancers. Cancer Cell 2006;9(6):473.
41. Davis IJ, McFadden AW, Zhang Y, et al. Identification of the receptor tyrosine kinase c-Met and its ligand, hepatocyte growth factor, as therapeutic targets in clear cell sarcoma. Cancer Res 2010;70(2):639.
42. Patel RM, Downs-Kelly E, Weiss SW, et al. Dual-color, break-apart fluorescence in situ hybridization for EWS gene rearrangement distinguishes clear cell sarcoma of soft tissue from malignant melanoma. Mod Pathol 2005;18(12):1585.
43. Noujaim J, Jones RL, Swansbury J, et al. The spectrum of EWSR1-rearranged neoplasms at a tertiary sarcoma centre; assessing 772 tumour specimens and the value of current ancillary molecular diagnostic modalities. Br J Cancer 2017;116(5):669–78.
44. Panagopoulos I, Mertens F, Isaksson M, et al. Absence of mutations of the BRAF gene in malignant melanoma of soft parts (clear cell sarcoma of tendons and aponeuroses). Cancer Genet Cytogenet 2005;156(1):74.
45. Zembowicz A, Granter SR, McKee PH, et al. Amelanotic cellular blue nevus: a hypopigmented variant of the cellular blue nevus: clinicopathologic analysis of 20 cases. Am J Surg Pathol 2002;26(11):1493.
46. Ferrari A, Casanova M, Bisogno G, et al. Clear cell sarcoma of tendons and aponeuroses in pediatric patients: a report from the Italian and German Soft Tissue Sarcoma Cooperative Group. Cancer 2002;94(12):3269.
47. Wright S, Armeson K, Hill EG, et al. The role of sentinel lymph node biopsy in select sarcoma patients: a meta-analysis. Am J Surg 2012;204(4):428.
48. Pea M, Bonetti F, Zamboni G, et al. Clear cell tumor and angiomyolipoma. Am J Surg Pathol 1991;15(2):199.
49. Zamboni G, Pea M, Martignoni G, et al. Clear cell "sugar" tumor of the pancreas. A novel member of the family of lesions characterized by the presence of perivascular epithelioid cells. Am J Surg Pathol 1996;20(6):722.
50. Folpe AL, Mentzel T, Lehr HA, et al. Perivascular epithelioid cell neoplasms of soft tissue and gynecologic origin: a clinicopathologic study of 26 cases and review of the literature. Am J Surg Pathol 2005;29(12):1558.
51. Folpe AL, Kwiatkowski DJ. Perivascular epithelioid cell neoplasms: pathology and pathogenesis. Hum Pathol 2010;41(1):1.
52. Thway K, Fisher C. PEComa: morphology and genetics of a complex tumor family. Ann Diagn Pathol 2015;19(5):359.
53. de Saint Aubain Somerhausen N, Gomez Galdon M, Bouffioux B, et al. Clear cell 'sugar' tumor (PEComa) of the skin: a case report. J Cutan Pathol 2005;32(6): 441.
54. Mentzel T, Reisshauer S, Rutten A, et al. Cutaneous clear cell myomelanocytic tumour: a new member of the growing family of perivascular epithelioid cell

tumours (PEComas). Clinicopathological and immunohistochemical analysis of seven cases. Histopathology 2005;46(5):498.

55. Tan J, Peach AH, Merchant W. PEComas of the skin: more common in the lower limb? Two case reports. Histopathology 2007;51(1):135.

56. Liegl B, Hornick JL, Fletcher CD. Primary cutaneous PEComa: distinctive clear cell lesions of skin. Am J Surg Pathol 2008;32(4):608.

57. Chaplin A, Conrad DM, Tatlidil C, et al. Primary cutaneous PEComa. Am J Dermatopathol 2010;32(3):310.

58. Charli-Joseph Y, Saggini A, Vemula S, et al. Primary cutaneous perivascular epithelioid cell tumor: a clinicopathological and molecular reappraisal. J Am Acad Dermatol 2014;71(6):1127.

59. Llamas-Velasco M, Mentzel T, Requena L, et al. Cutaneous PEComa does not harbour TFE3 gene fusions: immunohistochemical and molecular study of 17 cases. Histopathology 2013;63(1):122.

60. Wambacher-Gasser B, Zelger B, Zelger BG, et al. Clear cell dermatofibroma. Histopathology 1997;30(1):64.

61. Zedek DC, Murphy BA, Shea CR, et al. Cutaneous clear-cell granular cell tumors: the histologic description of an unusual variant. J Cutan Pathol 2007; 34(5):397.

62. Magro CM, Crowson AN, Mihm MC. Unusual variants of malignant melanoma. Mod Pathol 2006;19(Suppl 2):S41.

63. Hornick JL, Fletcher CD. PEComa: what do we know so far? Histopathology 2006;48(1):75.

64. Calder KB, Schlauder S, Morgan MB. Malignant perivascular epithelioid cell tumor ('PEComa'): a case report and literature review of cutaneous/subcutaneous presentations. J Cutan Pathol 2008;35(5):499.

65. Harris GC, McCulloch TA, Perks G, et al. Malignant perivascular epithelioid cell tumour ("PEComa") of soft tissue: a unique case. Am J Surg Pathol 2004;28(12): 1655.

66. Enzinger FM, Weiss SW, Liang CY. Ossifying fibromyxoid tumor of soft parts. A clinicopathological analysis of 59 cases. Am J Surg Pathol 1989;13(10):817.

67. Donner LR. Ossifying fibromyxoid tumor of soft parts: evidence supporting Schwann cell origin. Hum Pathol 1992;23(2):200.

68. Schofield JB, Krausz T, Stamp GW, et al. Ossifying fibromyxoid tumour of soft parts: immunohistochemical and ultrastructural analysis. Histopathology 1993; 22(2):101.

69. Min KW, Seo IS, Pitha J. Ossifying fibromyxoid tumor: modified myoepithelial cell tumor? Report of three cases with immunohistochemical and electron microscopic studies. Ultrastruct Pathol 2005;29(6):535.

70. Hirose T, Shimada S, Tani T, et al. Ossifying fibromyxoid tumor: invariable ultrastructural features and diverse immunophenotypic expression. Ultrastruct Pathol 2007;31(3):233.

71. Folpe AL, Weiss SW. Ossifying fibromyxoid tumor of soft parts: a clinicopathologic study of 70 cases with emphasis on atypical and malignant variants. Am J Surg Pathol 2003;27(4):421.

72. Gebre-Medhin S, Nord KH, Moller E, et al. Recurrent rearrangement of the PHF1 gene in ossifying fibromyxoid tumors. Am J Pathol 2012;181(3):1069.

73. Graham RP, Weiss SW, Sukov WR, et al. PHF1 rearrangements in ossifying fibromyxoid tumors of soft parts: a fluorescence in situ hybridization study of 41 cases with emphasis on the malignant variant. Am J Surg Pathol 2013;37(11): 1751.

74. Antonescu CR, Sung YS, Chen CL, et al. Novel ZC3H7B-BCOR, MEAF6-PHF1, and EPC1-PHF1 fusions in ossifying fibromyxoid tumors–molecular characterization shows genetic overlap with endometrial stromal sarcoma. Genes Chromosomes Cancer 2014;53(2):183.

75. Kao YC, Sung YS, Zhang L, et al. Expanding the molecular signature of ossifying fibromyxoid tumors with two novel gene fusions: CREBBP-BCORL1 and KDM2A-WWTR1. Genes Chromosomes Cancer 2017;56(1):42.

76. Kilpatrick SE, Ward WG, Mozes M, et al. Atypical and malignant variants of ossifying fibromyxoid tumor. Clinicopathologic analysis of six cases. Am J Surg Pathol 1995;19(9):1039.

77. Zamecnik M, Michal M, Simpson RH, et al. Ossifying fibromyxoid tumor of soft parts: a report of 17 cases with emphasis on unusual histological features. Ann Diagn Pathol 1997;1(2):73.

78. Schneider N, Fisher C, Thway K. Ossifying fibromyxoid tumor: morphology, genetics, and differential diagnosis. Ann Diagn Pathol 2016;20:52.

79. Miettinen M, Finnell V, Fetsch JF. Ossifying fibromyxoid tumor of soft parts–a clinicopathologic and immunohistochemical study of 104 cases with long-term follow-up and a critical review of the literature. Am J Surg Pathol 2008;32(7):996.

80. Atanaskova Mesinkovska N, Buehler D, McClain CM, et al. Ossifying fibromyxoid tumor: a clinicopathologic analysis of 26 subcutaneous tumors with emphasis on differential diagnosis and prognostic factors. J Cutan Pathol 2015;42(9):622.

81. Graham RP, Dry S, Li X, et al. Ossifying fibromyxoid tumor of soft parts: a clinicopathologic, proteomic, and genomic study. Am J Surg Pathol 2011; 35(11):1615.

82. Doyle LA, Wang WL, Dal Cin P, et al. MUC4 is a sensitive and extremely useful marker for sclerosing epithelioid fibrosarcoma: association with FUS gene rearrangement. Am J Surg Pathol 2012;36(10):1444.

83. Hornick JL, Fletcher CD. Cutaneous myoepithelioma: a clinicopathologic and immunohistochemical study of 14 cases. Hum Pathol 2004;35(1):14.

84. Flucke U, Palmedo G, Blankenhorn N, et al. EWSR1 gene rearrangement occurs in a subset of cutaneous myoepithelial tumors: a study of 18 cases. Mod Pathol 2011;24(11):1444.

85. Antonescu CR, Zhang L, Shao SY, et al. Frequent PLAG1 gene rearrangements in skin and soft tissue myoepithelioma with ductal differentiation. Genes Chromosomes Cancer 2013;52(7):675.

86. Laskin WB, Fetsch JF, Lasota J, et al. Benign epithelioid peripheral nerve sheath tumors of the soft tissues: clinicopathologic spectrum of 33 cases. Am J Surg Pathol 2005;29(1):39.

87. Hart J, Gardner JM, Edgar M, et al. Epithelioid schwannomas: an analysis of 58 cases including atypical variants. Am J Surg Pathol 2016;40(5):704.

88. Miettinen M, McCue PA, Sarlomo-Rikala M, et al. Sox10–a marker for not only schwannian and melanocytic neoplasms but also myoepithelial cell tumors of soft tissue: a systematic analysis of 5134 tumors. Am J Surg Pathol 2015; 39(6):826.

89. Billings SD, Giblen G, Fanburg-Smith JC. Superficial low-grade fibromyxoid sarcoma (Evans tumor): a clinicopathologic analysis of 19 cases with a unique observation in the pediatric population. Am J Surg Pathol 2005;29(2):204.

90. Folpe AL, Weiss SW. Pleomorphic hyalinizing angiectatic tumor: analysis of 41 cases supporting evolution from a distinctive precursor lesion. Am J Surg Pathol 2004;28(11):1417.

91. Carter JM, Sukov WR, Montgomery E, et al. TGFBR3 and MGEA5 rearrangements in pleomorphic hyalinizing angiectatic tumors and the spectrum of related neoplasms. Am J Surg Pathol 2014;38(9):1182.
92. Smith ME, Fisher C, Weiss SW. Pleomorphic hyalinizing angiectatic tumor of soft parts. A low-grade neoplasm resembling neurilemoma. Am J Surg Pathol 1996; 20(1):21.
93. Marshall-Taylor C, Fanburg-Smith JC. Hemosiderotic fibrohistiocytic lipomatous lesion: ten cases of a previously undescribed fatty lesion of the foot/ankle. Mod Pathol 2000;13(11):1192.
94. Browne TJ, Fletcher CD. Haemosiderotic fibrolipomatous tumour (so-called haemosiderotic fibrohistiocytic lipomatous tumour): analysis of 13 new cases in support of a distinct entity. Histopathology 2006;48(4):453.
95. Hallor KH, Sciot R, Staaf J, et al. Two genetic pathways, t(1;10) and amplification of 3p11–12, in myxoinflammatory fibroblastic sarcoma, haemosiderotic fibrolipomatous tumour, and morphologically similar lesions. J Pathol 2009;217(5): 716.
96. Antonescu CR, Zhang L, Nielsen GP, et al. Consistent t(1;10) with rearrangements of TGFBR3 and MGEA5 in both myxoinflammatory fibroblastic sarcoma and hemosiderotic fibrolipomatous tumor. Genes Chromosomes Cancer 2011; 50(10):757.
97. Solomon DA, Antonescu CR, Link TM, et al. Hemosiderotic fibrolipomatous tumor, not an entirely benign entity. Am J Surg Pathol 2013;37(10):1627.
98. Zreik RT, Carter JM, Sukov WR, et al. TGFBR3 and MGEA5 rearrangements are much more common in "hybrid" hemosiderotic fibrolipomatous tumor-myxoinflammatory fibroblastic sarcomas than in classical myxoinflammatory fibroblastic sarcomas: a morphological and fluorescence in situ hybridization study. Hum Pathol 2016;53:14.
99. Elco CP, Marino-Enriquez A, Abraham JA, et al. Hybrid myxoinflammatory fibroblastic sarcoma/hemosiderotic fibrolipomatous tumor: report of a case providing further evidence for a pathogenetic link. Am J Surg Pathol 2010; 34(11):1723.
100. Enzinger FM, Zhang RY. Plexiform fibrohistiocytic tumor presenting in children and young adults. An analysis of 65 cases. Am J Surg Pathol 1988;12(11):818.
101. Fetsch JF, Miettinen M, Laskin WB, et al. A clinicopathologic study of 45 pediatric soft tissue tumors with an admixture of adipose tissue and fibroblastic elements, and a proposal for classification as lipofibromatosis. Am J Surg Pathol 2000;24(11):1491.

Inflammatory Dermatopathology for General Surgical Pathologists

Emily H. Smith, MD[a,b], May P. Chan, MD[a,b,*]

KEYWORDS

- Dermatitis • Lichenoid • Spongiotic • Psoriasiform • Vasculopathic
- Granulomatous • Vesiculobullous • Neutrophilic dermatosis

KEY POINTS

- Classification of inflammatory skin diseases based on tissue reaction patterns helps guide differential diagnosis and facilitates effective communication with dermatologists.
- Certain inflammatory skin diseases may mimic neoplastic conditions and vice versa. Correct diagnosis requires recognition of important diagnostic clues and appropriate use of ancillary tools.
- Understanding of the clinical presentations of common dermatitides is imperative in the diagnosis of these conditions.

INTRODUCTION

Inflammatory dermatopathology is often viewed as an intimidating subject among surgical pathologists and even dermatopathologists. This article follows a basic and practical approach to inflammatory skin diseases. Most inflammatory conditions of the skin can be classified into one of the following patterns: lichenoid, spongiotic, psoriasiform, vascular, granulomatous, vesiculobullous, and diffuse. Further classification requires observation of additional histopathologic features and clinical correlation. The importance of the latter cannot be overemphasized; many inflammatory conditions cannot be diagnosed with certainty without knowledge of the clinical presentation. This article focuses on the most common inflammatory diseases involving the epidermis and dermis, as well as those with important clinical implications. Important diagnostic pitfalls are highlighted, and recommendations are provided when additional work-up is indicated.

Conflict of Interest Disclosure: None declared.
[a] Department of Pathology, University of Michigan, 1301 Catherine Street, Medical Science I, M3261, Ann Arbor, MI 48109, USA; [b] Department of Dermatology, University of Michigan, 1500 East Medical Center Drive, Ann Arbor, MI 48109, USA
* Corresponding author. Department of Pathology, University of Michigan, 1301 Catherine Street, Medical Science I, M3261, Ann Arbor, MI 48109.
E-mail address: mpchan@med.umich.edu

Clin Lab Med 37 (2017) 673–696
http://dx.doi.org/10.1016/j.cll.2017.05.008
0272-2712/17/© 2017 Elsevier Inc. All rights reserved.

labmed.theclinics.com

LICHENOID PATTERN

The lichenoid pattern is subclassified into lichenoid interface dermatitis and vacuolar interface dermatitis, both characterized by lymphocyte-mediated destruction of the basal layer. In lichenoid interface dermatitis there is a dense bandlike lymphocytic infiltrate, whereas vacuolar interface dermatitis shows sparse lymphocytes tagging along the dermoepidermal junction with associated vacuolar change of the basal layer. Both result in necrotic keratinocytes in the forms of eosinophilic cytoid bodies and dyskeratotic/apoptotic cells. Degeneration of the basal layer also leads to melanin incontinence. Subclassification of lichenoid and vacuolar interface dermatitides is shown in **Fig. 1**.

Lichen Planus and Other Lichenoid Lesions

Lichen planus (Fig. 2A)
Acanthosis with wedge-shaped hypergranulosis
Orthohyperkeratosis (compact hyperkeratosis without retained nuclei)
Lichenoid interface dermatitis with frequent cytoid bodies and melanophages
Pointed rete ridges with sawtooth appearance

Lichen planus (LP) is the prototype of lichenoid interface dermatitis. Clinically, LP presents as pruritic, polygonal, purple, flat-topped papules (4 Ps) with white, reticulated scale known as Wickham striae. Histopathologically, interface damage of the dermoepidermal junction may be so robust as to produce an artifactual subepidermal cleft known as Max-Joseph space. The lichenoid infiltrate consists predominantly of

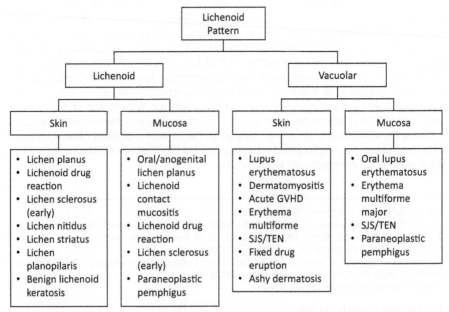

Fig. 1. Subclassification of selected entities with lichenoid pattern. GVHD, graft-versus-host disease; SJS, Stevens-Johnson syndrome; TEN, toxic epidermal necrolysis.

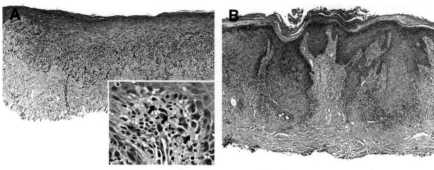

Fig. 2. Lichenoid interface dermatitis. (*A*) Lichen planus. Arrows show cytoid bodies (*inset*). (*B*) Hypertrophic lichen planus (H&E, original magnification ×40).

lymphocytes. Parakeratosis and eosinophils are uncommon; when present, a lichenoid drug reaction should be suspected. In oral specimens, the most common causes of lichenoid mucositis are LP, lichenoid drug eruption, and lichenoid contact reaction to amalgam or cinnamon.[1] Note that parakeratosis is seen in oral LP. The squamous mucosa of oral LP lacks the hypergranulosis of cutaneous LP.

Hypertrophic lichen planus (Fig. 2B)
Prominent acanthosis and hyperkeratosis (pseudoepitheliomatous hyperplasia)
Lichenoid inflammation concentrated at base of bulbous rete ridges
Eosinophils commonly present

Hypertrophic lichen planus (HLP) is a variant of LP typically presenting on the shins as multiple erythematous to violaceous nodules or plaques. Pseudoepitheliomatous hyperplasia in HLP can be difficult to distinguish from well-differentiated squamous cell carcinoma (SCC). Concentration of lymphocytes at the tips of the bulbous rete ridges and the presence of eosinophils favor HLP.[2] Diagnosis of multiple SCCs on the legs should at least raise suspicion for HLP and prompt a search for lichenoid inflammation in those specimens. Complicating matters, SCC can arise within lesions of HLP, and therefore close clinical follow-up and low threshold for biopsy is necessary.

Benign lichenoid keratosis
Orthohyperkeratosis and/or parakeratosis
Epidermis may be acanthotic or of normal thickness
Lichenoid infiltrate consisting of lymphocytes, plasma cells, neutrophils, and/or eosinophils

Benign lichenoid keratosis is also known as LP-like keratosis. It presents as a solitary lesion on the trunk (most commonly chest) or proximal extremities. Acanthotic lesions may have identical histology to LP, although close examination often reveals parakeratosis and a more mixed inflammatory cell infiltrate.[3] If similar histology is encountered in the context of multiple lesions, the possibility of LP or another lichenoid eruption should be entertained.

Connective Tissue Diseases

Most connective tissue diseases involving the skin share the common feature of vacuolar interface dermatitis, with varying degrees of dyskeratosis, perivascular and periadnexal inflammation, and dermal mucin.

Discoid lupus erythematosus (Fig. 3A)
Atrophic epidermis with vacuolar interface dermatitis
Epidermal and follicular hyperkeratosis
Thickened basement membrane
Periadnexal and perivascular lymphoplasmacytic infiltrate
Increased dermal mucin

Discoid lupus erythematosus (DLE) presents as discrete scaly erythematous plaques, usually on sun-exposed skin. Patients may have DLE lesions confined to the skin, or it may present in the setting of systemic lupus erythematosus. Other forms of lupus erythematosus and dermatomyositis are variations on the same histopathologic spectrum. Plasmacytoid dendritic cells, as highlighted by CD123 immunostain, are increased in number with formation of clusters in connective tissue diseases; in contrast, they tend to be sparse and singly dispersed in other inflammatory conditions.[4]

Similar to HLP, the hypertrophic variant of cutaneous lupus erythematosus may be easily misinterpreted as SCC because of pseudoepitheliomatous hyperplasia (Fig. 3B).[5] Recognition of other typical features of lupus erythematosus, namely vacuolar interface change, perivascular and periadnexal inflammation, increased dermal mucin, as well as correlation with clinical history of lupus erythematosus, is crucial in achieving the correct diagnosis. An immunostain for CD123 may also be used to aid in the diagnosis, because the infiltrate in cutaneous lupus erythematosus often has clusters of CD123-positive plasmacytoid dendritic cells.[6]

Graft-Versus-Host Disease

Acute graft-versus-host disease (Fig. 3C)
Vacuolar interface dermatitis involving epidermis and follicular epithelium
Occasional dyskeratotic keratinocytes associated with lymphocytes (satellite cell necrosis)

Cutaneous graft-versus-host disease is a common complication of allogeneic stem cell transplant. The acute form usually occurs within 90 days of transplant or on weaning of immunosuppression. The eruption is morbilliform and typically involves the face, trunk, and extremities. The differential diagnosis often includes an interface drug reaction. However, no histologic criterion, including the presence of eosinophils, has been shown to reliably distinguish between the two.[7] In these instances, a comment regarding the need for clinicopathologic correlation is appropriate.

Erythema Multiforme, Stevens-Johnson Syndrome, and Toxic Epidermal Necrolysis

Although erythema multiforme (EM) and Stevens-Johnson syndrome (SJS)/toxic epidermal necrolysis (TEN) are clinically distinct entities, they exist on a histopathologic spectrum.

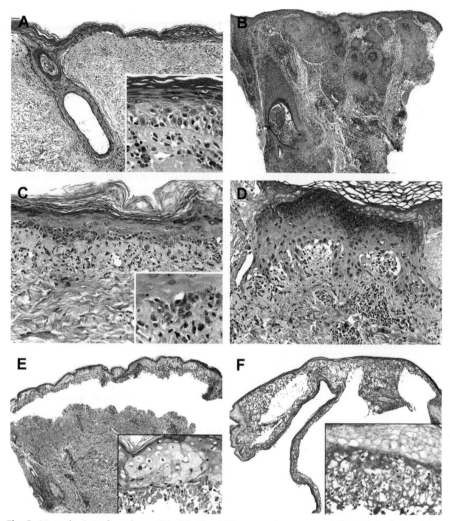

Fig. 3. Vacuolar interface dermatitis. (*A*) Discoid lupus erythematosus (H&E, original magnification, ×40). (*B*) Hypertrophic lupus erythematosus (H&E, original magnification, ×40). (*C*) Acute graft-versus-host disease (H&E, original magnification, ×100). (*D*) Erythema multiforme (H&E, original magnification, ×100). (*E*, *F*) SJS/TEN. Frozen section of rolled desquamated skin (H&E, original magnification, ×40) (*F*) shows predominantly necrotic epidermis (H&E, original magnification, ×40). ([*F*] Courtesy of Drs Thomas Bander and Stephanie Chen, University of Michigan, Ann Arbor, MI, USA)

Erythema multiforme (Fig. 3D)
Vacuolar interface dermatitis with prominent dyskeratoses
Superficial perivascular lymphocytic infiltrate
Variable number of eosinophils

Lesions of EM are targetoid and frequently affect the palmar surfaces, classically preceded by herpes simplex virus infection.[8] Significant basal degeneration may result in bullous EM, but the degree of epidermal necrosis is usually limited compared with SJS/TEN.

Stevens-Johnson syndrome/toxic epidermal necrolysis (Fig. 3E)
Robust vacuolar interface dermatitis
Full-thickness epidermal necrosis and detachment
Sparse dermal inflammatory infiltrate

Most cases of SJS/TEN are drug induced.[9] Clinically, SJS/TEN manifests as a desquamative dusky eruption on the trunk and extremities. Mucosal involvement is almost always present. Skin sloughing in SJS/TEN may raise clinical consideration for staphylococcal scalded skin syndrome (SSSS). Because SJS/TEN is a dermatologic emergency, prompt diagnosis may be achieved by rolling the desquamated skin onto a cotton-tipped applicator and submitting it for frozen section analysis. However, this technique can be difficult. A punch biopsy submitted for frozen section often yields better results. Visualization of full-thickness necrotic epidermis indicates a subepidermal split, thus supporting a diagnosis of SJS/TEN (**Fig. 3**F). In contrast, SSSS is characterized by a subcorneal split in which the desquamated skin consists of mostly stratum corneum and only a few superficial keratinocytes (discussed later).[10]

Pseudomelanocytic Nests

Pseudomelanocytic nests (Fig. 4)
Nested aggregates of macrophages, lymphocytes, and rare melanocytes at dermoepidermal junction
Constituent cells appear dyshesive and contain variably pigmented cytoplasm and small bland nuclei
Interface change and melanin incontinence

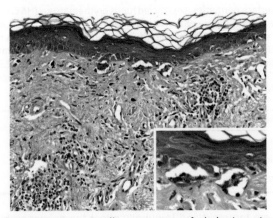

Fig. 4. Pseudomelanocytic nests. Small aggregates of dyshesive pigmented cells and lymphocytes are found at the basal layer. Dermal fibrosis and melanophages suggest a burnt-out interface dermatitis (H&E, original magnification ×100). (*Courtesy of* Dr Lori Lowe, University of Michigan, Ann Arbor, MI.)

Lichenoid dermatitis may result in pseudomelanocytic nests of mostly nonmelanocytic cells, notorious for their resemblance to true melanocytic nests. In combination with other features of lichenoid dermatitis, pseudomelanocytic nests readily raise concern for an atypical melanocytic lesion with regression. To add to the diagnostic challenge, constituent cells in pseudomelanocytic nests may contain degraded melanosomes, resulting in nonspecific cytoplasmic staining for certain melanocytic markers.[11] To avoid this pitfall, nuclear markers (MiTF and SOX10) are generally preferred when evaluating junctional melanocytes. Because clusters of cytoid bodies are unusual in melanocytic lesions, their presence serves as a clue to pseudomelanocytic nests. The importance of clinicopathologic correlation cannot be overstated. Recognition of this phenomenon would avoid overdiagnosis of atypical melanocytic lesions, in particular melanoma in situ.

SPONGIOTIC PATTERN

The spongiotic reaction pattern is defined by intraepidermal edema resulting in increased spacing between keratinocytes and prominent desmosomal spines (intercellular bridges). Langerhans cell microabscesses and lymphocyte exocytosis are common. These changes may be accompanied by parakeratosis and a dermal inflammatory infiltrate depending on the specific entity. A list of common spongiotic dermatitides is shown in **Box 1**.

Eczematous Dermatitis

Eczema (Fig. 5A)
Spongiosis
Parakeratosis and/or serum crust
Superficial dermal perivascular lymphocytic infiltrate
Eosinophils are common

Eczema is a common condition that presents as pruritic, ill-defined, erythematous, and often scaly papules and plaques. The lesions can be classified as acute, subacute, or chronic based on the degree of spongiosis, acanthosis, inflammation, and scale formation (**Table 1**). In eczematous dermatitis, lymphocyte exocytosis should be mild and confined to areas of spongiosis. In contrast, mycosis fungoides (a form

Box 1
Examples of spongiotic and psoriasiform dermatitides

Spongiotic pattern	*Psoriasiform pattern*
• Eczema (atopic dermatitis) • Nummular dermatitis • Contact dermatitis • Eczematous drug reaction • Id reaction (autoeczematization) • Seborrheic dermatitis • Pityriasis rosea	• Psoriasis • Psoriasiform drug reaction • Chronic candidiasis/dermatophytosis • Secondary syphilis • Sebopsoriasis • Pityriasis rubra pilaris • Nutritional deficiency • Bazex syndrome • Reiter syndrome

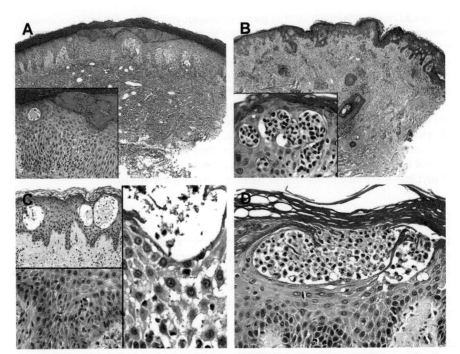

Fig. 5. Spongiotic dermatitis (vs mycosis fungoides). (*A*) Eczema (H&E, original magnification ×40). (*B*) In mycosis fungoides, the number of intraepidermal lymphocytes is out of proportion to the degree of spongiosis. Pautrier microabscesses (*inset*) consist of atypical lymphocytes with little cytoplasm and hyperchromatic nuclei (H&E, original magnification ×40). (*C*) Allergic contact dermatitis with intraepidermal spongiotic vesicles (*left upper*), eosinophilic spongiosis (*left lower*), and prominent intercellular bridges (*right*) (H&E, original magnification ×600). (*D*) A Langerhans cell microabscess in spongiotic dermatitis opens to the epidermal surface and consists of large cells with abundant cytoplasm (H&E, original magnification ×200).

of cutaneous T-cell lymphoma) shows more frequent lymphocyte exocytosis out of proportion to the degree of spongiosis, and may comprise collections of atypical intraepidermal lymphocytes known as Pautrier microabscesses (**Fig. 5**B). Wiry fibrosis in the upper dermis is another clue to mycosis fungoides. Immunohistochemical workup and/or T-cell receptor gene rearrangement study should be performed when these atypical features are present.[12]

Contact Dermatitis

Allergic contact dermatitis (Fig. 5C)
Acute spongiotic dermatitis with Langerhans cell microabscesses
Intraepidermal eosinophils
Superficial dermal lymphocytic and eosinophilic infiltrate

Contact dermatitis is most often classified in the category of acute spongiotic dermatitis, although subacute and chronic forms do exist. The presence of Langerhans cell microabscesses (**Fig. 5**D) is reportedly more reliable (although not entirely

Table 1
Histopathologic spectrum of spongiotic dermatitis

	Acute	Subacute	Chronic
Spongiosis	Prominent, with spongiotic vesicles	Mild	Mild to absent
Scale	Normal basket-weave stratum corneum	Mild parakeratosis	Prominent orthokeratosis or parakeratosis
Acanthosis	Absent	Mild to moderate	Prominent
Inflammatory infiltrate	Prominent	Mild to moderate	Mild to minimal

specific) than the density of eosinophils in this diagnosis.[13] Therefore, when present, the possibility of allergic contact dermatitis should be raised in the report. Because scabies infestation may share similar histopathologic features, it should also be considered in the correct clinical setting and prompt careful examination for mite parts.

PSORIASIFORM PATTERN

This pattern encompasses conditions with psoriasiform hyperplasia: elongation of thin rete ridges of roughly equal width and length, often likened to the shape of a comb.

Psoriasis (Fig. 6A)

Confluent parakeratosis with neutrophils

Regular elongation of thin, club-shaped rete ridges

Hypogranulosis (loss of granular layer)

Thinning of suprapapillary plates

Dilated capillaries at tips of dermal papillae

Minimal perivascular infiltrate without eosinophils

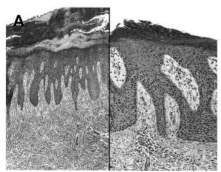 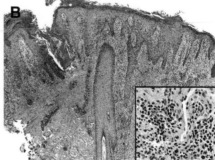

Fig. 6. Psoriasiform dermatitis. (*A*) Psoriasis. (*B*) Secondary syphilis with abundant plasma cells (*inset*) (H&E, original magnification (*A*) ×100 (*left*), ×200 (*right*), (*B*) ×100).

Classic plaque-type psoriasis presents as well-demarcated beefy red plaques with overlying silvery scale on extensor surfaces. The confluent parakeratosis in psoriasis is typically devoid of serum, corresponding with the dry silvery scale noted clinically. Similarly, the epidermis typically lacks significant spongiosis. However, should a psoriatic lesion be biopsied at an early stage of development or after treatment, some of the aforementioned features may be attenuated or absent.

The differential diagnosis of the psoriasiform pattern is broad (see **Box 1**). When psoriasiform features are observed in combination with spongiosis and eosinophils, the possibility of a psoriasiform drug eruption should be considered. Many drugs have been implicated (eg, β-blockers, statins, nonsteroidal antiinflammatory drugs, lithium, interferon alfa), with tumor necrosis factor alpha inhibitors becoming an increasingly common cause.[14]

Secondary syphilis (Fig. 6B)

Psoriasiform hyperplasia with slender rete ridges

Bandlike or interstitial inflammatory infiltrate containing plasma cells

Endothelial swelling

An important differential diagnosis to recognize is secondary syphilis. The histopathologic spectrum of secondary syphilis is wide, with a subset of cases showing a psoriasiform pattern. However, unlike psoriasis, secondary syphilis typically displays more robust and mixed inflammation.[15] Psoriasiform lesions from the oral/perioral and genital areas should raise suspicion for syphilis. The diagnosis can be easily confirmed by the use of spirochete immunostain, which highlights helical rods near the dermoepidermal junction and around blood vessels.

Candidiasis and dermatophytosis

Variable degree of spongiosis and psoriasiform hyperplasia

Neutrophils and/or serum in stratum corneum

Fungal hyphae present between an upper layer of normal basket-weave keratin and a lower layer of compact orthokeratosis or parakeratosis (sandwich sign)

Psoriasiform hyperplasia may also be seen in chronic candidiasis and dermatophytosis. Grocott methenamine silver or periodic acid–Schiff stain can be used to confirm the diagnosis.

VASCULAR PATTERN

This group of diseases may be subdivided into perivascular, vasculitic, and vasculopathic patterns based on the presence/absence and the type of vascular damage (**Fig. 7**).

Perivascular Dermatitis

Many diseases display a perivascular inflammatory infiltrate, either alone or in combination with other reaction patterns. This category refers to those with a pure perivascular pattern.

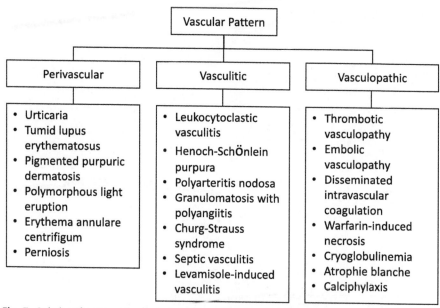

Fig. 7. Subclassification of selected entities with vascular pattern.

Urticaria (Fig. 8A)
Scant perivascular and some interstitial eosinophils and neutrophils
Intravascular neutrophilic margination
Mild dermal edema

The most common entity in this category is urticaria. It presents as erythematous and edematous papules and plaques without surface changes, commonly described as hives or wheals, developing and resolving within 24 to 48 hours. The histopathologic changes are usually subtle, giving the impression of normal skin (one of the so-called invisible dermatoses); however, sparse inflammation can be appreciated on closer examination.

Vasculitis

Cutaneous vasculitides are a group of immune complex–mediated diseases involving small or medium-sized vessels. The size of the involved vessels determines the clinical presentation, ranging from palpable purpura in small vessel vasculitides to deeper dermal nodules or even ulcerative and necrotic lesions in medium-vessel vasculitides.

Leukocytoclastic vasculitis (Fig. 8B)
Fibrinoid necrosis of small vessel walls
Perivascular and transmural neutrophilic inflammation with leukocytoclasia (nuclear fragments of neutrophils)
Extravasation of erythrocytes

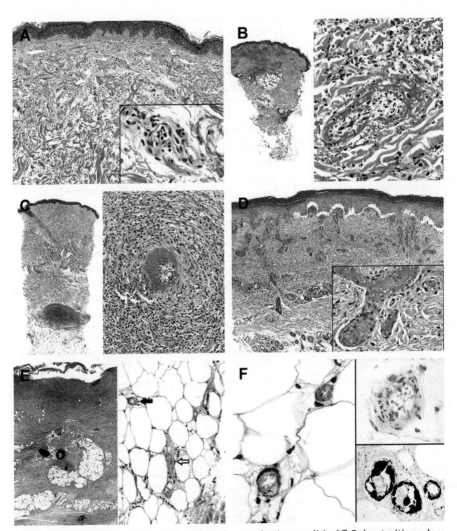

Fig. 8. Vascular pattern. (*A*) Urticaria. (*B*) Leukocytoclastic vasculitis. (*C*) Polyarteritis nodosa. (*D*) Thrombotic vasculopathy. (*E, F*) Calciphylaxis. Vascular calcification (*E, black arrow*; *F, left*) and microthrombus (*E, white arrow*) are present. von Kossa stain highlights fine stippled (*F, right upper*) and chunky (*F, right lower*) calcifications in vessel walls (H&E, original magnification (*A*) ×40, (*B*) ×10 (*left*), ×400 (*right*), (*C*) ×10 (*left*), ×200 (*right*), (*D*) ×40, (*E*) ×20 (*left*), ×200 (*right*), (*F*) ×600).

Leukocytoclastic vasculitis (LCV) involves small vessels and most commonly manifests in the lower legs. The histopathologic features are best appreciated when a lesion is biopsied within 24 to 48 hours. A second lesional biopsy submitted for direct immunofluorescence can confirm immune complex deposition, especially in the diagnosis of immunoglobulin A (IgA) vasculitis (Henoch-Schönlein purpura).[16] However, other forms of LCV generally do not require direct immunofluorescence to establish the diagnosis. Note that identical vascular changes may also be seen in secondary vasculitis (unrelated to immune complex deposition) near an ulcer or in association with an infection.

> **Polyarteritis nodosa (Fig. 8C)**
>
> Fibrinoid necrosis of medium-sized vessels in deep dermis and subcutis
>
> Perivascular and transmural neutrophilic and lymphocytic inflammation
>
> Wreathlike appearance of the thickened vessels

Diagnosis of medium-vessel vasculitis requires a deep punch biopsy to visualize the deep dermis and subcutis. The changes in polyarteritis nodosa are mostly confined to the walls of the medium-sized vessels. In contrast, antineutrophil cytoplasmic antibody–associated vasculitides (granulomatosis with polyangiitis/Wegener granulomatosis and eosinophilic granulomatosis with polyangiitis/Churg-Strauss syndrome) may show LCV, extravascular granulomas, and necrosis in addition to medium-vessel vasculitis.[17]

Vasculopathy

Vasculopathy refers to occlusion of the vascular lumen and may be subclassified based on cause. Possible causes include various coagulopathies, fibrin or cholesterol emboli secondary to recent vascular procedures, cryoglobulinemia, and calciphylaxis.[18] Clinically these lesions are sharply angulated purpuric patches with or without eschar.

> **Thrombotic vasculopathy (Fig. 8D)**
>
> Fibrin thrombi in vascular lumen
>
> Epidermal, eccrine, and/or dermal necrosis (infarction) may be present

Thrombotic vasculopathy secondary to coagulopathy presents as retiform purpura (sharply angulated purpuric patches) with or without livedo reticularis. The lesions are typically pauci-inflammatory, although neutrophilic inflammation may ensue once necrosis and ulceration have developed. Cryoglobulinemia, levamisole-induced vasculitis,[19] and septic vasculitis are related conditions that may show a combination of vasculitis and vasculopathy. Because thrombotic vasculopathy can indicate a serious systemic illness (eg, disseminated intravascular coagulation), it is one of the most critical tissue reaction patterns to recognize.

> **Calciphylaxis (Fig. 8E)**
>
> Concentric medial calcification of small and/or medium-sized vessels
>
> Microthrombi and variable degree of fat necrosis commonly found in subcutis
>
> Ulceration and necrosis present in central eschar

Calciphylaxis is a life-threatening condition most commonly associated with end-stage renal disease. It presents as painful purpuric angulated plaques with central necrotic eschar. Histologic diagnosis relies on identification of calcified vessels and microthrombi, which can be subtle and requires adequate sampling of the subcutaneous fat. von Kossa or alizarin red stain helps to highlight concentric calcifications in small vessel walls, especially when fine and stippled (**Fig. 8**F). Extravascular and perieccrine calcifications may also be present.[20]

GRANULOMATOUS PATTERN

Granulomas in the skin can be subdivided into sarcoidal, tuberculoid, suppurative, palisading/interstitial, and foreign body types to narrow the differential diagnosis (**Fig. 9**).

Sarcoidal Granulomas

This type of granuloma is characterized by discrete aggregates of epithelioid histiocytes with minimal admixed lymphocytes. The prototype is sarcoidosis.

Sarcoidosis (Fig. 10A)

Discrete round aggregates of epithelioid histiocytes and occasional multinucleated giant cells

Minimal surrounding lymphocytes (naked granulomas)

Involvement of dermis and/or subcutis

Cutaneous sarcoidosis may manifest at sites of previous trauma (scar) or foreign body implantation (such as tattoos).[21] Rarely, granulomas in sarcoidosis contain small necrotizing foci. Because sarcoidal granulomas may also be found in infection, special stains for microorganisms are necessary in patients without a known history of sarcoidosis.

Tuberculoid Granulomas

Tuberculoid granulomas are loose to tight aggregates of epithelioid histiocytes surrounded by lymphocytes. This type of granuloma usually indicates infection.

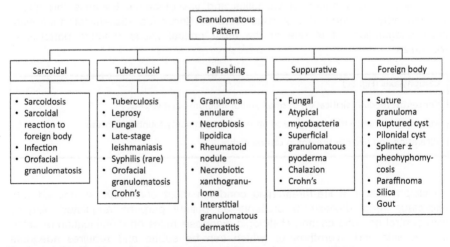

Fig. 9. Subclassification of selected entities with granulomatous pattern.

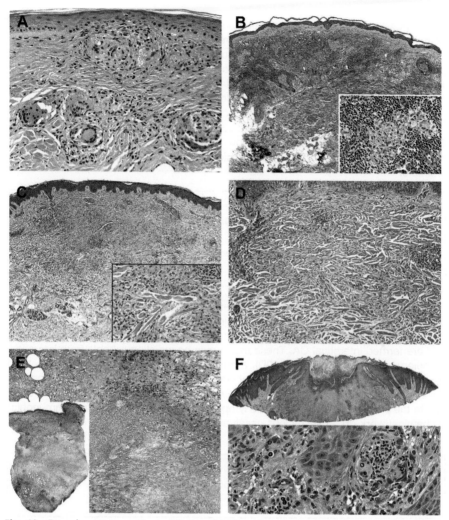

Fig. 10. Granulomatous pattern. (*A*) Sarcoidosis with naked granulomas. (*B*) Tuberculoid leprosy. (*C*) Granuloma annulare with palisading histiocytes around necrobiotic collagen (*inset*). (*D*) Interstitial granulomatous dermatitis. (*E*) Rheumatoid nodule with fibrinoid core. (*F*) Chromomycosis with pseudoepitheliomatous hyperplasia (*top*), suppurative granulomas, and pigmented fungal yeasts (*bottom*) (H&E. original magnification (*A, E*) ×100, (*B, C*) ×20, (*D*) ×40, (*F*) ×20 [*top*], ×400 [*bottom*]).

Tuberculoid leprosy (Fig. 10B)
Top-heavy infiltrate
Loose aggregates of epithelioid and multinucleated histiocytes
Granulomas surrounded by a brisk lymphoplasmacytic infiltrate

---

Tuberculoid granulomas are found in tuberculosis and leprosy, with perineural granulomas being more characteristic of the latter.[22] A modified acid-fast (Fite) stain is preferred to increase the sensitivity for atypical mycobacteria. Special stains are also needed to exclude fungal infection and, in some cases, syphilis.[23] Tuberculoid granulomas have also been reported in rare cases of late-stage leishmaniasis.[24]

Noninfectious causes of tuberculoid granulomas include Crohn disease and orofacial granulomatosis.[25] Orofacial granulomatosis is characterized by lip and facial swelling, with marked dermal edema and perivascular lymphocytic and granulomatous inflammation.[26] Exclusion of Crohn disease, sarcoidosis, and infection is necessary.

Palisading/Interstitial Granulomas

The granulomas in this group may show a predominantly palisading or interstitial pattern, or a combination of both. Granuloma annulare (GA) is the most common example.

Granuloma annulare (Fig. 10C)

Palisading pattern: histiocytes form a ring around a central zone of degenerated collagen (necrobiosis) and mucin

Interstitial pattern: histiocytes percolate between collagen bundles

Mild perivascular lymphocytic infiltrate

Classic GA presents as 1 or few annular plaques without surface changes, most frequently on the hands and feet. A combination of palisading and interstitial granulomas is usually present.[27] However, some cases show a purely interstitial pattern and are termed interstitial GA. These cases may be indistinguishable from interstitial granulomatous dermatitis (**Fig. 10**D), a condition associated with a wide variety of systemic diseases and drugs.[28] Clinical correlation is required for correct diagnosis. Another histologic mimicker of interstitial GA is interstitial mycosis fungoides.[29] Attention to the predominance of interstitial lymphocytes over histiocytes, and immunohistochemical work-up on suspicious cases avoids misdiagnosis.

Rheumatoid nodule (Fig. 10E)

Histiocytes palisade around an intensely eosinophilic fibrinoid core

Minimal interstitial pattern

Another example of palisading granulomas is rheumatoid nodule, which occurs as painless nodules near joints in patients with rheumatoid arthritis. An important differential diagnosis is epithelioid sarcoma, in which the epithelioid tumor cells are present around a central necrotic area (**Fig. 11**). The tumor cells in epithelioid sarcoma show at least mild atypia and pleomorphism. Demonstration of immunoreactivity for cytokeratin and loss of INI-1 expression confirm the diagnosis of epithelioid sarcoma.[30]

Suppurative and Foreign Body–type Granulomas

Suppurative granulomas are granulomas admixed with neutrophils. Like tuberculoid granulomas, these are most suggestive of infection, especially deep fungal and atypical mycobacterial infections. These infections may also result in pseudoepitheliomatous hyperplasia closely simulating SCC (**Fig. 10**F).[31] Chromomycosis and blastomycosis are especially notorious for this. The presence of any intraepidermal pustules and/or granulomas, especially of suppurative type, should raise concern for an infection in these cases.

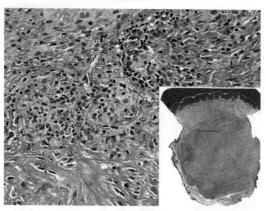

Fig. 11. Epithelioid sarcoma. Proliferation of atypical epithelioid tumor cells around a central necrotic area (H&E, original magnification ×400).

Neutrophils may also be seen in foreign body–type granulomas with or without superimposed infection. Examination under polarized light may help identify the foreign bodies. When a plant fragment is implanted, its surface should be inspected for evidence of phaeohyphomycosis.

VESICULOBULLOUS PATTERN

Conditions in this group are characterized by vesicle or blister formation. These conditions are subclassified based on the microscopic level of the split and any evidence of an autoimmune cause (**Fig. 12**).

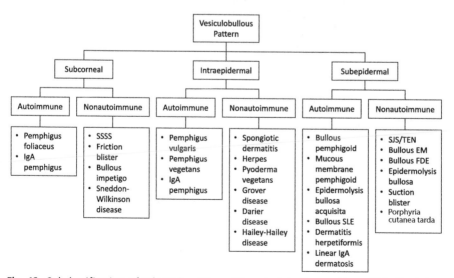

Fig. 12. Subclassification of selected entities with vesiculobullous pattern. FDE, fixed drug eruption; SLE, systemic lupus erythematosus.

Subcorneal Split

In this group, the split is located just below the stratum corneum, with or without acantholysis in the granular layer.

Staphylococcal scalded skin syndrome (Fig. 13A)
Broad subcorneal split
Some acantholytic keratinocytes within split
Scant to no neutrophils

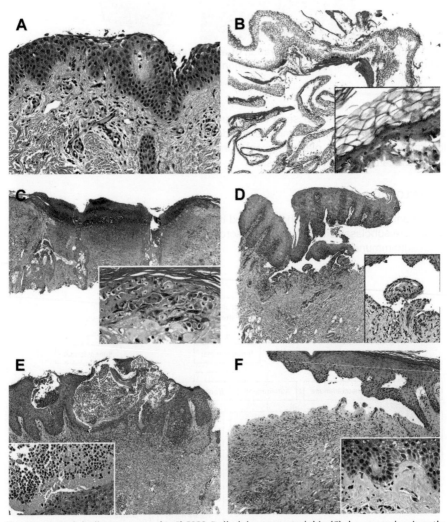

Fig. 13. Vesiculobullous pattern. (*A, B*) SSSS. Rolled desquamated skin (*B*) shows predominantly stratum corneum and a few superficial keratinocytes. (*C*) Ulcerated herpetic vesicle with necrosis of adnexal structures and viral inclusions adjacent to ulcer. (*D*) Pemphigus vulgaris. (*E*) Pemphigus vegetans. (*F*) Bullous pemphigoid. Prebullous phase shows eosinophils along dermoepidermal junction (*inset*) (H&E, original magnification (*A*) ×100, (*B*) ×20, (*C, D, E, F*) ×40).

As mentioned earlier, pathologists may receive frozen section requests for SSSS, which is a desquamative condition secondary to epidermolytic toxins produced by *Staphylococcus*. Rolled desquamated skin in SSSS consists predominantly of stratum corneum with only a few superficial keratinocytes and occasional neutrophils (**Fig. 13B**), in contrast with the full-thickness necrotic epidermis seen in SJS/TEN.[10]

Intraepidermal Split

This group of disorders shows separation of keratinocytes in the spinous layer. Common nonautoimmune causes include acute spongiosis and herpesvirus. Spongiotic vesicles contain intraepidermal edema fluid (discussed earlier), most frequently seen in eczema and contact dermatitis (**Fig. 5C**).

Herpetic vesicles (see Fig. 13C)
Acantholysis and necrosis of epidermis and adnexae
Infected keratinocytes display multinucleation, nuclear molding, and/or chromatin margination
Suppurative inflammation

Although herpetic vesicles with prominent viral inclusions pose little diagnostic difficulty, advanced lesions in which the epidermis is partially denuded and replaced by suppurative scale can be difficult to recognize. As a rule, exfoliated necrotic keratinocytes amid a suppurative scale crust should be carefully inspected for herpetic viral inclusions. Any inflamed or necrotic adnexal structures should also prompt examination for herpetic infection.[32] Immunostains for herpes simplex virus and varicella-zoster virus can be used to confirm the diagnosis.

Pemphigus vulgaris (Fig. 13D)
Suprabasilar acantholysis
Intact basal layer resembles a row of tombstones
Pauci-inflammatory cavity

Both pemphigus vulgaris and pemphigus vegetans are examples of autoimmune intraepidermal bullous disorders. Pemphigus vulgaris is the most common type of pemphigus and manifests as flaccid bullae on the skin and/or oral mucosa.

Pemphigus vegetans (Fig. 13E)
Intraepidermal collections of neutrophils and/or eosinophils
Papillomatous epidermal hyperplasia
Minimal acantholysis

Pemphigus vegetans presents as vegetative plaques in intertriginous areas, and is often difficult to discern as a vesiculobullous process both clinically and histopathologically.[33] Because pemphigus vegetans closely mimics pyodermatitis vegetans and cutaneous infections with pseudoepitheliomatous hyperplasia, correlation with any history of inflammatory bowel disease and special stains for microorganisms are recommended.[31,34] Immunofluorescence and/or serologic studies are required to confirm the diagnosis.

Subepidermal Split

In this group of disorders, the split is located at the dermoepidermal junction (basement membrane zone). It can be caused by robust interface dermatitis causing significant basal layer damage and eventual separation of the epidermis. As mentioned earlier, the most important example to recognize is SJS/TEN (discussed earlier).

Bullous pemphigoid (Fig. 13F)
Clean split between epidermis and dermis
Abundant eosinophils present in dermis and sometimes epidermis

The prototype of autoimmune subepidermal bullous disorder is bullous pemphigoid (BP). The blisters are tense and typically affect the skin of elderly patients. Its mucosal variant is known as mucous membrane pemphigoid. Biopsy of the early prebullous phase (urticarial BP) shows eosinophils aligning along the dermoepidermal junction and within the epidermis (see **Fig. 13F**, inset).[35] Appreciation of these findings should prompt immunofluorescence or serologic studies to confirm the diagnosis.

Dermatitis herpetiformis
Foci of subepidermal split
Neutrophilic microabscesses in dermal papillae

Recognition of dermatitis herpetiformis may help identify patients with gluten sensitivity. These patients present with multiple pruritic erythematous papules on the extensor surfaces. Because the vesicles are often excoriated, a vesiculobullous disorder may not be suspected clinically. Papillary dermal microabscesses are an important clue, although identical features may be seen in linear IgA disease and sometimes BP. Distinction of these conditions requires immunofluorescence or serologic studies.[36]

DIFFUSE PATTERN

This pattern refers to a diffuse inflammatory infiltrate in the dermis. Conditions with this pattern are subclassified based on the predominant cell type (**Fig. 14**).

Neutrophilic

The prototypes of neutrophilic dermatosis are pyoderma gangrenosum (PG) and Sweet syndrome.

Pyoderma gangrenosum (Fig. 15A)
Ulcer
Sheets of neutrophils in dermis
Neutrophils undermine the epidermis at the ulcer edge
Neutrophils are gradually replaced by lymphocytes and plasma cells further away from the ulcer

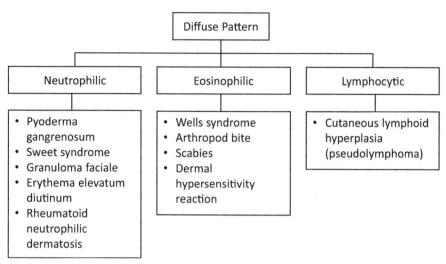

Fig. 14. Subclassification of selected entities with diffuse pattern.

The classic presentation of PG is a large ulcer with violaceous rolled border. It may occur in association with inflammatory bowel disease, hematologic disorders, or other systemic diseases. Caused by pathergy, PG has a tendency to occur at sites of trauma or surgery.[37] Histopathologically, PG is indistinguishable from infection, although it usually lacks basophilic necrosis and vascular changes away from the ulcer bed. Distinction from infection has important clinical implications. First, unnecessary debridement of PG for presumed infection results in more extensive PG caused by pathergy.[38] In contrast, misdiagnosis of cellulitis as PG may lead to steroid treatment and exacerbation of infection. Tissue cultures and careful clinical correlation are therefore imperative.

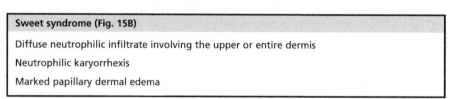

Sweet syndrome (Fig. 15B)

Diffuse neutrophilic infiltrate involving the upper or entire dermis

Neutrophilic karyorrhexis

Marked papillary dermal edema

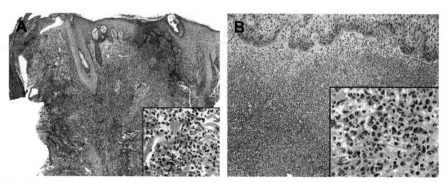

Fig. 15. Diffuse pattern. (A) PG. (B) Sweet syndrome (H&E, original magnification (A) ×40, (B) ×100).

Classic Sweet syndrome presents as nonulcerated, erythematous, and edematous papules or nodules. It has various clinical associations, most notably myeloid disorders. Again, diagnosis requires exclusion of infection. Variants of Sweet syndrome often present a diagnostic challenge. The subcutaneous form needs to be distinguished from other types of neutrophilic panniculitis.[39] Necrotizing Sweet syndrome involves deep soft tissue and closely mimics necrotizing fasciitis; tissue cultures and correlation with history of hematologic malignancy are key to its diagnosis.[40] Histiocytoid Sweet syndrome is composed of histiocytoid mononuclear myeloid cells (rather than mature neutrophils), which often raise concern for leukemia cutis, especially in patients with known leukemia. Fluorescence in situ hybridization may help in the correct diagnosis.[41]

Eosinophilic

A marked eosinophilic infiltrate often indicates a hypersensitivity reaction, such as to an arthropod bite, scabies infestation, or drug. Wells syndrome is a prototype of eosinophilic dermatosis that is commonly thought to be a robust hypersensitivity reaction to an unknown trigger.

Lymphocytic

An exuberant reaction to various localized insults (eg, tattoo, ear piercing, arthropod bite) may result in a lymphomatoid reaction, better known as cutaneous lymphoid hyperplasia. Such lesions typically present as erythematous nodules at the site of insult.

Cutaneous lymphoid hyperplasia
Dense dermal sheetlike or nodular lymphocytic infiltrate
Some admixed histiocytes, plasma cells, and eosinophils

Immunophenotyping and gene rearrangement studies are often needed to distinguish reactive lymphoid infiltrate from lymphoma. When T cells predominate, the main differential diagnosis is primary cutaneous CD4+ small/medium T-cell lymphoproliferative disorder.[42] When B cells predominate, the differential diagnosis includes extranodal marginal zone lymphoma and primary cutaneous follicle center lymphoma.[43]

SUMMARY

Most skin biopsies performed for rashes can be classified by tissue reaction patterns. Efforts should be made to obtain clinical information, if not already provided, to ensure accurate diagnosis. The tissue reaction pattern and additional histopathologic features should be included in the pathology report. Special stains should be used whenever an infection is suspected. In addition, recommendations on any additional work-up, such as tissue cultures, direct immunofluorescence, and serology, should be conveyed to the clinicians to help guide clinical management.

REFERENCES

1. DeRossi SS, Ciarrocca K. Oral lichen planus and lichenoid mucositis. Dent Clin North Am 2014;58(2):299–313.
2. Alomari A, McNiff JM. The significance of eosinophils in hypertrophic lichen planus. J Cutan Pathol 2014;41(4):347–52.

3. Morgan MB, Stevens GL, Switlyk S. Benign lichenoid keratosis: a clinical and pathologic reappraisal of 1040 cases. Am J Dermatopathol 2005;27(5):387–92.
4. Tomasini D, Mentzel T, Hantschke M, et al. Plasmacytoid dendritic cells: an overview of their presence and distribution in different inflammatory skin diseases, with special emphasis on Jessner's lymphocytic infiltrate of the skin and cutaneous lupus erythematosus. J Cutan Pathol 2010;37(11):1132–9.
5. Arps DP, Patel RM. Cutaneous hypertrophic lupus erythematosus: a challenging histopathologic diagnosis in the absence of clinical information. Arch Pathol Lab Med 2013;137(9):1205–10.
6. Ko CJ, Srivastava B, Braverman I, et al. Hypertrophic lupus erythematosus: the diagnostic utility of CD123 staining. J Cutan Pathol 2011;38(11):889–92.
7. Weaver J, Bergfeld WF. Quantitative analysis of eosinophils in acute graft-versus-host disease compared with drug hypersensitivity reactions. Am J Dermatopathol 2010;32(1):31–4.
8. Sokumbi O, Wetter DA. Clinical features, diagnosis, and treatment of erythema multiforme: a review for the practicing dermatologist. Int J Dermatol 2012;51(8):889–902.
9. Dodiuk-Gad RP, Chung WH, Valeyrie-Allanore L, et al. Stevens-Johnson syndrome and toxic epidermal necrolysis: an update. Am J Clin Dermatol 2015;16(6):475–93.
10. Amon RB, Dimond RL. Toxic epidermal necrolysis. Rapid differentiation between staphylococcal- and drug-induced disease. Arch Dermatol 1975;111(11):1433–7.
11. Maize JC Jr, Resneck JS Jr, Shapiro PE, et al. Ducking stray "magic bullets": a Melan-A alert. Am J Dermatopathol 2003;25(2):162–5.
12. Wilcox RA. Cutaneous T-cell lymphoma: 2016 update on diagnosis, risk-stratification, and management. Am J Hematol 2016;91(1):151–65.
13. Rosa G, Fernandez AP, Vij A, et al. Langerhans cell collections, but not eosinophils, are clues to a diagnosis of allergic contact dermatitis in appropriate skin biopsies. J Cutan Pathol 2016;43(6):498–504.
14. Laga AC, Vleugels RA, Qureshi AA, et al. Histopathologic spectrum of psoriasiform skin reactions associated with tumor necrosis factor-α inhibitor therapy. A study of 16 biopsies. Am J Dermatopathol 2010;32(6):568–73.
15. Flamm A, Parikh K, Xie Q, et al. Histologic features of secondary syphilis: a multicenter retrospective review. J Am Acad Dermatol 2015;73(6):1025–30.
16. Elston DM, Stratman EJ, Miller SJ. Skin biopsy: biopsy issues in specific diseases. J Am Acad Dermatol 2016;74(1):1–16 [quiz: 17-8].
17. Chen KR. Skin involvement in ANCA-associated vasculitis. Clin Exp Nephrol 2013;17(5):676–82.
18. Llamas-Velasco M, Alegría V, Santos-Briz Á, et al. Occlusive nonvasculitic vasculopathy: a review. Am J Dermatopathol 2016. [Epub ahead of print].
19. Roberts JA, Chevez-Barrios P. Levamisole-induced vasculitis: a characteristic cutaneous vasculitis associated with levamisole-adulterated cocaine. Arch Pathol Lab Med 2015;139(8):1058–61.
20. Mochel MC, Arakaki RY, Wang G, et al. Cutaneous calciphylaxis: a retrospective histopathologic evaluation. Am J Dermatopathol 2013;35(5):582–6.
21. Kluger N. Sarcoidosis on tattoos: a review of the literature from 1939 to 2011. Sarcoidosis Vasc Diffuse Lung Dis 2013;30(2):86–102.
22. Nirmala V, Chacko CJ, Job CK. Tuberculoid leprosy and tuberculosis skin: a comparative histopathological study. Lepr India 1977;49(1):65–9.

23. Rysgaard C, Alexander E, Swick BL. Nodular secondary syphilis with associated granulomatous inflammation: case report and literature review. J Cutan Pathol 2014;41(4):370–9.
24. Ridley DS, Ridley MJ. Late-stage cutaneous leishmaniasis: immunopathology of tuberculoid lesions in skin and lymph nodes. Br J Exp Pathol 1984;65(3):337–46.
25. Emanuel PO, Phelps RG. Metastatic Crohn's disease: a histopathologic study of 12 cases. J Cutan Pathol 2008;35(5):457–61.
26. Marcoval J, Penin RM. Histopathological features of orofacial granulomatosis. Am J Dermatopathol 2016;38(3):194–200.
27. Piette EW, Rosenbach M. Granuloma annulare: clinical and histologic variants, epidemiology, and genetics. J Am Acad Dermatol 2016;75(3):457–65.
28. Peroni A, Colato C, Schena D, et al. Interstitial granulomatous dermatitis: a distinct entity with characteristic histological and clinical pattern. Br J Dermatol 2012;166(4):775–83.
29. Reggiani C, Massone C, Fink-Puches R, et al. Interstitial mycosis fungoides: a clinicopathologic study of 21 patients. Am J Surg Pathol 2016;40(10):1360–7.
30. Orrock JM, Abbott JJ, Gibson LE, et al. INI1 and GLUT-1 expression in epithelioid sarcoma and its cutaneous neoplastic and nonneoplastic mimics. Am J Dermatopathol 2009;31(2):152–6.
31. Zayour M, Lazova R. Pseudoepitheliomatous hyperplasia: a review. Am J Dermatopathol 2011;33(2):112–22.
32. Crowson AN, Saab J, Magro CM. Folliculocentric herpes: a clinicopathological study of 28 patients. Am J Dermatopathol 2017;39(2):89–94.
33. Ruocco V, Ruocco E, Caccavale S, et al. Pemphigus vegetans of the folds (intertriginous areas). Clin Dermatol 2015;33(4):471–6.
34. Clark LG, Tolkachjov SN, Bridges AG, et al. Pyostomatitis vegetans (PSV)-pyodermatitis vegetans (PDV): a clinicopathologic study of 7 cases at a tertiary referral center. J Am Acad Dermatol 2016;75(3):578–84.
35. Schmidt E, della Torre R, Borradori L. Clinical features and practical diagnosis of bullous pemphigoid. Dermatol Clin 2011;29(3):427–38.
36. Smith EP, Zone JJ. Dermatitis herpetiformis and linear IgA bullous dermatosis. Dermatol Clin 1993;11(3):511–26.
37. Ahronowitz I, Harp J, Shinkai K. Etiology and management of pyoderma gangrenosum: a comprehensive review. Am J Clin Dermatol 2012;13(3):191–211.
38. Wong WW, Machado GR, Hill ME. Pyoderma gangrenosum: the great pretender and a challenging diagnosis. J Cutan Med Surg 2011;15(6):322–8.
39. Chan MP. Neutrophilic panniculitis: algorithmic approach to a heterogeneous group of disorders. Arch Pathol Lab Med 2014;138(10):1337–43.
40. Kroshinsky D, Alloo A, Rothschild B, et al. Necrotizing sweet syndrome: a new variant of neutrophilic dermatosis mimicking necrotizing fasciitis. J Am Acad Dermatol 2012;67(5):945–54.
41. Chavan RN, Cappel MA, Ketterling RP, et al. Histiocytoid sweet syndrome may indicate leukemia cutis: a novel application of fluorescence in situ hybridization. J Am Acad Dermatol 2014;70(6):1021–7.
42. Lan TT, Brown NA, Hristov AC. Controversies and considerations in the diagnosis of primary cutaneous CD4+ small/medium T-cell lymphoma. Arch Pathol Lab Med 2014;138(10):1307–18.
43. Baldassano MF, Bailey EM, Ferry JA, et al. Cutaneous lymphoid hyperplasia and cutaneous marginal zone lymphoma. Am J Surg Pathol 1999;23(1):88–96.

Moving?

Make sure your subscription moves with you!

To notify us of your new address, find your **Clinics Account Number** (located on your mailing label above your name), and contact customer service at:

Email: journalscustomerservice-usa@elsevier.com

800-654-2452 (subscribers in the U.S. & Canada)
314-447-8871 (subscribers outside of the U.S. & Canada)

Fax number: 314-447-8029

Elsevier Health Sciences Division
Subscription Customer Service
3251 Riverport Lane
Maryland Heights, MO 63043

*To ensure uninterrupted delivery of your subscription, please notify us at least 4 weeks in advance of move.

Printed and bound by CPI Group (UK) Ltd, Croydon, CR0 4YY

03/10/2024

01040491-0010